REFERENCE

DO NOT REMOVE FROM LIBRARY

CONGENITAL DISORDERS SOURCEBOOK

Health Reference Series

Volume Twenty-nine

CONGENITAL DISORDERS SOURCEBOOK

Basic Information about Disorders Acquired during Gestation, Including Spina Bifida, Hydrocephalus, Cerebral Palsy, Heart Defects, Craniofacial Abnormalities, Fetal Alcohol Syndrome, and More, along with Current Treatment Options and Statistical Data

Edited by
Karen Bellenir

Omnigraphics, Inc.
Penobscot Building / Detroit, MI 48226

BIBLIOGRAPHIC NOTE

This volume contains documents and excerpts from publications issued by the following government agencies: Centers for Disease Control and Prevention (CDC), Food and Drug Administration (FDA), and subagencies of the National Institutes of Health (NIH) including the National Institute on Alcohol Abuse and Alcoholism (NIAAA), National Institute of Allergy and Infections Diseases (NIAID), National Institute of Child Health and Human Development (NICHD), and the National Institute of Neurological Disorders and Stroke (NINDS). This volume also contains copyrighted documents from the following organizations: American College of Obstetricians and Gynecologists (ACOG), Children's National Medical Center, Cleft Palate Foundation, Environmental Research Foundation, Hydrocephalus Association, Hydrocephalus Research Foundation, John's Hopkins University Press, Let's Face It, The National Association for the Craniofacially Handicapped, Sturge-Weber Foundation, and United Cerebral Palsy Research and Educational Foundation. Copyrighted articles from the following journals are also included: *Archives of Neurology*, *American Family Physician*, *Journal of the American Medical Association*, *Medical Sciences Bulletin*, *Neurology*, *Ostomy Quarterly*, and *Twins Magazine*. All copyrighted material is reprinted with permission. Document numbers where applicable and specific source citations are provided on the first page of each chapter. Every effort has been made to secure all necessary rights to reprint the copyrighted material. If any omissions have been made, contact Omnigraphics to make corrections for future editions.

Edited by Karen Bellenir
Peter D. Dresser, Managing Editor, *Health Reference Series*

Omnigraphics, Inc.

Matthew P. Barbour, *Production Manager*
Laurie Lanzen Harris, *Vice President, Editorial*
Peter E. Ruffner, *Vice President, Administration*
James A. Sellgren, *Vice President, Operations and Finance*
Jane J. Steele, *Marketing Consultant*

Frederick G. Ruffner, Jr., *Publisher*

Copyright © 1997, Omnigraphics, Inc.

Library of Congress Cataloging-in-Publication Data

Congenital disorders sourcebook : basic information about disorders acquired during gestation, including spina bifida, hydrocephalus, cerebral palsy, heart defects, craniofacial abnormalities, fetal alcohol syndrome, and more, along with current treatment options and statistical data / edited by Karen Bellenir.
    p. cm. -- (Health reference series : v. 29)
    Includes bibliographical references and index.
    ISBN 0-7808-0205-5
    1. Abnormalities, Human--Popular works. 2. Developmental disabilities--Popular works. I. Bellenir, Karen. II. Series.
RG626.C597   1997   97-17092
616'.043--dc21   CIP

∞

This book is printed on acid-free paper meeting the ANSI Z39.48 Standard. The infinity symbol that appears above indicates that the paper in this book meets that standard.

Printed in the United States

Contents

Preface ix

Part I: Introduction

Chapter 1—Decreasing the Chance of Birth Defects 3
Chapter 2—How Folate Can Help Prevent Birth Defects 11
Chapter 3—Prenatal Testing 19
Chapter 4—How to be an Assertive Parent on the
             Treatment Team 25

Part II: Spina Bifida and Hydrocephalus

Chapter 5—Answering Your Questions about
             Spina Bifida 33
Chapter 6—Children with Hydrocephalus 67
Chapter 7—Social Skills Development in Children
             with Hydrocephalus 75
Chapter 8—Eye Problems Associated with
             Hydrocephalus 79
Chapter 9—Seizures in Children with Congenital
             Hydrocephalus 83
Chapter 10—Third Ventriculostomy 97
Chapter 11—The Variable Pressure Programmable Valve 103

Chapter 12—Prenatal Onset Hydrocephalus:
    Fetal Diagnosis 107
Chapter 13—Pregnancy and Maternal Hydrocephalus
    Survey 111

Part III: Cerebral Palsy

Chapter 14—Cerebral Palsy: Hope Through Research 119
Chapter 15—Cerebral Palsy: Statistics and Risk Factors 149
Chapter 16—Treating Muscle Spasticity in Cerebral Palsy ... 155
Chapter 17—Surgical Treatment of Drooling 163
Chapter 18—Current Research Initiatives in Cerebral
    Palsy 165
Chapter 19—Magnesium Linked to Lower Incidence of
    Cerebral Palsy 175

Part IV: Fetal Alcohol Syndrome

Chapter 20—Clinical Recognition of Fetal Alcohol
    Syndrome 181
Chapter 21—Critical Periods for Prenatal Alcohol
    Exposure 195
Chapter 22—Effects of Paternal Exposure to Alcohol
    on Offspring Development 209
Chapter 23—Comparative Teratogenicity of Alcohol
    and Other Drugs 223
Chapter 24—A Long-Term Perspective of Fetal Alcohol
    Syndrome 241
Chapter 25—Tracking the Prevalence of Fetal Alcohol
    Syndrome 259

Part V: Other Congenital Disorders

Chapter 26—Congenital Heart Defects 273
Chapter 27—Twin-Twin Transfusion Syndrome 305
Chapter 28—Hirschsprung's Disease 309
Chapter 29—Clubfoot and Other Pediatric Foot
    Deformities 315
Chapter 30—Cleft Lip and Cleft Palate 325

Chapter 31—Sturge-Weber Syndrome 351
Chapter 32—Hemangiomas 357

Part VI: Chemicals, Medications, and Infectious Organisms Linked to Congenital Disorders

Chapter 33—Chemicals and Birth Defects 363
Chapter 34—The Thalidomide Tragedy 391
Chapter 35—Accutane 399
Chapter 36—ACE Inhibitors and Birth Defects 405
Chapter 37—Outcomes of Pregnancy Associated with
              Antiepileptic Drugs 407
Chapter 38—Rubella 419
Chapter 39—Streptococcus B Infection of the Newborn 423
Chapter 40—Toxoplasmosis 425
Chapter 41—Cytomegalovirus Infection 435
Chapter 42—Syphilis 439

Part VII: Research Initiatives

Chapter 43—Maternal Heat Exposure and Neural
              Tube Defects 447
Chapter 44—Investigating Prenatal Causes of Mental
              Retardation and Developmental Disabilities..... 459
Chapter 45—Assessment of Outcomes Following
              Neonatal Asphyxia 465
Chapter 46—Long-Term Outcome in Birth Asphyxia—
              The Role of Encephalopathy in Prediction 483
Chapter 47—Research Update: Pre-Term and Low
              Birthweight Infants 497
Chapter 48—Perinatal Emphasis Research Centers
              (PERCS) 513

Part VIII: Resources for Further Help and Information

Chapter 49—National Directory of Hydrocephalus
              Support Groups 523
Chapter 50—Hydrocephalus Association on the Internet
              and the World Wide Web 533

Chapter 51—United Cerebral Palsy Associations
 on the Internet 537
Chapter 52—Resources for People with Facial
 Differences 541
Chapter 53—Resources for Other Congenital Disorders 559

Index **569**

Preface

About This Book

According to statistics compiled by the Centers for Disease Control and Prevention, birth defects are the leading cause of infant mortality in the United States resulting in more than 8,000 infant deaths each year. In addition, another 40,000 babies are born and live with congenital disorders that result in a wide variety of disabilities ranging from treatable anomalies to life-long challenges. For example, each year 2,500 to 3,000 babies are born with spina bifida or other neural tube defects, and more than 4,500 American babies and infants are diagnosed with cerebral palsy. Although recent advances in medical technology have increased the chance of survival for children with birth defects, their disabilities may be lifelong.

Most congenital disorders begin early in gestation—before the twelfth week of pregnancy—but many are not diagnosed until birth or shortly after birth. This book offers information about congenital disorders related to the effects of toxic substances, disease organisms, birth trauma, spontaneous malformations, and other disorders of unknown origin. Information on disorders with a known genetic basis is included in the *Genetic Disorders Sourcebook* (Volume 13 of the *Health Reference Series*).

How to Use This Book

This book is divided into parts and chapters. Parts focus on broad areas of interest. Chapters are devoted to single topics within a part.

Part I: Introduction provides basic information about birth defects, their causes, and some steps prospective parents can take to reduce their risk of having a child born with a congenital disorder. Parents seeking information about the medical management of birth defects will also find practical advice on how to work effectively with health care providers.

Part II: Spina Bifida and Hydrocephalus offers information and answers to questions about two of the most commonly occurring, and often co-occurring, congenital disorders. Issues related to physical and social development in affected children are addressed along with information about treatments and current research efforts.

Part III: Cerebral Palsy provides an overview of the different types and symptoms of cerebral palsy and their treatment options. It dispels popular myths and presents information on possible causes along with research updates.

Part IV: Fetal Alcohol Syndrome gives readers information about recognizing and preventing fetal alcohol syndrome, a congenital disorder first officially defined in the 1970s. According to the Centers for Disease Control and Prevention, alcohol is the most common known cause of fetal damage in the United States, and it is the leading cause of preventable mental retardation. This section offers diagnostic aids, statistical data, and an explanation of the cellular events that are disrupted by alcohol.

Part V: Other Congenital Disorders gives readers information on a wide variety of specific congenital disorders. Many of these develop from unknown causes and their ability to respond to treatment varies considerably. Cleft palate and club foot, two of the more common birth defects, can be surgically repaired. Many—but sadly not all—heart malformations can also be treated surgically so that children can live normal or near-normal lives. Other disorders addressed in this section include twin-twin transfusion syndrome, Hirschsprings disease, Sturge-Weber Syndrome, and hemangiomas (the most common type of tumor found in infants).

Part VI: Chemicals, Medications, and Infectious Organisms Linked to Congenital Disorders provides current information about some agents known to cause birth defects. These include industrial chemicals, prescription drugs, and infectious diseases such as rubella and syphilis.

Part VII: Research Initiatives reports on the results of recent and ongoing research into prenatal and perinatal health. The relationship between maternal exposure to heat (in hot tubs and saunas) and neural tube defects, prenatal causes of mental retardation, the effects of birth asphyxia, and the problems faced by low-birthweight and preterm infants are among the topics addressed.

Part VIII: Resources for Further Help and Information offers lists of places that can provide encouragement, support, print literature, and answers to questions about many congenital disorders. Readers unable to find an appropriate resource here may wish to consult the appendix of *Genetic Disorders Sourcebook* (Volume 13, *Health Reference Series*, Omnigraphics) or contact the National Organization for Rare Disorders (NORD), P.O. Box 8923, New Fairfield, CT 06812; (203) 746-6518; (203) 746-6481 fax; (800) 999-6673 toll-free.

Acknowledgements

This book would not have been possible without the assistance and cooperation of many individuals and organizations. Special thanks go to Ann Marie Liakos of the Hydrocephalus Research Foundation and Emily Fudge of the Hydrocephalus Association for providing information about neural tube defects and hydrocephalus. The Children's National Medical Center, Cleft Palate Foundation, Let's Face It, The National Association for the Craniofacially Handicapped, the Sturge-Weber Foundation, and United Cerebral Palsy Research and Educational Foundation also graciously provided much of the information that has been reproduced here. In addition, thanks go to Margaret Mary Missar for obtaining many of the documents included in this volume, Jenifer Swanson for searching the internet, and to Bruce the Scanman for doing so much more than merely scanning.

Note from the Editor

This book is part of Omnigraphics' *Health Reference Series*. The series provides basic information about a broad range of medical concerns. It is not intended to serve as a tool for diagnosing illness, in prescribing treatments, or as a substitute for the physician/patient relationship. All persons concerned about medical symptoms or the possibility of disease are encouraged to seek professional care from an appropriate health care provider.

Part One

Introduction

Chapter 1

Decreasing the Chance of Birth Defects

When Tammy Troutman of Knoxville, Tenn., was planning her first pregnancy, she had a good reason to be concerned about birth defects.

Born with a mild form of spina bifida, Troutman worried her child would also have the condition. So she did what health-care experts say is the best first step toward preventing birth defects: She visited her physician for an exam well before she and her husband tried to conceive.

"Before I decided to have children, I went to the doctor to make sure everything would be OK," Troutman remembers.

He advised her to take a daily multivitamin supplement containing folic acid, a B vitamin that would decrease her chances of having a baby with spina bifida. Troutman took the vitamins for five months before conceiving her son, Evan, who was born in August 1993 with a normal, healthy spine.

"Even if he had been born with spina bifida," Troutman says, "I felt secure knowing that I had done everything I could to prevent it."

Of the 4 million infants born annually in the United States, about 3 to 5 percent are born with birth defects, according to the March of Dimes. Birth defects account for 20 percent of all infant deaths in the United States, more than from any other single cause.

"For the majority of birth defects, the cause is unknown," says Franz Rosa, M.D., a pediatrician with the Food and Drug Administration who monitors reports of prescription drugs causing birth defects. Rosa cites a list of drugs that are known to be birth-defect

---

FDA Consumer, November 1996.

causing, but he says they only account for a small percentage of all malformations.

"There's a lot we just don't know," Rosa says. "Most birth defects are not preventable and mothers should not feel guilty about causing defects that they really didn't. Worrying too much is not good for pregnancies."

What experts do know is that most birth defects occur in the first three months of pregnancy, when the organs are forming. It is in these crucial first few weeks—often before a woman even knows she's pregnant—that an embryo is most susceptible to teratogens, substances that can cause defects, However, some birth defects do occur later in pregnancy as well.

"The key is what your life is like at the time you become pregnant," says Deborah Smith, M.D., an obstetrician and gynecologist in FDA's Office of Women's Health. "Are you getting enough folic acid, are you immune to rubella, are you avoiding alcohol and smoking? These are some of the things we know are important."

Despite the benefits of seeing a doctor before conceiving, only 26 percent of women planning a pregnancy do so, according to the March of Dimes. Furthermore, health experts estimate more than 50 percent of pregnancies are unplanned. That's why a healthy lifestyle for all women who could become pregnant—even if they don't intend to—is the best way to minimize the risk of birth defects.

Healthy Diet

The maxim "You are what you eat" is sterling advice during the first three months of pregnancy.

Studies of women who had endured starvation during World War II illustrate the importance of diet early in pregnancy. Contrary to what researchers expected, it was not the babies *born* during food deprivation that had the most malformations, but those *conceived* during food deprivation.

One nutrient known to prevent birth defects is folic acid, the B vitamin Tammy Troutman took before her pregnancy. Folic acid is the chemical form of folate, which is found in green leafy vegetables, citrus fruits, and legumes. Folate aids in cell division, and taking extra folic acid reduces a woman's chance of having a child with spina bifida and other abnormalities of the spine and brain.

Spina bifida occurs when the vertebrae do not close completely. It is one of several conditions known as neural tube defects, because the neural tube is the portion of the embryo that develops into the brain

Decreasing the Chance of Birth Defects

and spinal column. In very mild cases, spina bifida causes few or minor problems, but in more severe cases, the spinal cord protrudes through the vertebrae into a sac outside the child's body. This impairs the child's mobility and other neurological functions and requires surgery to repair the opening.

To help prevent neural tube defects, the U.S. Public Health Service has recommended that all women of childbearing age who are capable of becoming pregnant consume 0.4 milligrams (mg) of folic acid per day. (For pregnant or lactating women, the daily value increases to 0.8 mg per day.) It is especially important that women take in sufficient folate before they become pregnant.

FDA recently published regulations requiring manufacturers to add folic acid to enriched grain products such as flour, noodles, bread, rolls, buns, farina, cornmeal, grits, and rice by January 1998. (See Chapter 2 "How Folate Can Help Prevent Birth Defects.")

Although the main challenge in pregnancy is getting enough nutrients, too much of a good thing is not good for a developing baby, either. Vitamins A and D are the most notable examples. Both can be toxic at levels higher than the recommended daily allowance. Such levels are rarely reached through food intake; however, women taking dietary supplements need to be aware of this risk and the amount of these vitamins they are taking. Women who take vitamin and mineral supplements should discuss with a health-care professional what vitamins are safe to continue taking during pregnancy.

Only a few foods are completely off-limits during pregnancy. These include raw or undercooked meat, such as "pink-in-the-middle" burgers, and raw or undercooked seafood. Bacteria from these can cause severe food poisoning, which is dangerous to a fetus and very unpleasant for the mother.

Soft drinks, coffee, tea, and other caffeinated drinks can be used in moderation. Although large doses of caffeine have caused skeletal defects in rats, one or two cups of coffee daily are not considered dangerous for developing fetuses.

Alcohol should be avoided at all times during pregnancy because it leads to low birth weight and can cause deformities as well.

According to the March of Dimes, alcohol is the most common known cause of fetal damage in the country and the leading cause of preventable mental retardation. Pregnant women who drink alcohol, especially in large amounts, put their babies at risk for fetal alcohol syndrome, which causes growth retardation, facial deformities such as a small head, thin upper lip, and small jaw bone, an underdeveloped thymus gland, and mental deficiencies or developmental delays.

If a woman has had a glass or two of wine before finding out she was pregnant, she probably has not harmed her child. But since no one knows the exact amount of alcohol that is dangerous, it's best to avoid alcohol when pregnancy is possible.

Healthy Mothers, Healthy Babies

A pregnant woman who has a serious medical condition may face a greater than normal risk that her child will have a birth defect.

Diabetes, for example, can complicate a pregnancy in many ways. Women who must take insulin daily to control their blood sugar are three or four times more likely to have a baby with major birth defects than are other mothers. That's not to say they should abandon insulin, however. Without it, many diabetic women and their babies wouldn't survive pregnancy at all.

Birth defects among diabetics can be greatly reduced if women get their blood sugar levels under control before becoming pregnant and strictly manage their diets throughout pregnancy. Gestational diabetes, which develops during pregnancy, can also be harmful to mother and child, but it can be controlled through diet or medication.

Epilepsy also increases a woman's chance of having a baby with a birth defect. It's not clear whether the disease itself or the drugs used to control it cause malformations, but in either case, the woman's neurologist and obstetrician should work together to find the safest course of treatment for the epilepsy and pregnancy.

Rubella, toxoplasmosis, cytomegalovirus, and syphilis can cause birth defects in the infants of women who have these infectious diseases. Rubella infection during early pregnancy can cause abnormalities of the heart, eyes and ears. Any woman planning a pregnancy should be tested for rubella immunity and vaccinated if necessary. She must wait three months after vaccination before becoming pregnant, however, because the vaccine itself can endanger a developing fetus.

Toxoplasmosis is transmitted only through raw meat and cat feces, both of which pregnant women should try to avoid. The disease causes malformations of the brain, liver and spleen if a fetus becomes infected in the first trimester.

If a woman has syphilis, she should be treated with antibiotics before pregnancy. If not treated by at least the fourth month, syphilis can cause bone and tooth deformities in the baby, as well as nervous system and brain damage.

Decreasing the Chance of Birth Defects

Cytomegalovirus (CMV) is a herpes virus that causes no real problem—and sometimes not even symptoms—for adults and children. In pregnancy, however, it can damage the fetus' brain, eyes or ears. Because most people contract the infection, whose symptoms are much like a cold, when they are children, most adults are immune to it. Pregnant women who do not know if they've had CMV and who work with large groups of young children should discuss the situation with their health-care provider.

Sometimes it is not a disease that causes birth defects, but the medication used to treat it. Unfortunately, no one knows for certain how most drugs will affect a developing fetus. Historically, most women of childbearing age have been excluded from clinical trials of new drugs, and, although that is changing, drug manufacturers are understandably reluctant to involve pregnant women in clinical trials for new drugs. Therefore, the effects of many drugs are not known until they are in wider use after market approval.

To be on the safe side, a pregnant woman shouldn't take any drug unless it is absolutely necessary and not until she's checked with her health-care provider. However, even physicians have little information when prescribing medication for pregnant women. What is known about most drugs in pregnancy is based either on animal studies or on reports of problems after the drug is on the market. To give guidance about pregnancy safety, FDA requires that manufacturers include in the professional labeling for each drug which one of several categories, reflecting known or unknown danger to the fetus, the drug is in. The categories also provide guidance on weighing the benefits and risks of use in pregnancy.

Two examples: Taxol (paclitaxel), used to treat ovarian and breast cancer, may in some instances be appropriate in pregnancy even though it causes birth defects in animals and is therefore believed to cause fetal harm in humans. The benefits of its use to fight life-threatening cancers may outweigh the potential harm to a fetus.

Accutane (isotretinoin) should never be used in pregnancy. It is highly effective for treating severe cystic acne, but it causes serious birth defects. There are other drugs available to treat acne, and the disease is not life-threatening to the mother (see Chapter 35).

Who Should Paint the Nursery?

Chemicals—whether it's paint in the nursery or exhaust fumes in a parking garage—have long been suspected of causing birth defects.

It's important for pregnant women to realize that most birth defects are not caused by a single factor, nor are they usually caused by faint traces of toxins. Scientists believe it takes a combination of factors to trigger a congenital malformation.

"Most birth defects have one or more genetic factors and one or more environmental factors," explains Richard Leavitt, director of science information at the March of Dimes.

Most of the chemicals a pregnant woman encounters pose little threat compared with the harm in smoking, drinking alcohol, or eating a poor diet.

"Most environmental exposure is at a low level compared to things you put in your mouth or inhale purposefully into your lungs," Leavitt says. "Public health warnings are aimed at the many to help the relatively few avoid a problem."

Daily, heavy exposure to chemicals may be dangerous, however. If a pregnant woman must work around fumes or chemicals, such as in a dry-cleaning business, art studio, or factory, she should use gloves, masks and adequate ventilation. But if she just gets a whiff of dry-cleaning fluid while picking up her laundry from the cleaners, there's little need to worry, Leavitt says.

Some environmental toxins such as lead are best avoided at any time, but especially during pregnancy. Scraping leaded paint off an old house window, drinking water from a pipe soldered with lead, or drinking out of decorative pottery containing lead can all potentially cause lead poisoning—and mental retardation—in a fetus.

Radiation is also dangerous to developing babies. A pregnant woman who works in an x-ray department of a hospital must take precautions to avoid exposure. Elective dental x-rays should be postponed until delivery, and any nonpregnant woman who has an x-ray should have her reproductive organs shielded with a lead apron.

Taking hot baths, using saunas, or exercising in hot, humid weather can raise a woman's core temperature and have the potential to cause birth defects, especially in the first trimester. Lukewarm baths and moderate exercise are fine, however.

And what about computers or video display terminals? Although they have at times been accused of causing harm, there's probably no need to worry. Recent studies have not found any relationship between computer terminals and miscarriages.

And as for who should paint the nursery—today's paints don't contain lead and therefore probably aren't dangerous. But there are other reasons to find someone else to do this task. The repetitive motion of painting can be a strain on back muscles already under pressure from

Decreasing the Chance of Birth Defects

the extra weight of pregnancy, and standing on your feet for hours can make advanced pregnancy miserable. If someone else can do it, pass this chore along.

Of all the environmental harms, undoubtedly the most harmful is one women can control—smoking. Although there is no evidence smoking causes birth defects, it deprives the fetus of oxygen and leads to a number of problems. If all pregnant women avoided smoking, the United States would see a 5 percent reduction in miscarriages, a 20 percent reduction in low-birth-weight births, and an 8 percent reduction in premature deliveries in this country, according to the March of Dimes.

In the Family

Finally, a number of birth defects are inherited. They are usually triggered when the child inherits a matching pair of disease-causing genes, one from each parent. This is most often an issue for couples of similar ethnic or geographic origins.

For example, African-American couples are most at risk for having a child with sickle cell anemia. According to the March of Dimes, couples of Ashkenazic Jewish or French Canadian descent may be carriers of Tay-Sachs disease. People who know of genetic disorders in their families, or those who have already had one child with a disorder are also at a greater risk, as are couples who are closely related, such as first cousins. Genetic testing is available to determine the risk of passing some genetic disorders to an unborn child. Once a pregnancy begins, prenatal testing is available to detect a number of disorders, as well.

Some genetic abnormalities, such as Down syndrome (a genetic abnormality that causes mental retardation, short stature, and flattened features), increase with the parents' ages. Women over 35 are at higher risk of having a child with Down syndrome—about 1 in 100 for a 40-year-old, compared to 1 in 10,000 for a 20-year-old mother or 3 in 1,000 for a 35 year-old mother. And it's not always just the mother's age that matters. An estimated 25 percent of Down syndrome cases can be attributed to increased age of the father.

Finally, it's important to remember that for most healthy women, the incidence of birth defects is very low—less than 3 percent. And of malformations that do occur, the most common are also the most treatable. Cleft palate and club foot, two of the more common birth defects, can be surgically repaired. Many heart malformations can be repaired with surgery so that children live normal lives.

For the most part, health experts say, a woman can do a lot to ensure the health of her child by maintaining a healthy lifestyle.

—by Rebecca Williams

Rebecca D. Williams is a writer in Oak Ridge, Tenn.

Chapter 2

How Folate Can Help Prevent Birth Defects

Preventing Spina Bifida and Other Neural Tube Defects

Each year in the United States, 2,500 to 3,000 infants are born with spina bifida or anencephaly, which are neural tube defects (NTDs) caused by the incomplete closing of the spine. However, the actual number of pregnancies affected by NTDs is likely to be greater, since birth defect surveillance programs do not detect birth defects among fetuses of less than 20 weeks' gestation.

All infants with anencephaly die shortly after birth, whereas most babies born with spina bifida grow to adulthood with varying degrees of paralysis. The annual medical care and surgical costs for persons with spina bifida in the United States exceed $200 million.

A Call to Action

The results of numerous studies have shown that folic acid, a B vitamin, is important in preventing NTDs. CDC estimates that half of all NTD-affected pregnancies could be prevented if all women of childbearing age consumed 0.4 mg of folic acid per day.

Although the specific mechanism of this preventive action is not known, the scientific evidence of its effectiveness is overwhelming and

---

This chapter contains information from "Preventing Spina Bifida and Other Neural Tube Defects," Centers for Disease Control and Prevention. August 1993; and "How Folate Can Help Prevent Birth Defects," *FDA Consumer*, September 1996.

is the basis for the following U.S. Public Health Service recommendation:

> *All women of childbearing age in the United States who are capable of becoming pregnant should consume 0.4 mg of folic acid per day for the purpose of reducing their risk of having a pregnancy affected with spina bifida or other NTDs. Because the effects of high intakes are not well known but include complicating the diagnosis of vitamin B_{12} deficiency, care should be taken to keep total folate consumption at <1 mg per day, except under the supervision of a physician. Women who have had a prior NTD affected pregnancy are at high risk of having a subsequent affected pregnancy. When these women are planning to become pregnant, they should consult their physicians for advice.*

How Folate Can Help Prevent Birth Defects

If you plan to have children some day, here's important information for the future mother-to-be: Think folate now.

Folate is a B vitamin found in a variety of foods and added to many vitamin and mineral supplements as folic acid, a synthetic form of folate. Folate is needed both before and in the first weeks of pregnancy and can help reduce the risk of certain serious and common birth defects called neural tube defects, which affect the brain and spinal cord.

The tricky part is that neural tube defects can occur in an embryo before a woman realizes she's pregnant. That's why it's important for all women of childbearing age (15 to 45) to include folate in their diets: If they get pregnant, it reduces the chance of the baby having a birth defect of the brain or spinal cord.

"Adequate folate should be eaten daily and throughout the childbearing years," said Elizabeth Yetley, Ph.D., a registered dietitian and director of FDA's Office of Special Nutritionals.

There are several ways to do this:

- Eat fruits, dark-green leafy vegetables, dried beans and peas, and other foods that are natural sources of folate.
- Eat folic acid-fortified breakfast cereals.
- Take a vitamin supplement containing folic acid.

Folate's potential to reduce the risk of neural tube defects is so important that the Food and Drug Administration is requiring that

How Folate Can Help Prevent Birth Defects

by 1998, food manufacturers fortify enriched grain products with folic acid. This will give women another way to get sufficient folate: by eating fortified breads and other grains.

Nutrition information on food and dietary supplement labels can help women determine whether they are getting enough folate, which is 400 micrograms (0.4 milligrams) a day before pregnancy and 800 micrograms a day during pregnancy.

Neural Tube Birth Defects

The technical names of the two major neural tube birth defects reduced by adequate folate intake are anencephaly and spina bifida. Babies with anencephaly do not develop a brain and are stillborn or die shortly after birth. Those with spina bifida have a defect of the spinal column that can result in varying degrees of handicap, from mild and hardly noticeable cases of scoliosis (a sideways bending of the spine) to paralysis and bladder or bowel incontinence. With proper medical treatment, most babies born with spina bifida can survive to adulthood. But they may require leg braces, crutches, and other devices to help them walk, and they may have learning disabilities. About 30 percent have slight to severe mental retardation.

The national Centers for Disease Control and Prevention estimate that about 2,500 infants with spina bifida and anencephaly are born each year in the United States.

Other maternal factors also may contribute to the development of neural tube defects. These include:

- family history of neural tube defects
- prior neural tube defect-affected pregnancy
- use of certain antiseizure medications
- severe overweight
- hot tub use in early pregnancy
- fever during early pregnancy
- diabetes.

Any woman concerned about these factors should consult her doctor.

Folate Link

Scientists first suggested a link between neural tube birth defects and diet in the 1950s. The incidence of these conditions has always been higher in low socioeconomic groups in which women may have poorer diets. Also, babies conceived in the winter and early spring are more likely to be born with spina bifida, perhaps because the mother's diet lacks fresh fruits and vegetables—which are good sources of folate—during the early weeks of pregnancy.

In 1991, British researchers found that 72 percent of women who had one pregnancy with a neural tube birth defect had a lower risk of having another child with this birth defect when they took prescription doses of folic acid before and during early pregnancy.

Another study looked at folic acid intake in Hungarian women. The evidence indicated that mothers who had never given birth to babies with neural tube defects and who took a multivitamin and mineral supplement with folic acid had less risk in subsequent pregnancies for having babies with neural tube defects than women given a placebo.

These studies led the U.S. Public Health Service in September 1992 to recommend that all women of childbearing age capable of becoming pregnant consume 0.4 mg of folate daily to reduce their risk of having a pregnancy affected with spina bifida or other neural tube defects.

That corresponds to FDA's Daily Value for folic acid, which is 400 micrograms for nonpregnant women, as well as children 4 and older and adult men. For pregnant women, the Daily Value jumps to 800 micrograms. Daily Values are dietary reference numbers used on the Nutrition Facts panel on food labels to show the amounts of various nutrients in a serving of food.

Many women between 19 and 50 get only 200 micrograms of folate a day, according to the U.S. Department of Agriculture.

Folate Sources

Folate occurs naturally in a variety of foods, including liver; dark-green leafy vegetables such as collards, turnip greens, and Romaine lettuce; broccoli and asparagus; citrus fruits and juices; whole-grain products; wheat germ; and dried beans and peas, such as pinto, navy and lima beans, and chickpeas and black-eyed peas.

Under FDA's folic acid fortification program, the agency is requiring manufacturers to add from 0.43 mg to 1.4 mg of folic acid per pound of product to enriched flour, bread, rolls and buns, farina, corn grits, cornmeal, rice, and noodle products. A serving of each product will provide about 10 percent of the Daily Value for folic acid. Whole-grain products do not have to be enriched because they contain natural

How Folate Can Help Prevent Birth Defects

folate. Some of the natural folate in non-whole-grain products is lost in the process of refining whole grains.

The fortification regulations become effective Jan. 1, 1998, although manufacturers may begin folic acid fortification immediately, as long as they adhere to the regulations.

Folate also can be obtained from dietary supplements, such as folic acid tablets and multivitamins with folic acid, and from fortified breakfast cereals.

A study reported in the March 9, 1996, issue of *The Lancet*, suggested that folic acid, the synthetic form of folate, may be better absorbed than folate found naturally in foods. Christine Lewis, Ph.D., a registered dietitian and special assistant in FDA's Office of Special Nutritionals, said, "This is a complex and poorly understood issue, and more data are needed."

Finding Foods with Folate

Certain information on food and dietary supplement labels can help women spot foods containing substantial amounts of folate. Some labels may claim that the product is "high in folate or folic acid," which means a serving of the food provides 20 percent or more of the Daily Value for folic acid. Or the label may say the food is a "good source" of folate, which means a serving of the food provides 10 to 19 percent of the Daily Value for folic acid. The exact amount will be given in the label's Nutrition Facts panel.

Some food and dietary supplement labels may carry a longer claim that says adequate folate intake may reduce the risk of neural tube birth defects. Products carrying this claim must:

- provide 10 percent or more of the Daily Value for folic acid per serving

- not contain more than 100 percent of the Daily Value for vitamins A and D per serving because high intakes of these vitamins are associated with other birth defects

- carry a caution on the label about excess folic acid intake, if a serving of food provides more than 100 percent of the Daily Value for folic acid. FDA has set 1 mg (or 1,000 micrograms) of folate daily as the maximum safe level. There are limited data on the safety of consuming more than 1 mg daily, and there may be a risk for people with low amounts of vitamin B_{12} in their bodies—for example, older people with malabsorption problems, and people on certain anticancer drugs or drugs for epilepsy whose effectiveness can diminish when taken with high intakes of folate.

- list on the label's Nutrition or Supplement Facts panel the amount by weight in micrograms and the %Daily Value of folate per serving of the product. This information, which appears toward the bottom of the panel, along with the listing of other vitamins and minerals, can be used to compare folate levels in various foods and supplements.

Table 2.1. Some Good Sources of Folate

Food	Serving Size	Amount (Micrograms)	%Daily Value*
Chicken liver	3.5oz	770	193
Breakfast cereals	½ to 1½ cup	100 to 400	25 to 100
Braised beef liver	3.5oz	217	54
Lentils, cooked	½ cup	180	45
Chickpeas	½ cup	141	35
Asparagus	½ cup	132	33
Spinach, cooked	½ cup	131	33
Black beans	½ cup	128	32
Burrito with beans	2	118	30
Kidney beans	½ cup	115	29
Baked beans with pork	1 cup	92	23
Lima beans	½ cup	78	20
Tomato juice	1 cup	48	12
Brussels sprouts	½ cup	47	12
Orange	1 medium	47	12
Broccoli, cooked	½ cup	39	10
Fast-food French fries	large order	38	10
Wheat germ	2 tbsp	38	10
Fortified white bread	1 slice	38	10

* based on Daily Value for folate of 400 micrograms
(Source: *Food Values of Portions Commonly Used*, 16th edition)

How Folate Can Help Prevent Birth Defects

Optional information may appear with the health claim to let consumers know about other risks associated with neural tube birth defects, when to consult a doctor, other foods that are good sources of folate, and other important messages about neural tube defects.

Other Considerations

The claim about folate cannot imply that adequate folate intake alone will ensure a healthy baby, since so many factors can affect a pregnancy.

Women should bear this in mind when contemplating pregnancy, advises Jeanne Latham, a registered dietitian and consumer safety officer in FDA's Office of Special Nutritionals. "Folate can make a significant contribution," she said, "but it's no guarantee of a healthy baby."

Genetics plays a role, as do other healthful prenatal practices, such as eating an all-around good diet. But unlike genetics, diet is a risk factor women can modify to their—and their baby's—advantage, said Jeanne Rader, Ph.D., director of the division of science and applied technology in FDA's Office of Food Labeling.

"Folic acid is one of many nutrients needed in a healthy diet for women of childbearing age," she said. "A well-balanced diet with a variety of foods can provide all those nutrients, including adequate amounts of folate."

Women have options for reaching the folate intake goal: They can get the necessary nutrients and calories both before and during pregnancy by eating a well-balanced diet, keeping in mind folate-rich foods, nutrition experts say. Folic acid-fortified grain products, including breakfast cereals, will help, too. Dietary supplements are another source of folate. Any one or a combination of these options for ensuring adequate folate can help assure women of childbearing age that, if they become pregnant, their babies will be off to a healthy start.

More Information

For more information on having a healthy baby, contact:

Maternal and Child Health Clearinghouse
5600 Fishers Lane, Room 18A-55
Rockville, MD 20857
(703) 821-8955

March of Dimes Birth Defects Foundation
1275 Mamaroneck Ave.
White Plains, NY 10605
(914) 428-7100
Voice mail only: (914) 997-4750
World Wide Web: http://server.triplesoft.com/marchofdimes/index.html

—by Paula Kurtzweil

Paula Kurtzweil is a member of FDA's public affairs staff.

Chapter 3

Prenatal Testing

Prenatal Peeks

Ultrasound

In an ultrasound exam, a device called a transducer passed over the abdomen or inserted into the vagina, bounces sound waves off the fetus, much like sonar locating a submarine. A computer converts the sound waves into an image. Many studies show it is very safe to mother and fetus.

Ultrasound can establish the date of conception, the presence of twins, and monitor development. By 8 weeks, an image resembling a lima bean with a pulsating blip in the middle is an assurance that a "viable fetus"—with its blip of a heartbeat—is there.

By 15 weeks, a trained eye can discern major organs. While the parents happily count toes and fingers, a physician may measure the length of the leg bones or check facial features for signs of Down syndrome.

By 20 weeks, a penis—or lack of one—may be apparent. By 35 weeks, calcium deposits in the placenta, the organ linking mother to child, signal lung maturity. As the birth day nears, ultrasound reveals the fetal position.

This chapter contains excerpts pertinent to contenigal disorders from "Genetic Screening—Fetal Signposts on a Journey of Discovery," *FDA Consumer*, December 1990, and "Statement on the Routine Use of Ultrasound Screening During Pregnancy," American College of Obstetricians and Gynecologists, Washington, DC, ACOG © September 15, 1993; Reprinted with permission.

Amniocentesis

Through amniocentesis, the amniotic fluid surrounding the fetus is sampled with a needle inserted into the woman's abdomen. Fetal cells floating in the fluid are grown and examined for chromosomal abnormalities, such as the extra chromosome 21 that causes Down syndrome. Biochemicals in the fluid also provide diagnostic clues to several inborn errors of metabolism. Approved since 1967, amniocentesis is offered to women over 35, the age when the risk of the procedure causing a miscarriage is equal to the risk of the woman carrying a fetus with a detectable chromosomal problem (this risk increases with age). Women younger than 35 may have the procedure if a relative has a detectable abnormality. Amniocentesis can rule out many disorders, but it cannot guarantee a healthy baby.

The major drawback of amniocentesis at present is that it cannot safely be performed until the 16th week of pregnancy, and it takes 10 days or longer for fetal cells to be cultured and results to be known. However, several medical centers are experimenting with performing amniocentesis as early as 12 weeks.

Another advance is the use of automated, computerized chromosome sorters that are programmed to scan for abnormalities. This replaces technicians cutting up photographs of chromosomes and arranging them into a standard chart, then searching visually for aberrations—a time-consuming process.

Yet another new approach to viewing chromosomes is "in situ hybridization," a technique that uses DNA probes (bits of DNA tagged with a chemical) to locate and highlight specific chromosomes with no need to culture them first. This approach, still for research use only, can identify the extra chromosome of Down syndrome in hours.

Chorionic Villus Sampling (CVS)

In CVS, recently approved by FDA, a catheter inserted through the vagina samples chorionic villi, finger-like structures that form the placenta by 10 weeks of prenatal development. Because villi cells descend from the fertilized egg, their chromosomes match those of the fetus.

The great advantage of CVS is that it can be performed as early as 8 weeks, and results are ready within days.

In the March 9, 1989, *New England Journal of Medicine*, George G. Rhoads, M.D., and co-workers at the National Institute of Child Health and Human Development reported on a seven-center study comparing CVS to amniocentesis. They conclude, "CVS is a safe and effective technique for the early prenatal diagnosis of cytogenetic abnormalities, but it probably entails a slightly higher risk of procedure failure and fetal loss than does amniocentesis." The risk of amniocentesis causing miscarriage is 0.5 percent; that of CVS is 1.3 percent. Miscarriages are more often associated when CVS is performed more than twice.

The Triple Test—AFP-Plus

In 1975, scientists found a link between high levels of alpha-fetoprotein (AFP) in pregnant women's blood and a type of fetal abnormality called a neural tube defect, which includes spina bifida (an open spine) and anencephaly (lack of higher brain structures). The open lesions of such defects allow AFP to leak faster than normal from the fetus' liver into the mother's bloodstream, causing the elevated levels.

In 1984, studies linked too little of the substance to Down syndrome. After this discovery, measuring AFP at 15 weeks for use as a prenatal warning greatly expanded. This helps in spotting Down syndrome in women under 35, who would usually not have amniocentesis. Abnormal AFP levels may also be associated with other birth defects and with late miscarriage, low birth weight, toxemia (very high blood pressure in a woman in the last trimester of pregnancy), premature delivery, and other birth defects.

How can one substance show so much? "We think the abnormal readings reflect something wrong with the placenta," says Washington Hill, M.D., director of maternal-fetal medicine at the Creighton University School of Medicine in Omaha.

AFP testing has a very high false-positive rate, because the level of AFP can be thrown off by such factors as a miscalculated due date, obesity, twins, or being black or diabetic. In 1987, accuracy was improved by considering levels of human chorionic gonadotropin, too, which is high in Down syndrome. The recent addition of a third measurement—unconjugated estriol—may make readings even more accurate.

By indicating a low risk, the use of this "triple test" could spare some women over 35 from amniocentesis recommended only because of their age. However, this is a screening test, not a diagnostic test, cautions George J. Knight, Ph.D., of the Foundation for Blood Research in Scarborough, Maine, where the test was developed. Women with abnormal results must undergo more definitive tests, such as ultrasound and amniocentesis, before the diagnosis is considered final.

Treating the Fetus

Blake Schultz' life was saved seven weeks before he was born. Early in 1990, ultrasound revealed a hole in his diaphragm, the muscle sheet dividing the chest from the abdomen. His stomach, intestines and spleen protruded into his chest, squashing his lungs. He would probably have suffocated shortly after birth, were it not for experimental surgery performed by Michael Harrison, M.D., and colleagues at the University of California at San Francisco.

They exposed part of the fetus, opened his left side, gently tucked the organs back into place, and repaired the hole with a patch of Goretex, a synthetic material used in warm-up suits. Blake was the first human success, following six others who didn't make it.

Other fetal treatments are more routine. For hydrocephalus ("water on the brain"), a shunt can drain the fluid buildup into the digestive tract, where it exits harmlessly. For too little amniotic fluid caused by a blocked fetal bladder, a catheter can be inserted to drain off the accumulating urine.

"Left untreated, this causes a backup of urine into the fetal genitourinary system, which leads to fetal kidney damage, too little amniotic fluid, and destruction of the lungs—which kills the baby," says Frank Craparo, M.D., who performs such surgery at Pennsylvania Hospital in Philadelphia.

Craparo samples fetal blood to detect anemia and rapidly analyze chromosomes, and can also enter the blood vessels of the umbilical cord to deliver drugs directly to the fetus while bypassing the mother. Called PUBS (percutaneous umbilical blood sampling), the procedure can also be used to provide a lifesaving transfusion when blood between mother and child is incompatible.

"In these cases, the fetus becomes severely anemic, and may die in utero, or be born prematurely," Craparo says. He is working on expanding the capabilities of PUBS. "We will be able to study blood gases, and perhaps see how well oxygenated a fetus is in cases of growth retardation. There are a whole host of tests on the horizon. Anything we can do on adult blood, we may be able to do on a fetus' blood." Still experimental, PUBS carries a risk of 1 to 1.5 percent of harming the fetus.

—*by Ricki Lewis, Ph.D.*

Ricki Lewis teaches biology at SUNY (State University of New York) Albany is a genetic counselor, and author of a book, *Beginnings of Life*.

The American College of Obstetricians and Gynecologists (ACOG) Statement on the Routine Use of Ultrasound Screening During Pregnancy

The American College of Obstetricians and Gynecologists (ACOG) does not recommend the routine use of ultrasound screening of all obstetrical patients, having stated in 1988 that more large clinical studies were needed in the United States to assess the role of routine ultrasound screening in pregnancy.[1] The College continues to advise that "ultrasound is not necessary for every woman or in every pregnancy."[2]

The study of the Routine Antenatal Diagnostic Imaging with Ultrasound (Radius) Study Group, a trial involving over 15,000 women, represents the largest U.S. study to date on the role of routine ultrasound, and provides the type of data called for by the College in its 1988 guidelines. The report's conclusion that routine ultrasound screening in low-risk pregnancy provides no apparent improvement in perinatal outcomes is an important addition to the medical literature on routine ultrasound.

In obstetrics, ultrasound is used to examine the growing fetus inside the mother's uterus, and can provide information regarding fetal viability, fetal age, whether the size of the fetus is right for its age, its rate of growth, the number of fetuses, the location of the placenta, the amount of amniotic fluid surrounding the fetus, and the detection of some types of birth defects. Targeted ultrasound exams, when an anomaly is suspected, can diagnose defects of the fetal head, spine, chest, limbs, and some heart defects.

Ultrasound may be indicated in cases where there is reason to suspect a problem or where additional information about the fetus is needed. Indications can include patients who, by history, clinical evaluation, or a prior ultrasound, are suspected of carrying a defective fetus; women with diabetes for whom the dating of gestational age becomes important to perinatal outcome; patients with a discrepancy between fetal size and onset of pregnancy; or patients with bleeding during pregnancy. In most cases, ultrasound will be used in conjunction with other exams and tests needed to diagnose and treat a problem.

The selective use of ultrasound screening for specific medical indications must be distinguished, however, from the routine use of ultrasound in all pregnancies. The conclusions of the RADIUS study are consistent with previous College recommendations against the routine use of ultrasound in pregnancy.

Notes

1. ACOG Technical Bulletin #116, May 1988.
2. *Ultrasound Exams in Ob/Gyn*, ACOG Patient Education Pamphlet, October 1988.

Chapter 4

How to be an Assertive Parent on the Treatment Team

Remember what you have that the professionals lack—a total commitment to the child and to your whole family, allied to uniquely complete knowledge of the child, and the responsibility of making decisions and choices in regard to every aspect of your child's management.

Remember what professionals bring to the case: a general desire to help achieve the best outcome utilizing variable amounts of specialized information and technique more or less relevant to the needs of all children sharing a particular problem; varying degrees of mental and administrative flexibility in applying their general knowledge to a particular case; and a variable degree of personal commitment to the knowledge-base and philosophy of a discipline.

You can bridge the gap! Share with the professionals your ability to be flexible, to take responsibility, and your knowledge of your child, all often much greater than theirs.

Demonstrate your knowledge and flexibility by active participation in the decision-making, planning and evaluation processes—by

---

The Information in this chapter was produced by the Hydrocephalus Association. It was adapted from an article by A. Mervyn Fox, M.D., B.S., F.R.C.P. (C), D.C.H, Developmental Pediatrician, Associate Professor, Pediatrics, University of Western Ontario, London, Canada, September 1986, and reviewed by Hydrocephalus Association's executive director, Emily Fudge, in 1996; reprinted with permission.

avoiding aggression and conflict through assuming responsibility and losing no chance to present your assertiveness.

You are already knowledgeable about your own child—but, like the professionals, you should acquire a documented data-base. They have their "chart" or "file"—so must you: First, make your own record of the facts, including specific details and times of behaviors (first words, how many words spoken, events leading up to misbehavior and your reactions to it, exact description of a seizure, etc.), diary of therapy sessions or results of interventions, tape recordings or videos of speech or movements patterns not exhibited in hospital or school: secondly, acquire your own copies of hospital discharge summaries, specialists consultation notes, psychologists reports, therapists recommendations, etc.

Make it clear from the first contact that you expect to be provided with such information—assertively but not aggressively—to help you ensure that you understand what the experts are doing and guarantee that you do everything to help their treatment plans work. When signing the authorization for reports to be shared among professional agencies, insert your own name in the distribution list. Ask the professionals to review what they have written with you. Make your own comments in writing if you wish and feed these back into the record system.

You need to become knowledgeable about your child's condition and the various means of helping that are available. You need not try to know as much as the professionals who will have had years of basic science preparation anyway, but you must be familiar with the jargon professionals use and with the basic mechanisms involved in causing and maintaining disability, and the range of treatment options.

If you are not given reading material, firmly indicate that you wish to know what books, articles or pamphlets the specialist or team would recommend. *Join the relevant parent/patient organization.* Review the reading material with the professionals who recommended it, having made notes of areas you find confusing, or about which you need to know more, or about which you have heard a conflicting opinion. In this regard use the professional as a student would a teacher—as a resource for information: but you are an adult, and in control of your own "curriculum", and entitled to the time and individual attention you are paying for.

How to be an Assertive Parent on the Treatment Team

If you come across information which you believe your professionals do not know, try to document it: insert a copy into your "file" or write down the name of the author, speaker or other original source.

Remember that most conflicts stem from failure to communicate: **aggression is an expression of poor communication, assertiveness is a means of effective communication** in itself. Work out in advance what it is you wish to get over to the treatment team, whether it be facts, plans and objectives, or feelings. Assertiveness implies initiating rather than reacting. Similarly try to work out in advance your own areas of doubt, confusion or ignorance and ensure that efforts are made to reduce these before trying to "build on a poor foundation". Whenever you meet with the professional team, or any individual member or professional, know your own "agenda"—a meeting without clear agenda will achieve nothing—and invite the team/professionals to state theirs too.

Use and take notes as much as possible. Bring written agenda to each meeting—"What I want to ask the doctor, therapist, etc.," "What I want to tell," and "What I want the meeting to achieve."

Do not hesitate to write or refer to notes during the meeting; good professionals do it the whole time. Write down answers to your questions if you are unlikely to remember them exactly, write down who is responsible for what, especially if you have been made responsible for something; write down definitions of words if necessary.

Be clear in your own mind what you want professional interventions to achieve for your child: ask directly if your objective and those of the team or medical professional are the same. If not, be sure you have come to a negotiated position in regard to what is happening, why, for how long, how the intervention will be evaluated, and what will happen next if the intervention does or does not work.

Be prepared to negotiate. Allow for the possibility that you may be wrong and the professionals right—and help them accept the reverse! Remember that every intervention is an experiment—it has never been tried before on your child. Remember that, with the exception of surgery, no intervention (therapy, special education, drugs, treatment-break, diet, exercise) is likely to do any harm over a short period, so it is safe to try anything provided you set down from the start the duration and evaluation and are objective in deciding whether the experiment has or has not worked. As a parent, be prepared to take the responsibility for your own experiments—whether of commission (we'll try it my way) or of omission (I can't and won't do it your way). Try to identify the obstacles to a proposed plan—yours or other team members—and suggest ways around them—compromise. You are much more able to be flexible than are the professionals—use this strength. Bargain—I'll do it your way if you'll do it mine later, or first, or in some other area. Never lose sight of the objective—short term (to walk, drink from a cup, read at grade level, speak intelligibly), or long term (to be independent, to use leisure time well, to get a decent job, to be able to leave home someday).

There is no need to feel intimidated. Professionals, to achieve their objectives, need your help just as much as you need theirs; within the professional relationship, you have hired their knowledge and time and it is up to you—not to them alone—to make the best use of what you are paying for. Be assertive—mutual respect is a great basis for a relationship! The professional may need help to respect you for your commitment, individual knowledge and flexibility. He will respond to your informed appreciation of his/her skills.

Make sure you understand the role of each member of the treatment team—as an individual and in terms of the discipline they represent. Who is the leader? Who is the most/least experienced? What exactly does an occupational therapist/kinesiologist/audiologist know and do? Are there disciplines relevant to the best outcome for your child not represented on the treatment team? If so, which, why not, where are they, who knows about them? Who will advise about nutrition, exercise, career-planning, educational placement, behavior management, or feelings (your child's, your own, your family's, your professionals)?

Make sure the team knows you—your expertise, the constraints upon you in terms of your own job (time, distance, shift-work), your involvement in recreation/voluntary/political activities, your sense of how your disabled child fits into the whole family system and its personal priorities and aspirations.

Do not avoid talking about feelings. If you feel intimidated, say so, and try to explain why—do you feel ignorant (about your child, you are anything but: about the rest, it is part of the professionals job to help you be well-informed)—but in the treatment situation you are the authority with the power to terminate the relationship. Does one member of the team make you feel uncomfortable? If so, you can determine just who is present at a meeting, or explore why that individual has that effect upon you. Change the situation to diminish your intimidation and assert your own control: state the agenda, making sure the professional agenda is not ignored. Take the head of the table; limit or increase the size of the group to your own comfort level; ask a particular team member to sit next to you; do not hesitate to bring in outside support from your family, church or other helping agencies.

If you feel angry, try to say so without acting out and try to pinpoint the source of the anger—is it relevant to the treatment, or are you still coping with earlier phases of the reaction to disability, or with quite different parts of your life? If you feel hopeless or depressed, seek appropriate support or help and share your mood with the treatment team. How does your mood affect your child, or his/her motivation to treatment/education/leisure? If you lack confidence in the treatment team, it is not fair to the professionals to hold this back. What changes would you make to give you confidence? Negotiate such change as is possible. Take responsibility for experiments and trials.

If you feel a second opinion would help, never hesitate to ask for one. Often the professionals would welcome this as much as you would but have not suggested it for fear of shaking your confidence. Make it quite clear, though, what you hope to gain from the second opinion: a diagnosis, a forecast for the future, a different plan of management, a check upon the team in whom you lack confidence. Discuss your objectives and what has lead up to your request. No good professional ever objects to being asked to arrange or provide date for a second opinion. If your team refuses to discuss a request for a second opinion, your lack of confidence is probably justified and you should consider seeking alternative sources of professionals anyway. Sometimes when you explain just what you are looking for from a second opinion the existing team will be able to provide this—as always, discuss and negotiate. Distinguish between asking for a second opinion in regard to an identified issue and what professionals call "shopping around" (making visits to a number of professionals in such a way that one visit follows another without resolution of a resolvable problem) which is a symptom of denial, insecurity, lack of either confidence or information, and is the signal for mutual re-assessment.

The assertive parent is not the "boss" of the treatment team, nor just their "client" (although use of this term reminds us who is hiring whom) but a "partner"—and the partner whose ultimate responsibility for the success of the whole project has the deepest roots and will be exercised long after the professionals have forgotten the case.

Aggressiveness will only produce defensive responses—professionals rarely dare show aggression in return—with eventual withdrawal from the case, or passive provisions of unimaginative routine procedures rather than the personal, enthusiastic, and individualized management that displays professionals skills, parental dedication and the strengths of your child to the best advantage and outcome.

Assertiveness yields mutual respect—and often, friendship. Your objectives will only be achieved if you say what they are. Professionals are well-informed, hardworking and highly motivated, and respond best to similarly endowed parents as their partners.

Balance your assertiveness with trust. Trust is greatest when best informed and quietly expressed. Trust has to grow out of experience; without taking a chance trust can never grow. As you show and express your trust in your professional partners, so will they grow in ability to trust you and accept your ability to exploit their skills to achieve the best outcome for your child, even if your plans are unorthodox or risky. The ability to trust in others springs from your ability to trust yourself—your own self-confidence and self-esteem as a mature adult. Know yourself and your limits, as well as your strengths and abilities. Do not hesitate to express your needs for yourself and your family as well as those for your disabled child. *If you do not look after yourself and your family, who will? If you do not know what is best for your child, who does?* If by discussion, negotiation, assertiveness and trust between sensible and well-informed people with appropriate resources one cannot arrive at the best possible outcome for your child, then we are all searching for miracles.

For More Information

Hydrocephalus Association
870 Market Street #955
San Francisco, California 94102
Telephone: (415) 732-7040; Fax: (415) 732-7044

Part Two

Spina Bifida and Hydrocephalus

Chapter 5

Answering Your Questions about Spina Bifida

Introduction

Spina Bifida is a complex birth defect recognized in man for thousands of years. It is the second most common birth defect and touches countless lives. Through this booklet we hope to provide information to help you understand the basic medical, educational and social issues which commonly affect people with spina bifida.

Until the early 1950s babies born with spina bifida rarely survived. Major medical advances in neurosurgery and urology have changed that. Today the majority of infants born with this birth defect will live into adulthood, and a better understanding of the social, educational and emotional aspects of spina bifida, along with significant changes in state and federal laws, have made it possible for many people with spina bifida to lead happy, productive lives.

There is still more work to be done and much more to be learned about this complex condition. By working together, medical and nonmedical specialists, families of those with spina bifida and individuals with spina bifida themselves will continue the impressive progress which has already been made.

The text and illustrations presented in this chapter are taken from *Answering Your Questions about Spina Bifida* ©1995 Children's National Medical Center; all rights reserved, reprinted with permission. Catherine Shaer, M.D., Editor; Martha Scheele Ross, Illustrator. For information on obtaining a copy of this publication, please contact The Spina Bifida Program, Children's National Medical Center, 111 Michigan Avenue, N.W., Washington, DC 20010-2970; (202) 884-3092. FAX (202) 884-2783.

Answering Your Questions about Spina Bifida

Prenatal/Genetic Issues

What is spina bifida? During the first 28 days of a pregnancy the brain and spinal cord of an embryo (developing baby) form. For reasons not well understood this development is interrupted in some babies and the birth defect spina bifida, also called myelomeningocele, occurs.

Spina bifida is actually one of a number of conditions called "neural tube defects" that occur when the central nervous system (the brain and spinal cord) of the developing baby fails to form normally at some point along its length. This can occur anywhere from the brain to the end of the spinal cord. When the brain itself is not completely developed the condition is called "anencephaly." When a portion of the spine is abnormally formed "spina bifida" results.

Spina bifida actually means split spine. This name comes from the fact that the bones or vertebrae of the spinal column which surround the developing spinal cord do not close as they normally would but, instead, remain open. Figure 5.1 compares the development of a fully formed spinal cord with the development of one with spina bifida.

Figure 5.1. Development of the spinal cord. This figure compares the development of a fully formed spinal cord with one where spina bifida results. Note the fluid cyst and open skin overlying the open neural tube in the spina bifida case (lower figure).

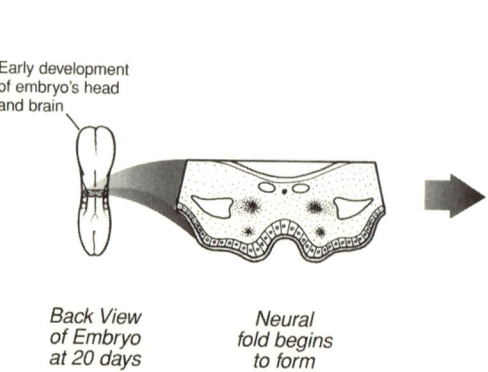

Early development of embryo's head and brain

Back View of Embryo at 20 days

Neural fold begins to form

20 days

Answering Your Questions about Spina Bifida

It is possible that only the bones of the spinal column will be incompletely developed and that the nervous tissue beneath will be normal. In these cases the skin of the back is also normal. This very different condition, called "spina bifida occulta," usually occurs at the lower end of the spine and rarely causes medical problems. Spina bifida occulta is a common variation of normal spinal cord development and is found in 10 to 15 percent of the general population. In some cases a "signature mark" on the skin of the back such as a dimple, hair patch, or red discoloration may be associated with spina bifida occulta. In these cases these may also be more significant abnormalities of the spinal cord. If one of these signs are present on the skin, the baby should be evaluated for abnormalities of the spinal cord.

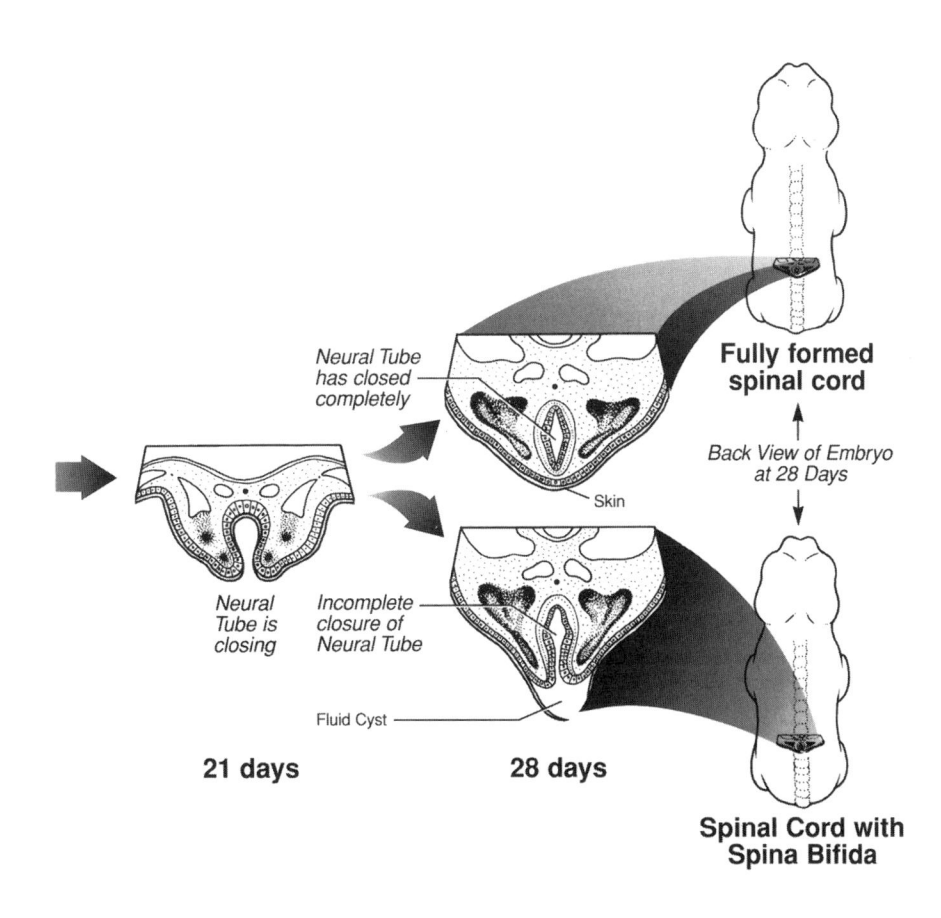

This chapter will deal with the most significant type of spina bifida, "myelomeningocele," in which a portion of the spinal cord is undeveloped, the overlying bones are not fully formed, and there is no skin covering the open bones or spinal cord. This can happen anywhere along the spine but is most common in the lower portions from the upper lumbar to the upper sacral areas. Figure 5.2 illustrates the various levels of the bones (vertebrae) and underlying spinal cord.

Why does spina bifida occur? Spina bifida occurs in the first month of pregnancy, before most women even know they are pregnant. At this time the cause (or causes) of spina bifida is not well understood. We do know, however, that it does not result from falling while pregnant, taking most commonly used medications during pregnancy or from common illnesses such as colds or urinary tract infections occurring during pregnancy.

The number of children born with spina bifida varies from country to country and has changed a great deal over time. Today spina bifida or anencephaly occur in approximately 1 out of every 1000 pregnancies in the United States. In most cases it is the first such birth defect to occur on either side of the family. Once a couple has one child with this birth defect, however, their risk of having a second affected child increases to between 1 and 5 out of 100. Remember, this also means that the chances for having a child without spina bifida are between 95 percent and 99 percent. If one parent has spina bifida, the chances of having an affected baby are between 1 percent and 5 percent. If both parents have spina bifida their chances of having a baby with this birth defect increase to 15 percent. Women taking certain anticonvulsant medications (medicines taken to control seizures) have a higher chance of having a baby with a neural tube defect. Genetic counselors are available in most large medical centers and can discuss the risk for each individual family.

Can spina bifida be found before a baby is born? There are several tests available to pregnant women which can be used to detect spina bifida before a baby is born (prenatally).

Blood drawn from pregnant women during the 16th week of pregnancy can be tested for alpha fetoprotein (AFP), a substance made by all developing babies. Abnormally high levels of this protein are found in the blood of women carrying babies with open central nervous systems and 85 percent of cases of spina bifida will be found with this simple screening test. This test is not specific for spina bifida, however. An error in the dates of the pregnancy, multiple babies, as well as other birth defects can all cause an abnormal reading. Therefore, further testing is recommended if the initial AFP reading is abnormal.

Answering Your Questions about Spina Bifida

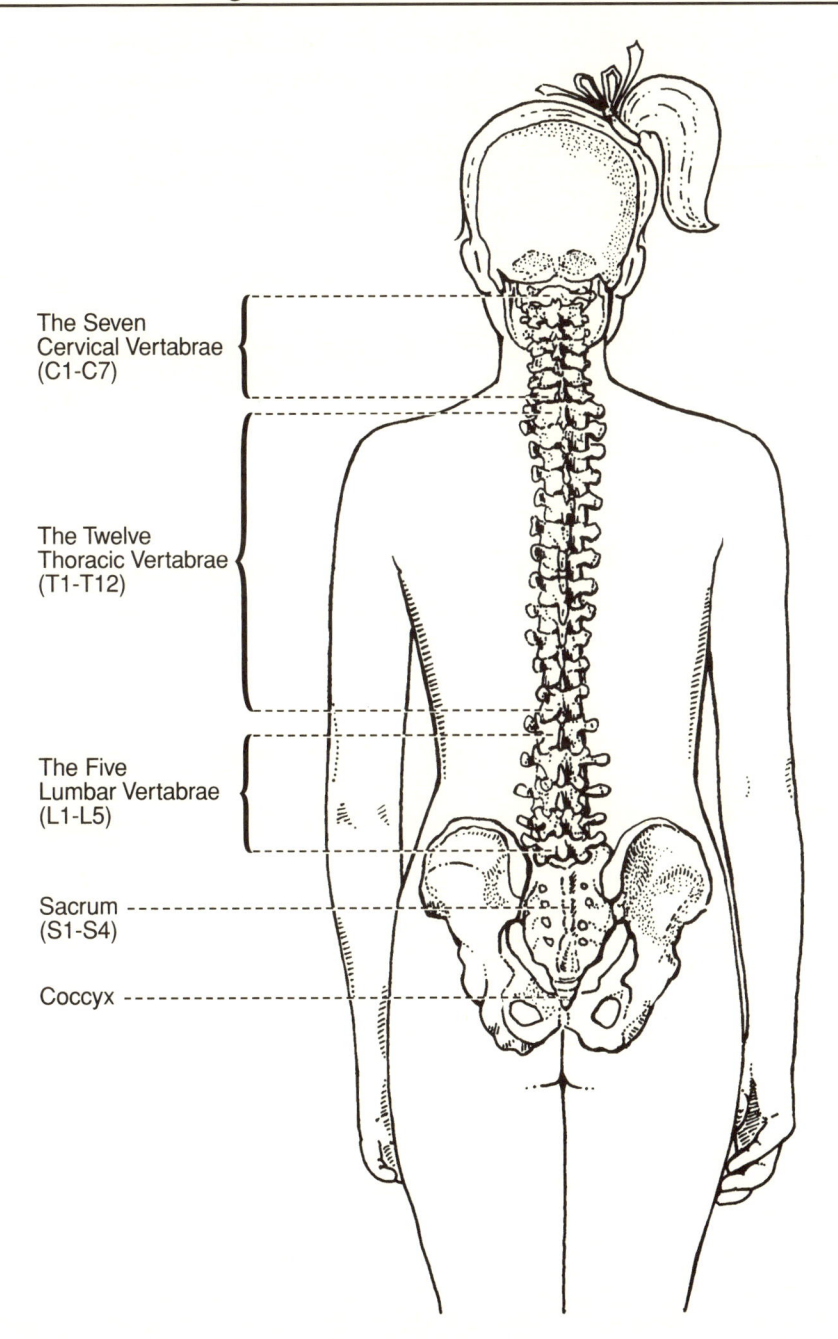

The Seven
Cervical Vertabrae
(C1-C7)

The Twelve
Thoracic Vertabrae
(T1-T12)

The Five
Lumbar Vertabrae
(L1-L5)

Sacrum
(S1-S4)

Coccyx

Figure 5.2. *Levels of the spinal column. This drawing shows the various levels of the spinal column. Spina bifida can occur at any level.*

Ultrasound (sonogram) can detect spina bifida by showing the defect in the spinal bones and certain changes in the brain. When this test is done between 18 and 20 weeks of pregnancy by experienced personnel, more than 90 percent of cases of spina bifida will be found.

Amniocentesis can also be used to detect spina bifida. Amniotic fluid (water surrounding the baby) is withdrawn from the womb between 14 and 17 weeks of pregnancy and is tested for AFP. This test is more accurate than screening the mother's blood. Amniocentesis carries a small risk of miscarriage and is usually offered only to women who are at increased risk for having a child with a birth defect. This includes women who are at increased risk for having a child with spina bifida (those who have already had an affected child, those with spina bifida themselves or whose partner has spina bifida, those with a strong family history of neural tube defects, and those taking certain medications to control seizures) as well as women over 35 years of age or those who have a significant medical or family history.

Women at increased risk of having a child with spina bifida will benefit from more extensive testing. A thorough ultrasound examination at 18 weeks along with either an AFP blood test or amniocentesis will provide the most reliable information. Again, genetic counselors can help families decide which tests are best for them, coordinate appropriate testing and interpret test results.

Can anything be done to prevent spina bifida? The cause or causes of spina bifida are unknown. In the late 1980s researchers around the world discovered that folic acid, a common B vitamin, can help reduce the risk of having a child with a neural tube defect including spina bifida and anencephaly. Women who take folic acid daily for at least one month before becoming pregnant and who continue to take it daily during the first three to four months of pregnancy will reduce their chances of having a baby with spina bifida and other neural tube defects.

There is still much to learn about the connection between neural tube defects and folic acid. At this time the Food and Drug Administration of the United States (FDA) recommends that all women of childbearing age take 0.4mg (400 micrograms) of folic acid every day. This is 100 percent of the recommended daily allowance and is found in many over-the-counter multivitamin supplements as well as in dark leafy green vegetables, whole grains and legumes (dried beans, soy beans, etc.). Those women at high risk of having a baby with a neural tube defect should take 0.4mg a day on a regular basis but should consult with their physicians about taking a higher daily dose when they are planning a pregnancy.

What effect does spina bifida have on the baby? Messages pass up and down the spinal cord carrying information between the brain and all areas of the body. When the spinal cord is not completely formed, these messages cannot be sent to or received from areas below the spina bifida. As a result, several body systems cannot function properly.

There are three primary areas of abnormal function: the central nervous system (brain and spinal cord), the urologic system (kidneys and bladder), and the musculoskeletal system (bones and muscles).

Neurosurgical Issues

How does spina bifida affect the spinal cord? The effect on the nervous system is very complicated. The entire central nervous system (the brain and spinal cord) is affected in individuals with spina bifida.

During the first weeks of pregnancy, the spinal cord begins to develop as a long flat area on the surface of the forming baby. Gradually the edges of this flat area fold together and form a structure called the neural tube. This process as shown in Figure 5.1 is normally completed by the 28th day of pregnancy. When the tube does not close at some point along the length of the developing spinal cord, the baby will have spina bifida. In addition, the bones of the spinal column (vertebrae) directly over the incompletely closed spinal cord do not come together and here is no skin over the open spinal cord. As a result, the infant has an open portion of the spinal cord protruding through the open bones and skin. Figure 5.3 compares the appearance of a fully developed spine to one where spina bifida has occurred. Figure 5.4 illustrates how a typical spina bifida defect at the mid-lumbar level would appear.

At the point of the spina bifida defect the normal passage of electrical impulses or messages from the brain to the nerves serving the rest of the body and from the body back to the brain is interrupted. A person with spina bifida will not be able to control muscles served by the abnormal nerves. In addition, there is usually no feeling in the skin below the defect. The point along the spinal cord where function is interrupted is referred to as the "level" of the spina bifida. The level

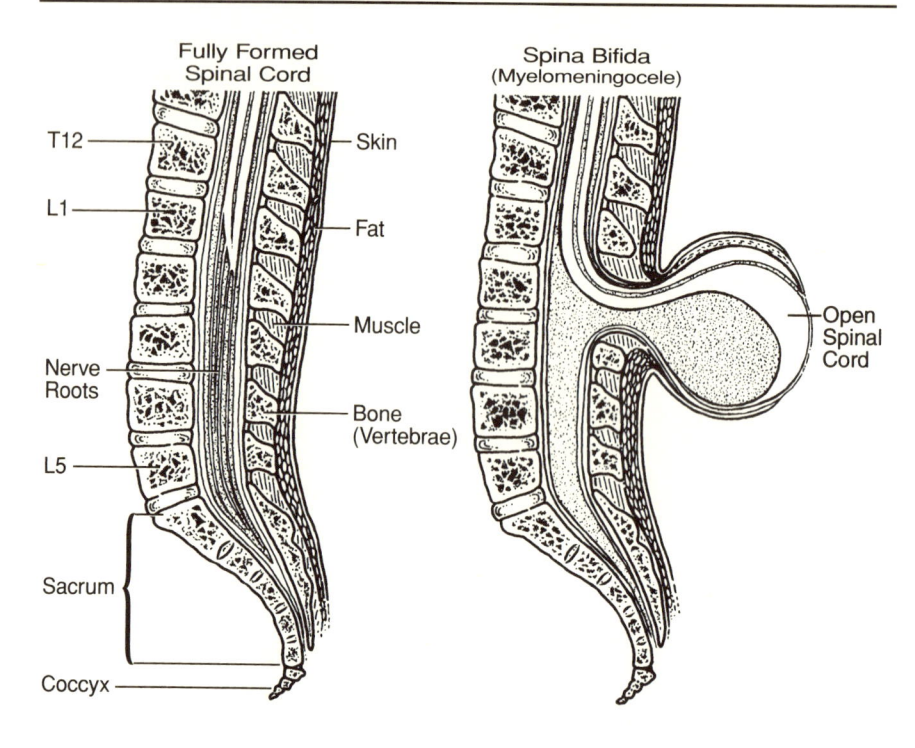

Figure 5.3. Side views of spinal cord. The left hand figure shows a fully formed spinal cord. The one on the right illustrates how the neural tube remains open and may protrude in cases of spina bifida.

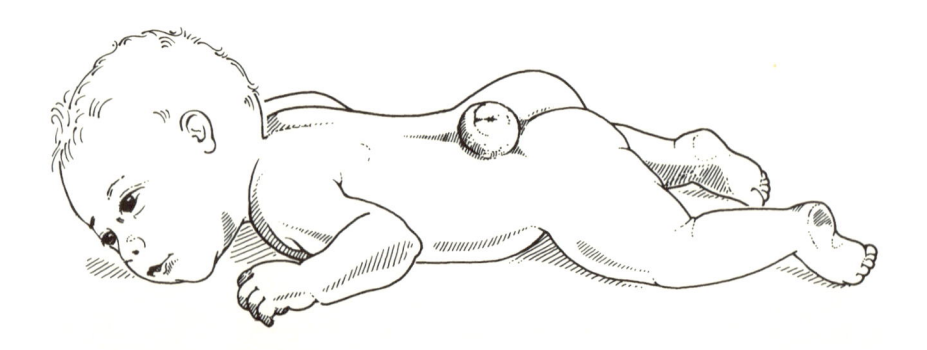

Figure 5.4. Infant with spina bifida before surgery. The open spinal cord can have a cyst-like appearance. This figure shows spina bifida in the mid to lower lumbar area.

of abnormal function cannot be fully determined by the location of the open area on the back of an infant. Examination of the baby by specialists is usually necessary to accurately determine the spina bifida level. Some individuals may have partial muscle function and patchy areas of feeling in their skin below the level of the spina bifida defect. This is called "sparing" of function or "spared" function.

Before birth, the womb and fluid surrounding the baby protect the open spine and exposed abnormal nerves from further damage and infection. During and after birth this open area can be further damaged and may become infected. In most cases, a neurosurgeon (a doctor specializing in surgery of the nervous system) will close the open back within 24 to 72 hours after birth. The purpose of the surgery is to return the spinal cord to as normal a position as possible and to protect any functioning nervous tissue from injury and infection. Currently there is no surgery or other treatment which can make an undeveloped spinal cord function normally. This operation, therefore, will not restore missing muscle control or skin sensitivity.

What is the effect of spina bifida on the brain? In virtually all individuals born with an open spinal cord there are abnormalities in the development of the brain, as well. In people with spina bifida the brain is positioned further down into the upper spinal column than it should be. This abnormal position of the brain, along with other internal differences in the brains of individuals with spina bifida, is called the Chiari II (also called Arnold Chiari) malformation. This malformation blocks the flow of the fluid which normally moves in and around the brain and results in an abnormal collection of fluid within the cavities or "ventricles" of the brain. This condition of overly filled ventricles is called hydrocephalus or, in common language, "water on the brain." Figure 5.5 shows both normal ventricles and ventricles enlarged by hydrocephalus.

Hydrocephalus is found on prenatal ultrasound testing in most infants with the myelomeningocele form of spina bifida. Severe collections of fluid frequently do not occur until after the open back is surgically closed, however. In 80 percent to 90 percent of individuals with spina bifida and hydrocephalus the neurosurgeon will need to implant a drainage device called a "shunt" to allow for the continuous drainage of spinal fluid and prevent severe hydrocephalus. Most commonly, the tube drains fluid from the ventricles to the abdominal cavity as shown in Figure 5.6. When severe hydrocephalus is present at birth, the back surgery and placement of the shunt may be done at the same time.

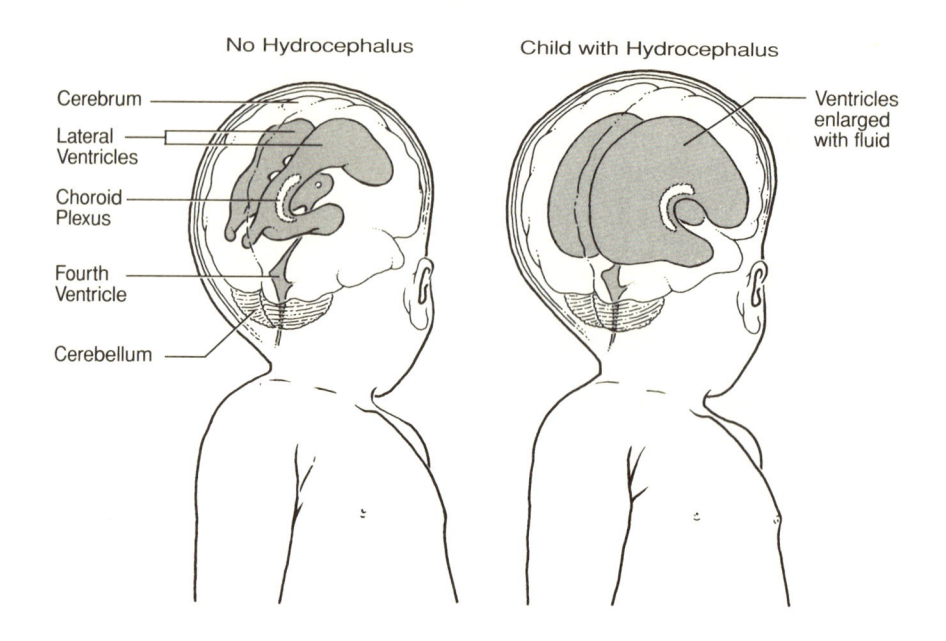

Figure 5.5. *The ventricular system of the brain. When the spinal fluid does not circulate normally the ventricles enlarge and hydrocephalus results.*

Although the reliability of shunts has steadily improved since the early 1950s, they are man-made devices which can fail. They can become clogged at either end, may break or be outgrown. The signs and symptoms of shunt malfunction vary with age and from individual to individual. The most common warning signs of shunt failure are listed on Table 5.1. When a shunt fails it will usually need to be replaced.

If shunt failure is suspected, the private physician or neurosurgeon should be notified without delay.

The Chiari II malformation can cause other problems with the brain. In a small percentage of cases the Chiari II malformation will lead to serious problems including an inability to regulate breathing, a loss of normal vocal cord function, difficulty swallowing, gagging with food or drink, or poor strength or function in the arms and hands. Children or adults with spina bifida exhibiting any of these problems may require surgery to relieve pressure on the back of the brain and should be seen by a neurosurgeon promptly.

Answering Your Questions about Spina Bifida

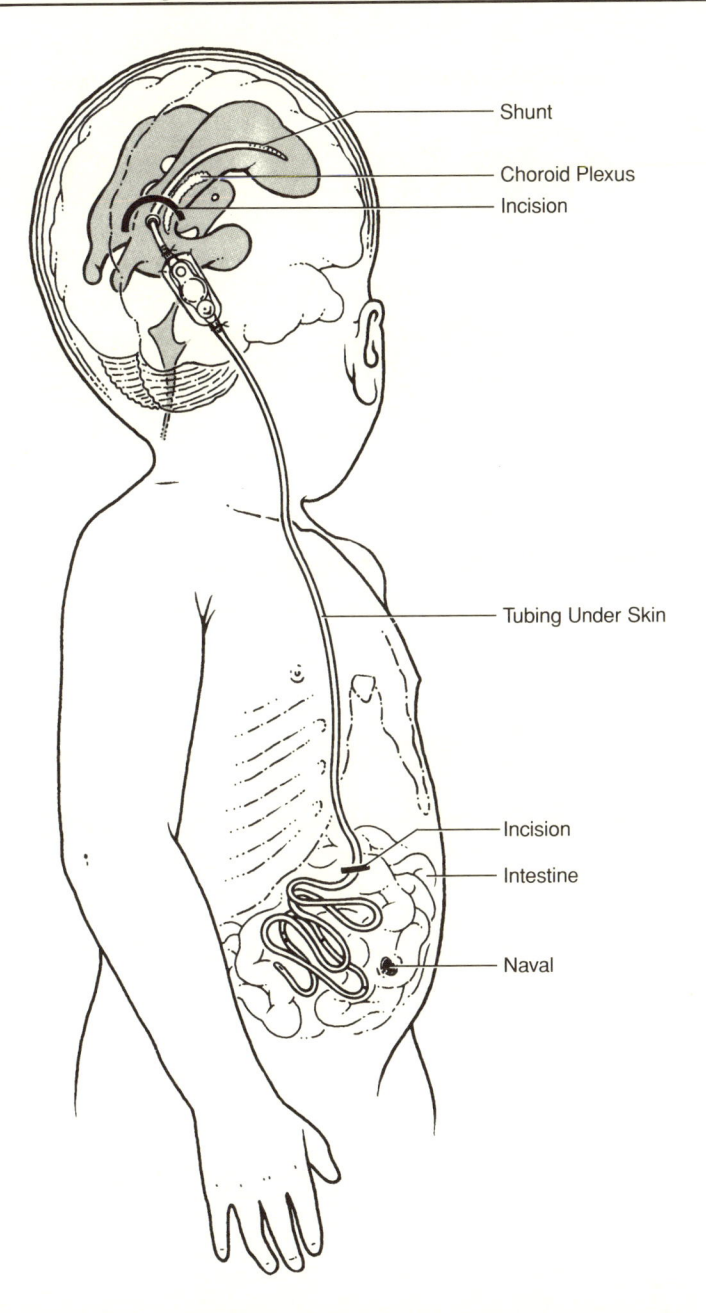

Figure 5.6. *Child after shunt surgery. The shunt, a thin straw-like device, is placed in the enlarged ventricles, tunneled under the skin, and placed in the abdominal cavity. This provides a pathway for the flow of spinal fluid, preventing the buildup of this fluid and controlling hydrocephalus.*

Table 5.1.

Age	Signs of Shunt Failure
Newborn to 1 year	Full or bulging fontanelle (soft spot) Enlarging head size Crossed eyes (new or worsening) Eyes looking downward Irritability Vomiting Increased sleepiness Swelling along shunt tract
2-3 years	Increased head size Irritability Personality changes Headache Vomiting Seizures Swelling along shunt tract Crossed eyes
4 years to adult	Personality changes Deterioration in school or job performance Headache Pain in spina bifida repair site Swelling along shunt tract Changes in vision

Urologic Issues

How does spina bifida affect the bladder and kidneys? Almost all newborn babies with spina bifida have normal kidney function. However, the nerves which control the bladder are almost always abnormal. As a result, normal bladder control is usually not possible. People with spina bifida are not able to feel when their bladders are full and many cannot empty their bladders of urine when needed. This can lead to several problems. If the bladder does not empty properly, urinary tract infections can occur. In addition, high pressure in the bladder may force urine backward toward the kidneys (a process called reflux). This can cause damage to the kidneys if the urine is infected. Figure 5.7 compares a healthy kidney with a kidney damaged by reflux. Kidney infections and damage can usually be prevented if the bladder is managed properly. Maintenance of healthy kidneys is best achieved with regular check-ups by a urologist, a doctor who specializes in the abnormalities of the kidneys and bladder.

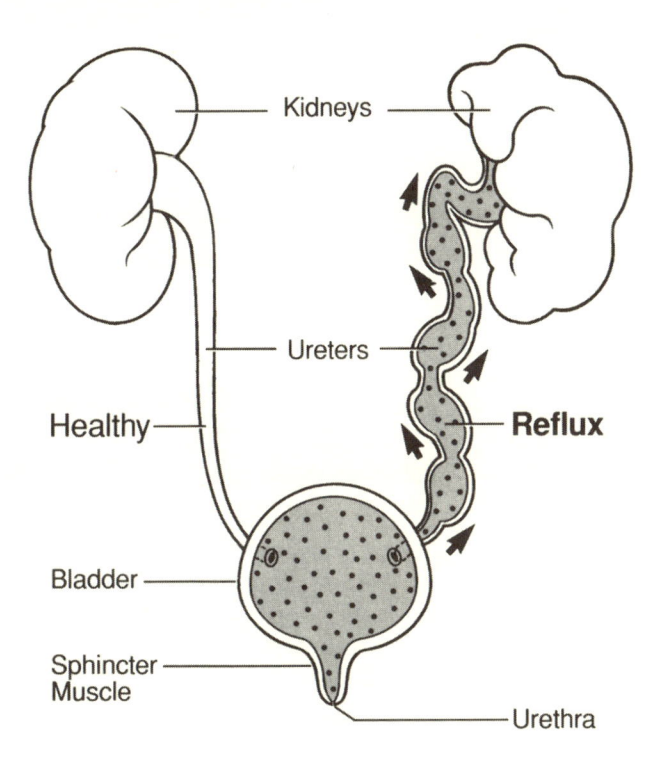

Figure 5.7. The kidneys and bladder. This figure compares a healthy kidney with one damaged by the back flow of urine (vesicoureteral reflux).

Testing is required to determine if the bladder is emptying properly, if abnormal backflow of urine (reflux) is present, and if the kidneys have become damaged. Because kidney and bladder problems usually cannot be detected on physical examination, and because the bladder can change as an individual ages, testing must be repeated periodically.

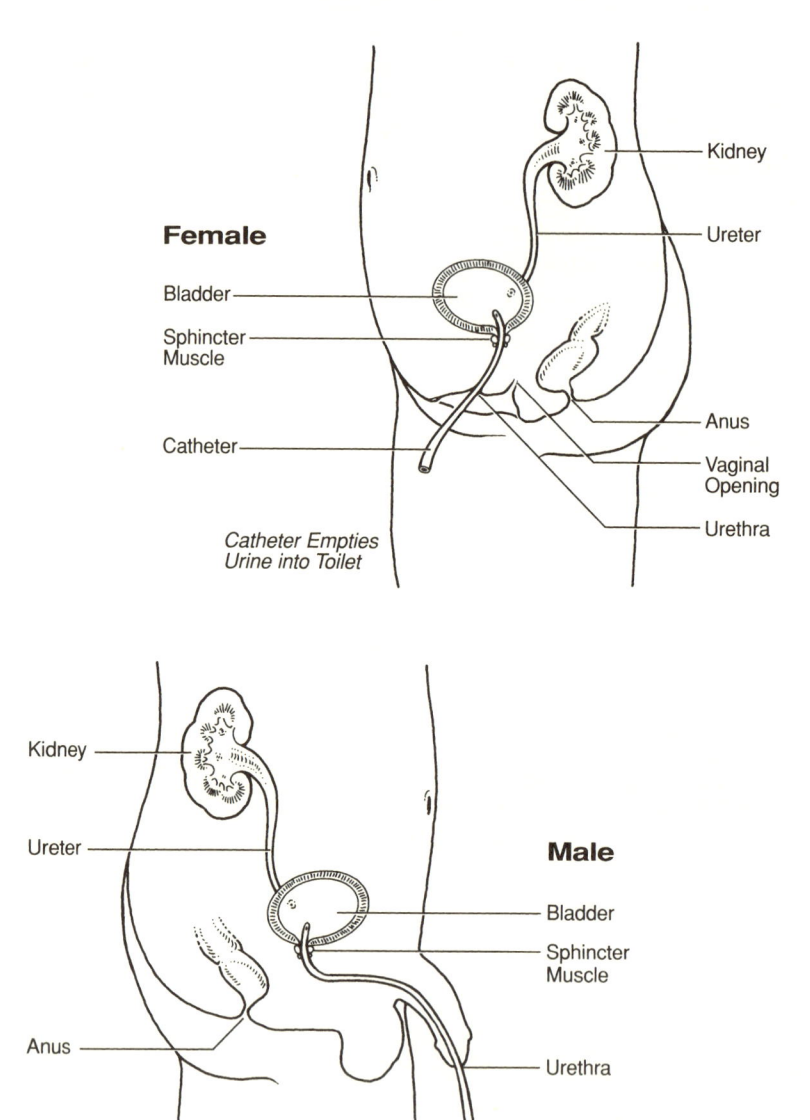

Figure 5.8. Catheterization in the male and female. In both males and females the catheter is inserted through the urethra and into the bladder. When urine flow stops and the bladder is empty the catheter is removed. The procedure is repeated at intervals prescribed by the urologist.

Since affected individuals will not have normal control of urination, children with spina bifida cannot be toilet trained in the usual sense. Most will learn to empty their bladders with a catheter, a small flexible straw-like device. During the day the catheter is inserted into the bladder every 2 to 4 hours and is removed when the bladder has been emptied. This program is usually started sometime between 3 and 5 years of age, although it may be started sooner in some children. The urologist will develop a specific plan tailored for each person's bladder. Parents or other adult caretakers will need to catheterize young children, but most children will be able to do the procedure themselves by the age of 7 or 8 years. They may require adult supervision for some time after they have learned the procedure, however. Figure 5.8 is a schematic representation of catheterization in a male and in a female. With the aid of catheterization and, in some cases medication, the vast majority of individuals with spina bifida will be dry and will not need to wear diapers to control wetness beyond early childhood. It is often recommended that boys with spina bifida be circumcised in order to make catheterization easier.

Bowel Control Issues

What about bowel control? The sacral nerves (refer to Figure 5.2) carry messages to and from the bowel and are usually undeveloped even in those individuals with a very low spina bifida defect. Therefore, most people with spina bifida cannot feel the need to move their bowels nor can they control when they have a bowel movement.

Food normally enters the stomach and moves into the small intestine where nutrients and minerals are absorbed. Stool then moves, in liquid form, into the large intestine. Here water is absorbed as it moves toward the rectum which is at the end of the large intestine. Figure 5.9 illustrates the various parts of the digestive tract. In many people with spina bifida liquid stool moves more slowly than it should through the colon and too much water is absorbed. This leads to firm, hard stools or constipation.

Hard stool may cause a partial or total blockage of the large intestine. Diarrhea can occur when liquid stool leaks around the blockage. It is important to keep stools soft because once hard stool forms, strong laxatives, enemas and occasionally hospitalization for a bowel clean-out may be needed. In addition, the lower portion of the rectum may stick out or "prolapse," past the anus. This tissue can be gently pushed back inside, but the prolapse will usually come back as long as the stools remain hard.

The sphincter, the muscle which surrounds the rectum, is normally tightened to hold stool in and relaxed when it is time to have a bowel movement. An individual with spina bifida will usually not have control of this muscle, and will therefore not have control of their bowel

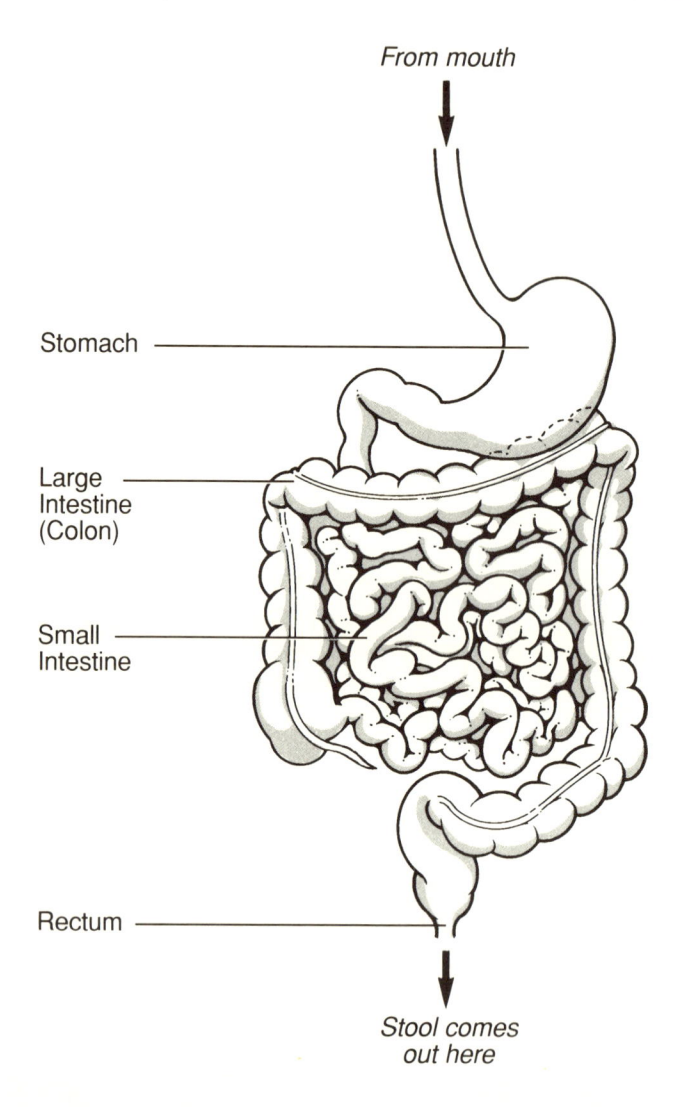

Figure 5.9. The digestive tract. Food and drink enter the stomach and pass into the small intestine as liquid stool. This stool then enters the large intestine and finally, passes out of the rectum. In many people with spina bifida liquid stool moves slowly through the large intestine and constipation often results.

movements. Bowel accidents—the passage of stool at inappropriate times—often occur and traditional toilet training is not possible. This may require the use of diapers into later childhood or even adulthood, making it difficult for affected individuals to separate from their parents and gain independence.

There are a variety of programs which may help individuals become bowel trained and achieve continence. Eating lots of fiber (fruits, vegetables, fiber supplements) will help the stool retain water as it passes through the large intestine and keep the stools soft. This will prevent hard, constipated stool from building up in the colon and stretching the muscles which line it. It is very important that parents pay attention to their child's bowel movements early on. Once a cycle of hard stool and constipation begins it is very difficult to reverse.

Suppositories, enemas, stool softeners or laxatives may sometimes be used to establish a pattern of regular bowel movements. This will take time and patience, but the rewards of success are tremendous. Remember, it is hard for a person to become independent if they have bowel accidents.

Orthopaedic Issues

How does spina bifida affect the muscles and bones of the body? Normal nerve development and function do not occur at or below the level of the abnormally developed spinal cord. The higher up the spinal cord the spina bifida defect, the greater the paralysis. Although each person must always be evaluated individually, Table 5.2 shows the typical amount of function found with different levels of spina bifida. There are a variety of tests which can be used to determine the level of paralysis.

Partial or complete paralysis of the legs does not necessarily mean a person cannot walk, but most people with spina bifida will need to wear leg braces in order to walk. Many will use braces along with crutches or canes. Even those with high, thoracic levels (see Figure 5.2) can be helped to move about in an upright position with the help of sophisticated braces and other devices. Those with levels at or above lumbar 3 (Figure 5.2) will often use braces for short distances and a wheelchair for more physically demanding activities such as shopping. Even children with good control of their legs may be fitted with braces in early childhood in order to support and protect weak muscles and vulnerable joints.

Many muscles work in pairs to keep bones in line and balance the movement of joints. In people with spina bifida it is not unusual for one muscle of a pair to have full function while the other member is partially or completely paralyzed. This imbalance can lead to a variety of problems including dislocated joints, misshapen bones and curvature of the spine. Early involvement of an orthopaedic surgeon—a doctor specializing in the evaluation and treatment of the bones and muscles—is important. Because of the imbalance of muscle pairs in the legs, many people with spina bifida will develop dislocated hips, bowed legs, curvatures of the spine and foot deformities. Some of these conditions are present at birth and others will develop over time. These conditions can sometimes be treated with exercise or splints but the orthopaedic surgeon will often need to do corrective surgery. Many individuals will need several orthopaedic operations, done over a period of years, to achieve the best possible body alignment.

Table 5.2.

Spina Bifida Level	Prognosis for Walking
S2-S4	Frequently walk without aides (braces or crutches). May need shoe inserts.
L5-S1	Usually need short leg braces to help with foot position and push off. May need crutches or cane.
L4	Usually need braces. May be above or below knee. May also use crutches or cane. Some use wheelchairs at older ages.
L2-L3	Long leg braces (up to thigh or waist) with crutches. May walk for exercise only in later years and use wheelchair for long distances.
L1	Long leg braces with a band around the waist. Uses crutches. Walks for exercise only. Wheelchair for any distances.
T12 and above	Can be braced to walk for short distances. Uses walker or crutches. Wheelchair for most activities even in childhood.

Answering Your Questions about Spina Bifida

Does the level of paralysis change over time? The level of actual paralysis should remain the same over time. As they grow, children with defects high on the spinal cord (mid- to upper lumbar and thoracic) will often choose to use a wheelchair for most of the day. This allows them to move more quickly and with much less energy and will free up their hands.

A condition called "tethered cord" can occur at any time during childhood or even into adulthood, however, and can cause additional damage to the spinal cord and nerves. When the opening in the spinal cord is surgically closed at birth, the tissues of the back may stick to the nervous system tissue during the healing process. As the child grows, the spinal cord may be stretched because it is stuck down or

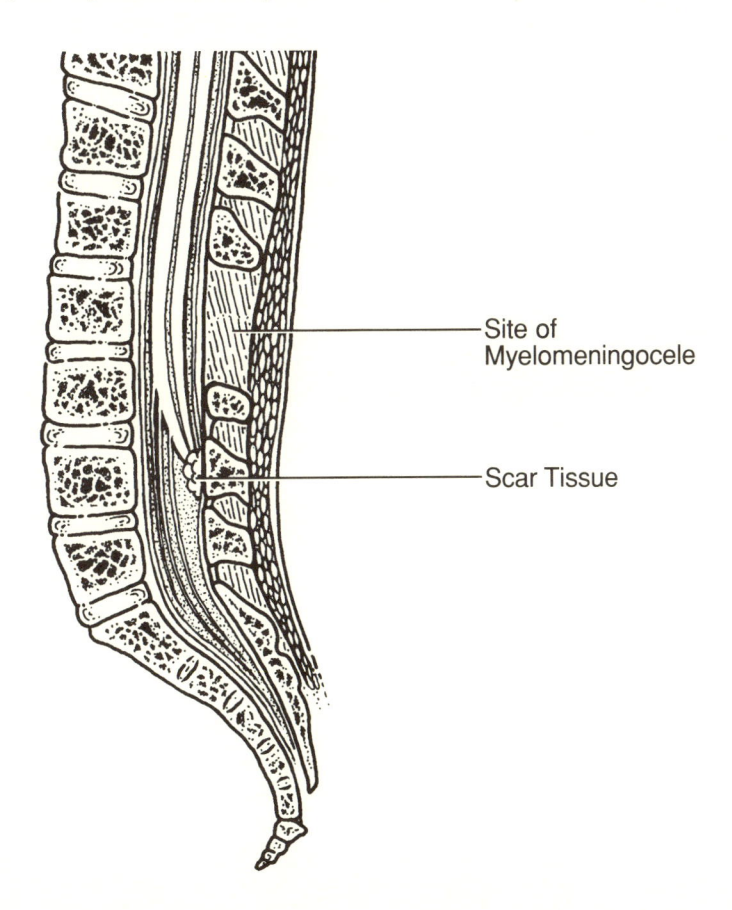

Figure 5.10. Tethered spinal cord. As shown in this drawing the spinal cord may become attached or "tethered" to nearby tissue. This may cause a loss of function.

tethered at the lower end. This is depicted in Figure 5.10. Significant stretching of the "stuck-down" spinal cord may occur during growth and cause new neurologic damage. Symptoms and signs of tethering include back pain, curvature of the spine (scoliosis), further loss of motor or sensory abilities, and changes in bowel or bladder function. When this occurs, an operation to release the spine (a de-tethering operation) can often prevent further damage and, in some cases, may even reverse some of the new damage. An MRI scan (a special diagnostic tool which creates a three-dimensional image of any part of the body) performed on the spinal cord can help determine if a de-tethering operation should be done. Symptoms of a tethered cord can also occur when the shunt used to control hydrocephalus fails to work properly. Shunt function may need to be investigated if symptoms of a tethered cord develop.

In some individuals abnormal pockets of fluid can form inside the spinal canal. These pockets are called syrinxes. Pressure from a syrinx can cause new paralysis anywhere along the spinal cord. People with spina bifida who show weakness in their arms or hands or an increase in scoliosis should be evaluated for a syrinx. An MRI of the spine is currently the most sensitive test available for diagnosing a syrinx.

Related Medical Issues

Can individuals with spina bifida participate in sports and other physical activities? Not only can they participate, it is important that a lifelong habit of regular physical exercise be developed at an early age. The decrease in activity resulting from partial or complete paralysis can lead to obesity and other medical problems such as high blood pressure, atherosclerosis (heart disease), and osteoporosis (weak bones).

A physical therapist or orthopaedic surgeon can help develop a safe and appropriate personalized exercise program. There are many local and national disability sports programs and organizations which provide opportunities to participate in tennis, horseback riding, swimming, basketball, baseball, track and field, skiing, and many other sports. Those individuals with shunts for controlling hydrocephalus are usually advised to avoid contact sports such as football and boxing. Information about what is available in your area can be obtained from your local recreational departments, Special Olympics office, county governments or Spina Bifida Association chapter.

Answering Your Questions about Spina Bifida

Are there any other problems commonly found in people with spina bifida? Yes. These are some of the most frequent problems:

- *Fractures*. People with spina bifida do not bear weight fully on their legs and, because of this, the bones of their lower extremities are often thin and easy to break. Because of decreased or absent feeling in the legs the individual may be unaware of their injury. Swelling, redness, deformity or fever may be the only signs of a significant fracture.

- *Seizures*. Seizures (epilepsy) occur in approximately 1 in every 500 children in the general population. This figure rises to about 1 in 20 individuals with spina bifida. The risk of developing a seizure disorder is greatest for those who have had central nervous system infections, have had their shunt fail a number of times, or have had episodes of respiratory insufficiency or arrest. Most seizure disorders are successfully treated with medication.

- *Eye problems*. Strabismus or lazy eye is a common disorder of children but is even more common in those with spina bifida. Without early treatment vision may be permanently impaired. If strabismus does not go away in the first six months of life it is recommended that the infant be evaluated by a pediatric ophthalmologist (eye specialist). Shunt failure may cause new strabismus or worsening of an already existing condition.

    Hydrocephalus may cause pressure on the optic nerve which can lead to poor vision. Children with spina bifida should be evaluated by an eye specialist by three years of age or earlier if eye problems are suspected.

- *Early Puberty (Precocious Puberty)*. The age of onset of puberty varies from child to child but, in the United States, it usually begins in girls at 10 to 11 years of age and at 11 to 12 years of age in boys. Puberty often begins early in children with abnormalities of the central nervous system including those with spina bifida and hydrocephalus. It may start as early as 7 or 8 years of age. During puberty growth stops in the longbones of the arms and legs. Therefore, when puberty occurs early, there are fewer years available for growth and affected individuals are shorter than average. There are medications which can be used to delay the start of puberty to a more appropriate time. A full evaluation by a specialist (usually an endocrinologist—a doctor specializing in the diagnosis and treatment of disorders of glands) must be done to determine if this treatment is right for an individual child.

- *Latex Allergy.* People with spina bifida are at high risk for the development of an allergy to latex (natural rubber). Although symptoms of latex allergy are frequently limited to a runny nose, itchy eyes, and hives, life-threatening reactions can occur. Experts recommend that individuals with spina bifida avoid exposure to latex.

  Synthetic catheters must be used by those on a catheterization program and only non-latex gloves should be used for medical, surgical and dental procedures. Contact with rubber balloons, balls, and other rubber toys should also be avoided.

- *Skin problems.* Spina bifida usually causes loss of sensation below the level of the spinal lesion. There may be partial or complete loss of normal skin sensitivity to pain, touch and temperature. Areas of affected skin also heal more slowly than areas with normal sensation. As a result, individuals with spina bifida are at risk for injury to their skin from many sources including extremes of temperature and pressure. Care must be taken to protect the skin from frostbite in the cold months and from burns from common sources such as hot bath water, radiators, and sunbaked blacktop.

  Redness and open areas, or pressure sores, can occur when the blood supply to the skin is cut off for more than ten minutes at a time. Pressure sores can be caused by not shifting weight frequently while sitting, using an improper wheelchair seat cushion, and wearing braces or shoes that don't fit well. Common pressure points are illustrated in Figure 5.11. Abrasions may occur with crawling on a rug or floor. If damaged skin is not treated early, deeper layers of the skin can become involved and serious infection of the skin or underlying bones may develop. It is important that good skin care and careful inspection of the skin be learned in early childhood and become part of a lifelong self-care routine.

What is the life expectancy of children born with spina bifida? This is a difficult question to answer since the treatment for

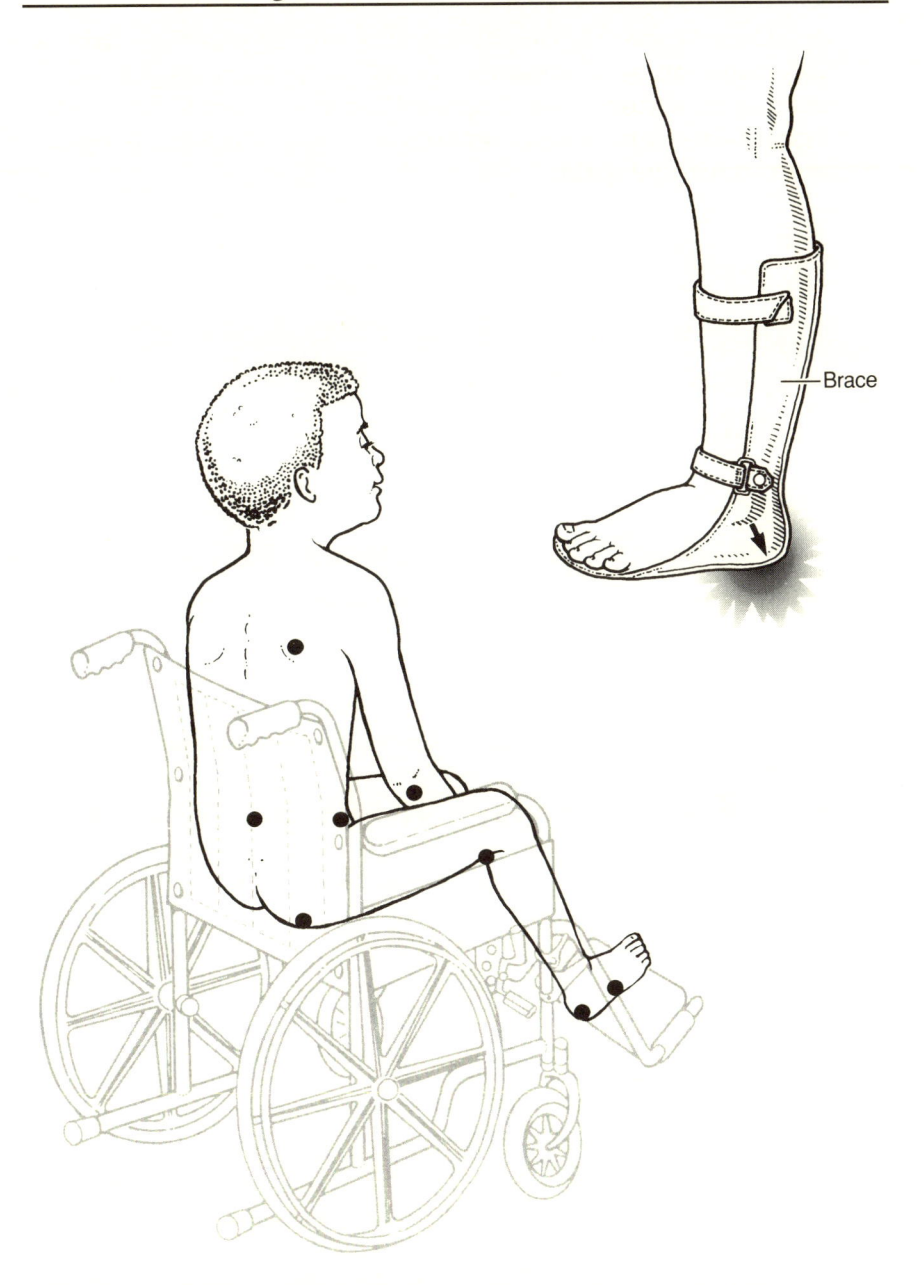

Figure 5.11. Possible pressure points. Common pressure points are located over the bones of the hip, buttocks, spine, ankles, and heels. When the bones and overlying skin rub or press against a surface for long periods of time the circulation to the skin will decrease and pressure sores may occur.

people with spina bifida has been improving steadily for the past several decades. It has only been since the late 1950s that most babies born with an open spinal cord survive beyond early childhood. In general, individuals who get early treatment and continue to have regular check-ups with specialists familiar with the medical problems of spina bifida patients do much better than those who do not. When there are no severe problems with hydrocephalus, unusual problems from the Chiari II malformation or significant kidney damage from uncontrolled pressure or infections, the vast majority of people with spina bifida will live into adulthood.

Non-Medical Issues

What are the important non-medical issues related to spina bifida? It is critical that adequate attention be paid to how having spina bifida can affect educational, social and psychological development.

- *Educational Needs.* The intelligence of individuals with spina bifida varies just as it varies with people in general. Although intelligence scores are usually in the low average range, verbal abilities are usually significantly higher than visual motor abilities. Therefore, many individuals with spina bifida have a specific pattern of learning disabilities.

  They often have poor short term memories and poor organizational skills. Tasks which are dependent on eye-hand coordination may be difficult and a grasp of verbal skills is often more advanced than that of mathematical concepts. Although some children with spina bifida will do well in regular classrooms without any special assistance, many will need support services in order to attend regular classes. Others will do best in a special educational setting. It is important that the abilities of each individual child be professionally assessed as early as possible, usually between the ages of two and five years. Psychological and neuropsychological strengths and weaknesses should be evaluated.

  Federal and state laws including the Americans with Disabilities Act (ADA) and Public Laws 94-142 and 99-457 require that individuals with disabilities be able to live, work and go to school in the least restrictive environment and receive those services necessary to help them benefit from their educational setting. It is important that parents be familiar with the various types of school programs available and, armed with the results of their child's psychological tests, advocate for appropriate placement. School entry can be made easier if parents meet with teachers and other school personnel before classes begin.

- *Social development.* In many cases infants and children with spina bifida require early and frequent hospitalization. This can interrupt normal social development and may lead parents and extended family members to try and "make it up to them" by shielding the child from the normal pressures and demands of life. In order to grow into confident, self-sufficient and independent adults it is critical that spina bifida be seen as just a part of what that child is all about. Each individual is unique and has strengths and weaknesses which they must learn to recognize and accept.

    It is very important that children with spina bifida be treated as normally as possible. They should have chores to do at home which are appropriate to their age and abilities and should learn to accept the consequences of their actions. They should have the opportunity to make choices and decisions, beginning with such simple things as what they will wear each day and how they will spend free time. It is very important that they play with children their own age and forge and maintain friendships with both disabled and non-disabled peers. Physical limitations may make adolescents and even young adults dependent on their parents for transportation to activities. Parents who make the extra effort to help their children maintain peer relationships are rewarded with more independent, well-balanced young men and women.

- *Psychological development.* As they grow and mature, children with any disability or special need will become aware of how they are different from others. This may not cause any difficulties until they start public school and are, for the first time, in a situation where their disability may make it difficult for them to participate fully. They may not be able to keep up at recess and, therefore, may be excluded from certain games or activities. This problem often escalates in pre-adolescence as other children move on to more grown-up social relationships. Children with special needs may rebel against a disability when they realize it cannot be wished away and may refuse to cooperate with medical treatments. This problem is not unique to children with spina bifida, but is seen in those with almost any special need or disability.

It is wise to consider counseling beginning in the pre-teen years, often around age nine or 10. Although parents can be very understanding, the opportunity to talk with a trained social worker, counselor, psychologist or psychiatrist about their inner fears, self-doubts and anger about their disability and the "normal" world can be very effective in helping the child come to terms with life and with themselves. Group sessions where they can interact with peers also dealing with a special need are often very effective. Once adolescent rebellion has become a problem it is much more difficult to treat.

- *Sexual function.* The nerves responsible for sexual sensation and function come from the lower portion of the spinal cord. As a result, most individuals with spina bifida will have some degree of sexual dysfunction. Females do not usually have sensation in the clitoris and, therefore, do not have orgasms with intercourse. However, they frequently have increased sensitivity in areas besides the genitalia and can have satisfying sexual lives. They are usually normally fertile. Those with high levels of paralysis may have severe curvature of the spine (scoliosis), small abdominal cavities, or other physical problems which make it difficult to carry a child for a full nine months. In addition, vaginal births will be difficult for these women. A gynecologist knowledgeable about spina bifida should be consulted when childbearing decisions are made. They will also be able to provide up-to-date information on the recommended dose of folic acid. Like their able-bodied peers, adult women with spina bifida require yearly gynecological examinations and should be screened for breast and cervical cancer.

    Some males with spina bifida can have erections. This ability is not always related to the level of paralysis. Ejaculation, or the discharge of sperm, does not always occur as it should and males may have difficulty fathering children. Like females with spina bifida males are able to enjoy sex. A sexual therapist or knowledgeable urologist can offer treatment to assist with both erection difficulties and infertility.

    As with all sexually active individuals, those with spina bifida are responsible for protecting themselves against unwanted pregnancy, AIDS and other sexually transmitted diseases. Latex condoms and diaphragms may cause severe allergic reactions.

Sheepskin condoms will not protect against AIDS. New products which are both latex free and do protect against sexually transmitted diseases are available. Consultation with a nurse or physician to determine the most appropriate form of birth control is recommended.

How can individuals with spina bifida get the medical care they need? Spina bifida is, indeed, a very complicated medical condition. Multidisciplinary clinics which bring together professionals from key specialties are able to provide up-to-date, comprehensive medical care as well as psychological and social support to people with spina bifida and their families. There are many clinics like this throughout the country. The Spina Bifida Association of America [see Resources at end of chapter] can give you information about the program nearest you. Individual programs will vary, but most multidisciplinary clinics have a neurosurgeon, orthopaedic surgeon, urologist, psychologist, social worker, dietitian, pediatrician, and physical therapist on the team. Visits are organized so that all of the doctors and other health professionals can be seen on the same day. X-rays and other required tests are often arranged for the day of the visit. Although the medical needs related to spina bifida may seem overwhelming, it is very important that children and adults with spina bifida have their own pediatrician, internist or family practitioner to provide routine check-ups, manage medical problems unrelated to the spina bifida, and be available to work with the specialty team in providing comprehensive care.

Does insurance cover this medical care? Finances are often a concern for families with children with special needs. In recent years there have been a lot of changes in what medical insurance will pay. It is best to check your policy and call your insurance representative if you have any questions. There are several state and federal programs such as Children's Medical Service and Social Security Supplemental Income (SSI) available. It is important to speak with a social worker or other member of the health care team about what is available in your state and from the federal government. In many areas there are also parent support networks and disability rights groups that have up-to-date information on resources.

At what age will a person with spina bifida no longer need specialized medical care? Spina bifida is a lifelong condition. In order to maintain their health and prevent avoidable complications it is important that adults with spina bifida continue to receive medical care from knowledgeable specialists including neurosurgeons, urologists and orthopaedic surgeons. Multidisciplinary clinics specializing in the treatment of adults with spina bifida are being developed in many areas of the country.

Final Thoughts

We have presented a lot of information. Absorbing and digesting it all will take some time. It may be helpful to read through this material several times and to write down any questions you may have. This may be especially helpful to parents of newborns with spina bifida or couples who have been told that their unborn child has a neural tube defect. Many local Spina Bifida Association chapters have parent-to-parent outreach programs and will provide support and information to parents, families and individuals with spina bifida. Most school districts will be available to provide detailed information on services available for children with special needs.

Parents, families and professionals alike should attend local and national spina bifida programs to obtain information about the latest advances in diagnosis, prevention and treatment. Medical researchers must continue their search for the cause or causes of spina bifida and other neural tube defects, and much more must be learned about their prevention. New methods and techniques for management of the medical, social and psychological needs of people with spina bifida must be sought after, found and brought to those who can benefit from them. There is much to be done, but with teamwork, dedication, and an increased national awareness of spina bifida this, and more is possible.

Glossary

AFO (*Ankle-foot orthosis*): A brace used to support the ankle and foot. It is L-shaped and fits behind the calf and runs under the foot.

AFP (*Alpha-feto-protein*): A substance made by all babies in the womb. If the baby has an open spina bifida or another neural tube defect, abnormally high levels are found in a pregnant woman's blood and in the fluid surrounding the baby.

Amniocentesis: A procedure where fluid surrounding a baby is removed from the womb and studied for a variety of possible birth

Answering Your Questions about Spina Bifida

defects. Open neural tube defects can be detected by abnormally high levels of AFP in this fluid.

Anencephaly: Lack of development of the brain. There is no treatment for this condition which is incompatible with life.

Catheterization: Process of inserting a thin, straw-like device (catheter) into the bladder to drain urine. Most individuals with spina bifida will be on a program where they catheterize every two to four hours during the day.

Clubfoot: A deformity of the foot where it is twisted out of shape or position. Frequently present in newborns with spina bifida, it may also develop later in life.

Decubitus: Another name for a pressure sore or skin ulcer.

Folic Acid: A common B vitamin. A daily dose of 0.4mg taken for three to four months prior to the start of a pregnancy and continued daily during the first three months of pregnancy will decrease the chances of having a baby with a neural tube defect.

Gibbus: Hump-like deformity of the spine which occurs in some individuals with a thoracic level of spina bifida.

Hydrocephalus: Dilatation of the fluid cavities of the brain.

KAFO (*Knee-ankle-foot orthosis*): A brace used to support the knee, ankle and foot. It is attached at the mid-thigh, the calf and the foot and supports the entire lower leg and foot.

Myelomeningocele: A synonym for the most severe form of spina bifida.

Neural Tube Defect: A group of birth defects in which the brain or a part of the spinal cord is not fully developed.

Neurosurgeon: Surgeon specializing in the treatment of disorders of the brain and spinal cord.

Orthopaedic Surgeon: Surgeon specializing in the treatment of disorders of the bones and muscles.

Parapodium: A frame-like device used to support children with high levels of spina bifida in a standing position. The device is jointed at the hips and knees to allow the child to be placed in a sitting position without removing them from the device.

Scoliosis: Curvature of the spine.

Shunt: Device implanted in the fluid cavities of the brain which allows for control of fluid buildup.

Sphincter: Circular muscle that normally controls the passage of stool or urine from the body.

Spina Bifida: Condition in which the bones covering the spinal cord (vertebrae) do not completely form somewhere along the length of the spine. Usually used to refer to a birth defect where the bones as well as the underlying spinal cord are not normally developed.

Standing Frame: A device used to help individuals with high levels of spina bifida be upright. It is very like a parapodium without joints at the hips or knees.

Syrinx: Dilatation of the usually tiny fluid cavity located within the spinal cord. A syrinx may cause weakness of the arms or hands, curvature of the spine or abnormalities of the regulation of breathing.

Tethered Cord: Abnormal attachment of the spinal cord to internal tissues. It can cause damage to the spinal cord and nerves.

Urologist: Surgeon specializing in the treatment of disorders of the kidneys and bladder.

Ventricles: Fluid cavities of the brain. Enlargement of the ventricles with fluid is called hydrocephalus.

Common Diagnostic Tests

Tests Used to Evaluate the Neurologic System

CT (CAT) scan: A highly sophisticated x-ray study which provides a three-dimensional image of the body part under examination. CT scans are frequently used to evaluate the size of the fluid cavities of the brain and to assess shunt function.

EEG: A test of the electrical activity of the brain. Used to evaluate an individual for seizures (epilepsy).

EMG testing: Used to determine which muscles of the body are working and how well they function. Needle electrodes are inserted into individual muscles and their activity is recorded.

MRI scan: A technique which uses a large magnet and radio waves to make a very detailed picture of the inside of the body. This test is excellent for evaluating the brain and spinal cord.

Tests Used to Evaluate the Kidneys and Bladder

IVP: A test which uses the injection of a special dye to enable doctors to examine the kidneys on x-ray.

Renal Scan: A study using injection of a substance that is filtered through the kidneys and which will show kidney size. function and any kidney damage.

Renal Sonogram: A test which uses sound waves to examine the kidneys and bladder. Kidney size and shape as well as abnormalities of the drainage system are seen well with this test.

Urodynamic Testing (CMG/EMG): Test done by a urologist or trained technician which determines how much the bladder will hold, and detects abnormal bladder contractions, increased bladder pressure and assesses sphincter activity.

VCUG: An x-ray study involving catheterization of the bladder and insertion of a substance which outlines the size and shape of the bladder and detects vesicoureteral reflux.

Other Frequently Used Tests

Laryngoscopy: Direct visualization of the vocal cords with a special flexible scope. Abnormal vocal cord motion may be symptomatic of a problem with the Arnold Chiari II malformation.

Sleep Study: The pattern of respirations and the ability of individuals to normally regulate the oxygen levels in their blood during sleep is recorded. An abnormal test may indicate a significant problem with the Arnold Chiari II malformation.

Resources

Alliance of Genetics Support Groups
35 Wisconsin Circle
Chevy Chase, MD 20815
800-336-4346
301-652-5553

Arnold Chiari Family Network
67 Spring Street
Weymouth MA 02188
617-337-2368

Association for the Care of Children's Health (ACCH)
7910 Woodmont Avenue, Suite 300
Bethesda, MD 20814
301-654-6549

Exceptional Parent Magazine
P.O. Box 300, Dept. EP
Denville, NJ 07834-9919
800-247-8080 (New Subscriptions)
800-562-1973 (Customer Service)

Guardians of Hydrocephalus Research Foundation
2618 Avenue Z
Brooklyn, NY 11235
718-743-4473

March of Dimes Birth Defects Foundation
1275 Mamaroneck Avenue
White Plains, NY 10605
914-428-7100

Answering Your Questions about Spina Bifida

National Center for Education and Maternal and Child Health
2000 15th Street N., Suite 701
Arlington, VA 22201-2617
703-524-7802

National Society of Genetic Counselors
233 Canterbury Drive
Wallingford, PA 19086
215-872-7608

Sibling Information Network
62 Washington Street
Middleton, CT 06457
203-344-7500

Spina Bifida Association of America
4590 MacArthur Boulevard, Suite 250
Washington, D.C. 20007-4226
202-944-3285

Chapter 6

Children with Hydrocephalus

Description

Hydrocephalus is a neurological disorder in which there is excessive accumulation of cerebrospinal fluid (CSF) within the ventricles of the brain. It may be caused by a birth defect, hemorrhage, viral infection, meningitis, a tumor, or head injury. Most forms of hydrocephalus are the result of obstructed CSF flow in the ventricular system. In infants, the most obvious symptom is an abnormally large head. Other symptoms include vomiting, sleepiness, irritability, an inability to look upwards, and seizures. In older children symptoms include headache, nausea, vomiting and, sometimes, blurred vision. There may be problems with balance, delayed development in walking or talking, and poor coordination. Irritability, fatigue, seizures, and personality changes such as an inability to concentrate or remember things may also develop. Lethargy, drowsiness and double vision are common symptoms as hydrocephalus progresses.

Treatment

Due to the multiple disorders and/or conditions resulting in the development of hydrocephalus, there is rarely a permanent cure. The

---

Information in this chapter is from "Childhood Hydrocephalus," National Institute of Neurological Disorders and Stroke, Bethesda, MD, July 1996, and "Primary Care Needs of Children with Hydrocephalus," Hydrocephalus Association, 870 Market Street #955, San Francisco, CA 94102, reprinted with permission.

most effective treatment is the surgical insertion of a shunt—a flexible, artificial tube—into the ventricular system of the brain to divert the flow of CSF into another area of the body, where the CSF can drain and be absorbed into the bloodstream.

Prognosis

The prognosis of hydrocephalus is determined by the cause, the presence or absence of associated anomalies, and the timeliness of diagnosis and treatment. Many children treated for hydrocephalus are able to lead normal lives with few, if any, limitations. In some cases, cognitive impairments in language and non-language function may occur. Occasionally, problems with shunts such as infection or malfunction will necessitate additional surgery.

Primary Care Needs of Children with Hydrocephalus

Children with hydrocephalus may have life-long special health care needs. These needs may alter their primary care. It is important that care-givers understand hydrocephalus in order to provide optimal primary health care to these children and their families.

Clinical Manifestations at Time of Diagnosis

Although the signs and symptoms of hydrocephalus may be somewhat varied by the specific cause of the condition, there are common clinical manifestations associated with increased intracranial pressure. If the accumulation of excessive CSF occurs slowly, the infant or young child may be asymptomatic until the hydrocephalus is quite advanced. Significant dilation of the ventricle may occur before abnormal head growth is apparent. Full or distended fontanels, frontal bossing, prominent scalp veins, vomiting, irritability, and even opisthotonic posturing may be observed before dramatic changes are noted in head circumference.

In the older child with fused cranial sutures, the development of hydrocephalus may result in the non-specific symptoms of headache, nausea, vomiting, and personality changes including irritability, lethargy and loss of interest in normal daily activities. Spasticity or ataxia of the lower extremities and urinary incontinence may occur. These children frequently complain of vision problems as increased intracranial pressures on the second, third or sixth cranial nerves result in extraocular muscular paresis and papilledema. Alterations in growth, sexual development and fluid and electrolyte imbalance may occur if increased pressure occurs at the site of the hypothalamus.

Implantation of a shunting device is usually the treatment of choice.

Associated Problems

Intellectual

Intellectual function is difficult to predict early in the disease process. The cause of hydrocephalus appears to be the most important determining factor of intellectual function. Uncomplicated hydrocephalus has a better cognitive prognosis than hydrocephalus associated with brain injury. In recent studies two thirds of children with hydrocephalus had normal or borderline normal intelligence. In children with intelligence quotient (IQ) scores above 70, performance IQ scores are lower than full-scale and verbal IQs. This discrepancy indicates a need for preschool and school counseling and testing to identify areas of learning disability.

Ocular

Ocular abnormalities are often found at the time of diagnosis or during episodes of shunt malfunction. Increased intracranial pressure results in optic nerve pressure, limited upward gaze, extraocular muscle paresis and papilledema.

Even though the shunt is functioning and hydrocephalus is controlled, these children commonly have visual problems. Gaze and movement problems such as strabismus, astigmatism, nystagmus and amblyopia are found in approximately 25-33% of children with hydrocephalus. Refractive and accommodation errors are found in approximately the same percentage of children but not necessarily in the same children. Abnormalities in vision are associated with lower performance scores but not with lower verbal intelligence scores.

Motor Disabilities

As many as 75% of children with hydrocephalus will have some form of motor disability. These disabilities vary from severe paraplegia to mild imbalance or weakness. The severity of the motor deficit is most often diagnosis-related; children with conditions such as porencephaly, Dandy-Walker malformation and meningomyelocele have more serious motor defects than children with simple congenital hydrocephalus.

Hydrocephalus also affects fine motor control. Kinesthetic-proprioceptive abilities of the hands are often affected negatively, and this, coupled with impaired bimanual manipulation and frequent visual deficits, may make it difficult for the child with hydrocephalus to perform well on time-limited, nonverbal intelligence tests.

Seizures

Seizures in infancy are not uncommon at the time of initial diagnosis of hydrocephalus because of increased intracranial pressure. About 20% of infants with hydrocephalus continue to have seizures after the first year of life. These seizures may be simple or complex and usually can be well managed with standard anticonvulsant therapy. Acquired hydrocephalus is more often associated with seizure activity caused by the underlying reason for the development of hydrocephalus (i.e. brain tumor, CNS trauma, or infection). These seizures may be more difficult to control and are usually more focal in origin.

Primary Care Management

Growth and Development

Both precocious puberty and short stature have been reported in children with hydrocephalus. Sexual development before the age of 8 in girls and 10 in boys is considered precocious and warrants further diagnostic study. Heights below the 5th percentile, if not compatible with family stature, indicate growth retardation. Treatment is available for both of these conditions, and children should be referred to an endocrinologist if symptoms occur.

In children suspected of having hydrocephalus, or who are known to have hydrocephalus, head circumference should be measured by experienced personnel. Until the cranial sutures are completely fused, which can be delayed in these children, growth of head size is a major diagnostic tool in evaluating the child's condition. Once a shunt has been placed, head circumference may decrease 1 to 2 cm as the pressure is relieved. After this initial decrease, the head should grow only in proportion of the child's body. The significance of head size

Children with Hydrocephalus

measurements in the child who has a shunt cannot be overestimated, and daily measurements may be necessary when evaluating the shunt-dependent infant for possible shunt malfunction.

Standard early infant developmental assessment tools used in primary care practice, such as the Denver Developmental Screening Tool, may be of little help in assessing infants with hydrocephalus. It is important for the practitioner to interpret developmental findings in light of other clinical observations to assist the parents in developing reasonable expectations for their infant. Some motor delays can be expected during infancy and childhood, given that approximately 75% of children with hydrocephalus have some form of motor disability. The primary care provider must document carefully motor skill acquisition because a loss of skill may indicate shunt malfunction or progression of the primary cause of hydrocephalus. This applies to older school-aged children as well. Ataxia, slurred speech, lack of progression in school, or incontinence also may indicate a deterioration neurologic status and the need for further evaluation.

Often children with hydrocephalus will benefit from infant stimulation programs or physical therapy, and the practitioner must be familiar with the programs available in the family's community to help them identify programs that would be most beneficial for their child.

Immunizations

Diphtheria, Tetanus, Pertussis (DPT). Pertussis can pose a special problem in infants with hydrocephalus as such children, with a history of seizures, are at increased risk of seizures after pertussis vaccination. Hence, deferral of DPT immunization may be prudent until neurologic stability is ascertained. The risk of contracting pertussis is low but because neurologically impaired children may be at an increased risk of morbidity and mortality from illness caused by *Bordetella pertussis*, immunization is not absolutely contraindicated, and in some patients (such as those with well-controlled seizures, corrected hydrocephalus or cerebral palsy) will be indicated. The primary care provider will need to weigh the risk of disease versus the risk of side effects of the vaccination. In these difficult situations, consultation with the child's neurosurgeon or neurologist may be advisable to help assess the child's potential for having seizures.

Measles. Measles vaccine also has been implicated in postvaccination seizures, with a higher incidence of this occurring in infants and children who have a history of convulsions. It is not believed these post-vaccine seizures produce permanent neurologic damage and the high ongoing risk of natural measles with its high morbidity rate justifies measles immunization in children with a personal history of convulsions.

***Haemophilus influenzae* type B.** Conjugated polysaccharide-diphtheria *Haemophilus influenzae* type B vaccination is recommended at 18 months for all children. The use of HIB vaccine is variable but generally this vaccine is given less often than other recommended vaccinations. Because of the increased risk of HIB CNS infections in children with shunts, children with hydrocephalus who have shunts should definitely receive the new conjugated vaccine as recommended. Children who have a history of documented HIB disease before 2 years of age may not produce adequate antibodies to prevent a second infection and therefore should be immunized.

Other Immunizations. Vaccination for polio, mumps and rubella should be given as routinely scheduled.

Screening

Visual Screening. Because of the high incidence of visual defects in children with hydrocephalus, special attention should be paid to visual screening. Hirschberg, cover test and funduscopic examinations should be performed during each office visit and the result carefully documented. At about six months of age, the child should be referred to a pediatric ophthalmologist for a thorough examination. Yearly examinations should be scheduled thereafter.

Hearing Screening. In addition to routine office screening for hearing acuity, infants with a history of CNS infection or antibiotic treatment with amino-glycosides should undergo auditory-evoked response testing. Subsequent shunt malfunctions or CNS infections require reassessment of hearing, and periodic evaluation by an audiologist is recommended.

Dental Screening. Routine dental care is advised. If the child is receiving phenytoin for seizure control, more frequent dental care may be needed because of the possibility of hyperplasia of the gums. If the child has a ventriculoatrial shunt, prophylaxis with penicillin is recommended for all dental work including adjustment of braces to prevent bacterial endocarditis.

Special Family Concerns

Parents of children with hydrocephalus constantly worry about continued shunt function. With every malfunction there is a need for surgery and the perceived threat of brain damage. This constant worry and the daily responsibility and stress of caring for a child who may have multiple medical problems is very difficult for families. Financial strain caused by numerous medical visits or surgical procedures may deplete a family's financial reserve, and private insurance may not be obtainable unless it is offered through a large group employment policy. Concerns about the child's ability to be self-supporting and independent in the future are also an issue for parents as the child grows into adolescence.

Depending on the child's condition, the number of specialists and community resources used, and the family's strengths or abilities, the parents may need assistance from the practitioner in case management. Coordination and communication between specialists, practitioners, family and school personnel can often become complex and overwhelming to parents. The practitioner can function as a central clearing house to help the parents understand the advised medical treatments, to follow-up on necessary referrals and to identify priorities for the family and child.

For More Information

This Information Sheet was produced by the Hydrocephalus Association. It was adapted from an article in the *Journal of Pediatric Health Care* written by Patricia Ludder Jackson, MS, RN, PNP, Program Coordinator of the Nursing Leadership in Pediatric Primary and Chronic Care Program at the University of California, San Francisco.

For more information contact:

Hydrocephalus Association
870 Market Street #955
San Francisco, California 94102
Telephone: (415) 732-7040
Fax: (415) 732-7044

Chapter 7

Social Skills Development in Children with Hydrocephalus

As the first generation of children shunted for hydrocephalus mature into young adulthood it has become apparent that some of these children have difficulties with development of their social skills. We know that the majority of children diagnosed with hydrocephalus will live and be smart enough to make it in this world. But will these children be happy?

For most of us, happiness means friends—the move from isolation to inclusion. It means comfort with social interaction so that other people are motivated to actively seek out our children, or at the very least, not ignore them. The acquisition of social skills is critical for social inclusion. And if some areas are weak we need to understand that these skills can often be broken down into component parts and taught like other skills such as addition or teeth brushing.

A recent study done by the National Institute of Health found that the greatest concerns of parents of special needs children regarding their social skills were:

- Talking over differences without getting angry
- Persistence when facing frustration
- Refusing requests politely

The information in this chapter was produced by the Hydrocephalus Association and reviewed by Executive Director, Emily Fudge in 1996. It was adapted from a talk given by Rochelle B. Wolk, Ph.D, a neuropsychologist with a specialty in working with children with hydrocephalus. Dr. Wolk, who has a private practice in Piedmont, California, is a member of the Medical Advisory Board of the Hydrocephalus Association; reprinted with permission.

- Taking turns while talking
- Understanding rules
- Following directions
- Waiting when necessary

Of course these problems are not limited to children with special needs. However, for most of us, learning the social skills necessary to handle these situations is automatic, while for children with learning disabilities and special needs, it often is not.

Most of our social learning is done automatically, by seeing, copying and conditioning. That is, social skills are learned incidentally, without formal instruction. However, many children with hydrocephalus have learning problems that make it difficult, or impossible, to pick up the verbal and non-verbal cues necessary for the acquisition of social skills.

Difficulty perceiving non-verbal cues can create serious social problems. Children with hydrocephalus often mis-estimate distance and spatial relationships. They get too close to other people (called "getting in your face"), or they stay back too far. Getting too close will cause others to back off and find an excuse to escape. Staying back too far makes eye contact difficult, puts them out of reach of voice range and is likely to cause others to ignore them.

These children may also have difficulty picking up other social cues, such as those from clothing for example. Someone dressed in a suit and carrying a briefcase tells us, "I am an authority." If a child doesn't pick up such cues, they might not figure out who is the authority, boss, teacher, or even the "boss kid." And, as a child, if you can't spot the leaders you may end up imitating the school nerd with the high probability that you will then be socially scorned or ignored.

Children who have a problem with non-verbal cues also often have difficulty perceiving intonation (the way in which the speaking voice emphasizes words). For example, consider the youngster who hears that a party is being planned and goes up to the 'boss kid' to ask if they can come. The 'boss' responds, "Yeah, sure, I *really* want *you* at my party." If the youngster shows up at the party, it is sure to be a heartbreaking experience. The child has heard the *words* ("I want you"), but not the *tone* ("I would rather hang by my thumbs than have you at my party"). Errors such as these can be incredibly painful for kids who are not attuned to such nuances as tone, rhythm or pitch.

Other important non-verbal cues are posture and facial expression. If a child can't read faces very well, he/she will likely interpret things

Social Skills Development in Children with Hydrocephalus

incorrectly. Often children with hydrocephalus perceive only two kinds of facial expressions, 'happy' and 'mad', and perhaps 'sad'. This understanding is not enough to get along in the world. They need to perceive such subtleties as 'quizzical', 'reflective', and others, and are expected to learn them incidentally.

It is known that some youngsters with hydrocephalus will be slower in acquiring such skills as walking, talking and hand-eye coordination. With time, remediation and early intervention however, these skills are often obtained. But what about social skills? If the child lags behind, will they eventually catch up on these skills on their own, or is intervention important at an early level?

It is believed by many neuropsychologists, especially those that have worked extensively with children with hydrocephalus, that intervention is vital because even if the child does catch up on their own, it will probably happen over time and some skills may always be missing. If undeveloped social skills do come later, by then a youngster may be exhausted, reclusive or self-defeating in interactions with others, having had so many rejections and bad experiences that they refuse to continue to extend themselves socially.

Parents do not need to wait for this self-defeating behavior to happen if they realize that many of these social skills can be taught. The first step in this process is a neuropsychological evaluation. An in-depth evaluation, conducted by an experienced neuropsychologist, can pinpoint areas of deficiency so that the most effective ways can be identified to teach youngsters the social skills they need. Although schools are now mandated to provide many types of evaluations, often the in-depth testing and remediation plans necessary to pinpoint areas of deficiency are best carried out by experienced specialists. Every child is guaranteed an appropriate education by federal law, but the law does not guarantee that a child will be evaluated in a way that pinpoints his/her strengths and weaknesses precisely so that an optimal remedial program can be formulated, and modified if necessary, to meet available resources.

Your child's neurosurgeon, neurologist or pediatrician may be able to recommend an experienced neuropsychologist. Sometimes the hospital social worker or a clinical nurse specialist has recommendations. And don't forget to ask other parents. Networking can often be the best way to gain information.

The cost of neuropsychological evaluation can run anywhere from $150.00 to $500.00. The cost is dependent on the number of tests given, amount of time spent in assessing data and preparation of the final report, which should include plans for remediation and intervention. Some insurance plans will cover the cost. Check your policy. Some policies will pay if the testing is for diagnostic purposes, others will not.

Unfortunately, the move from isolation to inclusion and the acquisition of social skills so necessary for our children's well being is not often well addressed in the school setting. At present, there are few good programs that teach social skills through the schools. Once an evaluation has been completed, and recommendations for intervention and remediation compiled, parents should contact their child's teacher or special education coordinator for help in implementing the program. As usual, parental involvement and advocacy will most likely be necessary.

There are no absolutes or guarantees that even with a thorough neuropsychological evaluation known interventions and strategies will work for all children. However, this is just one more way parents can help their children with hydrocephalus attain the high quality of life they desire for them, and that they deserve.

For More Information

Hydrocephalus Association
870 Market Street #955
San Francisco, California 94102
Telephone: (415) 732-7040
Fax: (415) 732-7044

Chapter 8

Eye Problems Associated with Hydrocephalus

Many children with hydrocephalus develop eye problems. For convenience they have been divided into three categories:

Eye Movements

An undue proportion of children with hydrocephalus will develop a squint—a turn to the eye, often inwards, and sometimes this starts when the child has problems with raised intracranial pressure. Once established, the squint will not disappear but may vary from time to time and often force the child to hold his/her head in an uncomfortable position. For example, if a child is in a stroller and needs to tilt his/her head backwards to see more clearly, it only adds to the child's difficulties. A squint may also compromise the useful field of vision. In addition, the child may look crosseyed. Squints usually require treatment by an eye surgeon (ophthalmologist).

Some children show a tendency for their eyes to "sunset"—their eyes turn downwards and the white shows above. This is essentially a feature seen in infancy and is often present before effective treatment of hydrocephalus. A sudden appearance of the "sunsetting" when it has been absent for some time may mean that the shunt is not working properly.

The information in this chapter was produced by the Hydrocephalus Association. It was adapted from an article by I.M. Rabinowic, M.A., R.R.C.S., D.O, for the Spina Bifida Association, and reviewed by Hydrocephalus Associations's Executive Director, Emily Fudge, in 1996; reprinted with permission.

Problems with Vision

Problems may arise from the effects of pressure on the pathways from the eye to the brain, but the exact mechanism is not yet fully understood although we already know a good deal about this. The visual problems vary from a subtle mild visual deterioration to, very rarely, a marked loss of vision. It appears that in most cases pressure is responsible and the signs are that early detection is important. How to detect it early? We all go to great lengths to stop our children from being introspective and over-dependent and frequently make light of minor complaints. The more intelligent the child, the less he/she may complain. Headaches arise from other causes than pressure and bumping into furniture may be part of your child's balance problems. However, if your child says he can't see well, if he/she is keen to sit closer to the television, if he/she is bumping into furniture when they didn't before, you should have them checked by an eye doctor. He/she may be near or farsighted, but it is hard for you to know that. If in doubt, talk to your doctor.

Perceptual Defects

Some children with hydrocephalus have perceptual problems. These represent an island of difficulty with recognizing and copying shapes, which is out of keeping with his/her other abilities. Some children have problems in picking objects out of a background. Parents often say, "He/she can see what he/she wants to see," or "He/she can see a bug on the carpet but he/she won't see me in a crowd." The importance of recognizing perceptual defects such as these is that they may make certain activities unduly difficult. To some, reading presents special problems. To others, writing or sorting things is difficult. If we suspect a perceptual problem, then we can test the child and find our his/her particular area of difficulty. Once we are aware of this, we can form guidelines of education and advice about areas of frustration.

Suggestions

- Every child with hydrocephalus should have his/her eyes checked regularly.

Eye Problems Associated with Hydrocephalus

- The appearance or reappearance of sunsetting, the sudden development of a turn to the eye, or a worsening of a squint should be reported. They may be unimportant, or may arise with other problems such as a shunt malfunction or urinary infection.

- If a child seems not to see as well as before, report it to your doctor.

- Perceptual defects can add to the child's frustrations both at school and in social situations. They can be assessed and strategies implemented.

Many of the eye problems occurring in children with hydrocephalus represent the effects of pressure both past and present. The eyes sometimes give an early warning of problems. If in any doubt, discuss the problems with the child's doctor.

For More Information

Hydrocephalus Association
870 Market Street #955
San Francisco, California 94102
Telephone: (415) 732-7040
Fax: (415) 732-7044

Chapter 9

Seizures in Children with Congenital Hydrocephalus

Seizures are a relatively common occurrence in children with congenital hydrocephalus.[1-4] Most studies have suggested that the etiology of the hydrocephalus, as well as shunt insertion or complications of shunting, may play a significant part in the origin of seizures in these patients.[2-7] However, long-term follow-up rarely has been provided and the outcome of seizures in children with congenital hydrocephalus is not well established. In addition, there is little information available concerning the prognosis for these children after discontinuation of antiepileptic drug therapy. The few studies that attempted to address these issues grouped together children with diverse causes for hydrocephalus, often including patients with acquired conditions.[2-6] Since long-term outcome in general correlates well with the specific etiology of hydrocephalus, the data generated in prior investigations may not be applicable to all subgroups of hydrocephalic patients. We therefore designed a combined prospective and retrospective study in which patients with congenital hydrocephalus not associated with myelomeningocele were evaluated to determine the frequency of seizures and the potential for long-term seizure control and remission. Previously we reported the results of a similar investigation examining seizures in our patients with myelomeningocele and hydrocephalus.[8]

"Seizures in Children with Congenital Hydrocephalus," Michael Noetzel, MD, and Jeffrey N. Blake, BA, *Neurology*, 42:1277-1279, July 1992; ©1992 Lippincott-Raven Publishers, New York, reprinted with permission.

Methods

The 68 patients in this study were followed in the Birth Defects Center at St. Louis Children's Hospital from 1965 to 1990 for congenital hydrocephalus not associated with myelomeningocele. All children required shunts for their hydrocephalus. The patients were born between 1962 and 1982; more than 90% of the children began to receive their care through the Birth Defects Center shortly after birth, being referred from the Children's Hospital newborn unit. All patients were followed through at least the age of 8 years, except for two children with intractable seizures who died at ages 18 months and 3.5 years. Hydrocephalus was diagnosed by ventriculography prior to 1976 and subsequently by CT. The criteria for shunting of CSF has been described.[8] During the prospective phase of the study (1980 to 1990), all children had at least one CT performed to evaluate the possibility of shunt obstruction. Seventy-two percent of the children had shunts before the age of 3 months; in more than 95% of the patients, the initial shunt was performed before 1 year of age. Excluded from investigation were children whose hydrocephalus was associated with myelomeningocele or was secondary to trauma, intracranial hemorrhage, meningitis, or tumor, as determined by history and radiologic findings.

The complete medical chart of all 54 children with congenital hydrocephalus being followed in the Birth Defects program in 1980 was examined in detail at the time of entry into the study. Information extracted from each child's record included sex, race, pre- and perinatal history, psychomotor development, performance in school, presence or absence of seizures, age at onset of seizures, findings on EEG, type and number of shunt procedures, presence of shunt infection, and family history of nonfebrile seizures. An additional 17 patients were prospectively enrolled in the investigation during 1980 to 1982 as they were referred to the center for ongoing management. All CTs were reviewed to determine the presence of CNS malformations involving the cerebral cortex, such as porencephaly, encephalocele, lobar holoprosencephaly, and disorders of neuronal migration.

Three patients were lost to follow-up at 6, 11, and 19 months after enrollment. They are not included in the analysis. None of these children had experienced a seizure at the time of his or her last examination. Their clinical and demographic characteristics were very similar to those obtained from the study patients. A retrospective review of 12 former patients whose care through the Birth Defects Center had ceased before 1979 was carried out. In addition, information on 10 patients with congenital hydrocephalus referred to the Birth Defects Center during 1983 to 1984 subsequently was collected. Analysis revealed no statistically significant differences in these 22 patients when compared with the 68 children enrolled in the protocol. Thus we believe that there was no obvious selection bias in the study. Our patient population would appear to reflect the characteristics commonly observed in children whose congenital hydrocephalus warrants management in a tertiary care setting.

The 68 study children were followed prospectively with serial neurologic evaluations and developmental testing for a 10-year period. The mean duration of prospective assessment was 8.9 ± 1.7 years, with a minimum of 5.5 years. Results of CTs obtained during the course of the study were reviewed. The onset of seizures in previously unaffected children was recorded, as were seizure frequency and characteristics in patients with previously documented convulsions. Detailed psychometric testing was performed on 46 (67.6%) of the children. The evaluation protocol and frequency of testing depended upon the age of the child. An age-appropriate general intelligence test, as described previously,[9] was administered to all children. Academic skills in children 5 years of age and older were evaluated by the Jastek Wide Range Achievement Test (1965); patients 2 years of age or older received the Peabody Picture Vocabulary Test (1965). Language development in children younger than 5 years was assessed with the Vineland Social Maturity Scale (1965). Psychometric testing was repeated in any child younger than the age of 2 years at the time of initial evaluation. This protocol of psychometric testing has been demonstrated to have predictive value for later intellectual development in children with hydrocephalus.[10] The use of serial evaluations minimized discrepant IQ scores. The diagnosis of mental retardation ([MR]; IQ <70) was based on at least one complete psychometric evaluation performed after the age of 3 years, except for the child who died at 18 months of age with severe lack of development. An additional 22 children (32.3%) were judged to be of average intelligence, based on their academic progress in school through at least the fifth grade, although some in this group were diagnosed as having mild-moderate learning disabilities.

The association between various clinical and demographic factors and the occurrence of seizures was assessed by Fisher's exact and chi-square tests. Multivariate analysis with logistic regression was carried out to test the independence of factors that were significantly related either to seizure occurrence or seizure remission. The analyses were two-tailed and were performed with PC SAS.[11]

Results

Seizures were documented in 33 (48.5%) of the 68 children with congenital hydrocephalus. The number, frequency, and characteristics of convulsions in each of these 33 children were consistent with a diagnosis of epilepsy. The minimum number of seizures in any patient was three. Most recurrences were observed after the institution of antiepileptic medication. Known precipitants of convulsions, such as acute shunt malfunction or high fever, were documented very infrequently. The age at onset of seizures varied but was rather uniformly distributed throughout the first 8 years of life. Seven children experienced their initial seizure within the first month of life. In each of these patients recurrent seizures were observed during later childhood, often after a 2- to 3-year seizure-free period.

Risk factors associated with the development of seizures included MR, which was diagnosed four times more frequently in children with seizures (Table 9.1). The presence on CT of cortical CNS malformations such as agenesis of the corpus callosum, encephalocele, porencephaly, and semilobar holoprosencephaly was also a statistically significant variable in predicting seizure occurrence (Table 9.1). Six children without seizures had malformations, including four with encephaloceles, one with porencephaly, and one with agenesis of the corpus callosum. Only two of these patients were mentally retarded and in general their malformations were not as severe as those demonstrated in patients with seizures, in whom, for example, two cases each of lobar holoprosencephaly and Walker-Warburg syndrome were observed. Congenital abnormalities within the posterior fossa consistent with the Dandy-Walker syndrome were not associated with an increase in seizure frequency in the absence of malformations of the cerebral cortex. Children with hydrocephalus and seizures could also be distinguished based upon a greater incidence of malformations not involving the CNS, such as congenital heart disease, tracheoesophageal fistula, and cleft lip/palate. Logistic regression analysis was used to determine the independent effects of factors that were related significantly to the development of seizures. MR was the only independent predictor of seizure occurrence ($p < 0.001$). Factors not associated with seizure occurrence included age at the time of shunt insertion, family history of nonfebrile seizures, and the number of shunt revisions and shunt infections preceding the initial convulsion, calculated either per patient or per patient-year. Finally, the distribution of the number of shunt revisions was statistically not different in patients with seizures compared with those without convulsions.

Seizures in Children with Congenital Hydrocephalus

Table 9.1. Variables Associated with Seizure Occurrence in Children with Congenital Hydrocephalus

	Seizures	No Seizures
Number	33 (48.5%)	35 (51.5%)
Duration of follow-up (yrs)	14.8 (±5.3)	13.6 (±6.0)
Mental retardation	25 (76%)*	6 (17%)
CNS malformation	16 (48%)†	6 (17%)
Non-CNS malformation	5 (15.2%)‡	1 (2.9%)
Shunt infection§	3 (9.9%)	7 (20%)
Shunt revision/ patient§	0.9	1.6
Age at shunt insertion (mean)	6.8 mos	8.9 mos
Family history of seizures	1 (3%)	1 (2.9%)

* $p < 0.001$.
† $p < 0.01$.
‡ $p < 0.05$.
§ Determined using only shunt complications that preceded initial seizure.

The outcome for our patients with congenital hydrocephalus and convulsions was not good. Only six (18.2%) of the 33 children had their antiepileptic medication successfully discontinued. Fourteen (42.4%) patients with chronic seizure disorders were judged to have adequately controlled convulsions while being maintained on one or two anticonvulsant drugs. In these patients, seizures have been occurring once every 4 months to 2 years. Tapering of antiepileptic drugs was unsuccessful in five patients in this group who had been seizure free for at least 3 years. Thus it was concluded that in these children, antiepileptic drug therapy was necessary to provide an acceptable degree of seizure control. The remaining 13 (39.4%) children have seizures that have not responded well to antiepileptic drug regimens consisting, for the most part, of two or three anticonvulsants. The seizure frequency in these children is at least one prolonged convulsion per month; unfortunately, most experience several seizures per week.

Total number of shunt revisions and infections, seizure type, number of seizures before the onset of treatment, family history of nonfebrile seizures, and age at the time of shunt insertion were not helpful in predicting either subsequent remission of seizures or good control on medication (Table 9.2). Several factors, however, did correlate with a lack of seizure remission, including the presence of MR, younger age at seizure onset, and paroxysmal EEG activity at seizure onset, consisting of focal or nonfocal abnormalities of the spike, spike wave, or slow-wave type (Table 9.2). The presence of a CNS malformation also was associated with an ongoing need for antiepileptic drug treatment, in particular predicting those children whose seizures would be poorly controlled despite anticonvulsant therapy (Table 9.2). There was no real difference in the severity of CNS malformation between those children controlled on medication and those with uncontrollable seizures. Logistic regression analysis was not helpful in determining the independent effects of these various factors on lack of seizure remission, as the variables segregated to the same patients.

In 11 children who had been seizure free on medication for a minimum of 2 years, an effort was made to discontinue treatment. In this group were three patients in whom withdrawal of medication was attempted on two separate occasions. Six patients successfully had their medication discontinued, including one child on his second attempt. These six children had been maintained on antiepileptic drugs for a mean of 2.9 seizure-free years before discontinuation of medication and have been followed for 7.6 ± 1.9 seizure-free years while off medication. Seven attempts to discontinue antiepileptic drugs in five children were followed by recurrent seizures, some occurring only after several years of being off medication. In these children, the mean time without seizures while on medication was 5.5 years (minimum, 3 years). Longer time without seizures while on medication clearly was not helpful in predicting which patients could successfully have their anti-convulsants withdrawn. Other variables, such as EEG results at time of first seizure, findings on CT, number of seizures before treatment, and age at onset of seizures, also did not correlate with seizure

Seizures in Children with Congenital Hydrocephalus

Table 9.2. Variables Related to Seizure Outcome

	1. Remission off medication	2. Controlled on medication	3. Uncontrolled on medication	p value
Number of cases	6	14	13	
Age at seizure onset (yrs)	3.4	1.9	1.5	<0.05 1 vs 2.3
Mental Retardation	0	13 (93%)	12 (92%)	<0.001 1 vs 2.3
CNS Malformation	0	5 (36%)	11 (85%)	<0.02 1 vs 2 <0.01 2 vs 3
Paroxysmal EEG at Seizure Onset	1 (17%)	9 (65%)	10 (77%)	<0.05 1 vs 2 <0.01 1 vs 3
Shunt Infection	2 (33%)	3 (21%)	3 (23%)	NS
Shunt Revisions/ Patient	2.5	2.0	1.5	NS
No. of Seizures Before Rx (mean)	2.2	2.3	3.1	NS

Seizure Type:
  Focal
  Generalized
	2 (33%)
	4 (67%)
		6 (43%)
		8 (57%)
			6 (46%)
			7 (54)
				NS
				NS

Family History of Seizures NS	0	1 (8%)	0	
Age at Shunt Insertion (mean)	6.2 mos	4.8 mos	8.3 mos	NS

NS Not significant.

remission when off medication (Table 9.3). In contrast, the presence of MR was highly predictive of subsequent seizure recurrence after removal of therapy ($p < 0.001$). None of the children successfully weaned from treatment was mentally retarded, although one child required two attempts to discontinue medicine. The five children who experienced recurrent seizures following discontinuation of medicine had IQs <70, including two patients in whom two attempts to withdraw anticonvulsants were made. One child had 7 and then 8 seizure-free years before medicine was withdrawn; the second patient experienced two 5-year seizure-free periods on therapy. On all four occasions, seizures recurred within 2 months of stopping medication.

Discussion

We attempted to determine whether any factors were predictive either of seizure control while on medication or seizure remission when off anticonvulsant therapy in children with congenital hydrocephalus. Previous reports have demonstrated that the frequency of seizures in children with hydrocephalus varies greatly, depending upon the etiology of the hydrocephalus.[1,2,4-6] In our study, therefore, we excluded patients with acquired hydrocephalus or myelomeningocele, reasoning that predictive factors might not be uncovered if the study group was too heterogeneous. In addition, our study would be more useful to other investigators if the results could be applied to a distinct but universally recognized category of patients with hydrocephalus.

The frequency of seizures in our patients with congenital hydrocephalus was 48.5%. Other investigators quote figures between 27 and 73%.[1-6] The increased frequency of seizures in patients with hydrocephalus may be secondary to the nervous system's pathologic condition producing hydrocephalus,[4,8] injury to the cortex as a result of shunt insertion,[2,3] or damage from shunt complications, such as infection or obstruction with resultant raised intracranial pressure.[2,5] Hosking[2] indicated that in children with seizures and hydrocephalus not accompanied by myelomeningocele, the average number of shunt revisions was greater than the figure determined in children without convulsions. The frequency of infection was not provided. In Blaauw's study,[5] by contrast, the number of valve revisions was not statistically higher in children with seizures, but the occurrence of epilepsy in patients with shunt infection was highly significant.

Table 9.3. Variables Related to Seizure Outcome Following Discontinuation of Medication.

	Seizure Remission	Seizure Recurrence
Number of cases	6†	5
Yrs without seizures *on* Rx	2.9 (±0.8)	5.5 (±1.8)
Yrs without seizures *off* Rx	7.6 (±1.9)	NA
Age at seizure onset (yrs)	3.4	2.9
Mental retardation	0*	5 (100%)
Malformation	0	2 (40%)
Paroxysmal EEG at seizure onset	1 (17%)	1 (20%)
Shunt infection	2 (33%)	1 (20%)
Shunt revisions/ patient	2.5	1.9
No. of seizures before Rx (mean)	2.2	1.6
Seizure type		
Focal	2 (33%)	2 (40%)
Generalized	4 (67%)	3 (60%)
Age at shunt insertion	6.2 mos	2.6 mos

* $p < 0.001$.
NA Not applicable.
† Includes one child who experienced a recurrent seizure following the first attempt to discontinue medication.

Stellman et al.[6] have suggested that seizures in their patients with hydrocephalus were not related to site of shunt insertion, number of shunt revisions, birth history, or physical handicap. Children with MR, however, were more likely to experience seizures than were those with normal intelligence.[6] Finally, Varfis et al.[3] postulated that the younger the patient at the time of shunt insertion, the greater the chance for the development of seizures.

The results of these studies are difficult to compare with our data. Hosking's[2] and Blaauw's[5] investigations included some children with acquired hydrocephalus, whereas in the study by Stellman et al.[6] all patients were grouped together regardless of the etiology of their hydrocephalus. In addition, all three studies included in their statistical evaluation shunt complications that occurred after the initial seizure. The findings of Varfis et al.[3] are also open to question since the selection criteria demanded an EEG recording before shunt placement, and thus the number of patients evaluated was rather small. In our study, the development of seizures in children with congenital hydrocephalus was statistically higher in patients with MR or the presence of a CNS malformation. Age at the time of shunt insertion, number of shunt revisions, number of shunt infections, and family history of seizures were not predictive of the occurrence of seizures. Our results are similar to the conclusions presented by Lorber et al.,[4] although they did not perform a statistical analysis of their findings.

The prognosis for children with seizures and congenital hydrocephalus has not been critically examined previously. No data are available concerning possible factors associated with good outcome or the frequency of relapse after adequate seizure control and withdrawal of therapy in these patients. In our study population, 39.4% of the 33 children with convulsions had poorly controlled seizures. An additional 42.4% had seizure disorders that necessitated chronic administration of antiepileptic medicine to provide an acceptable level of seizure control. Seizure remission and withdrawal of antiepileptic medications without recurrence was achieved in only six (18.2%) children. There were no potential risk factors, except cortical CNS malformation, which differentiated patients with seizures well controlled on medication from those with uncontrolled convulsions (Table 9.2). The most favorable outcome of seizure remission clearly correlated with a lack of MR, absence of CNS malformation on CT, older age at onset of seizures, and nonepileptiform EEG (Table 9.2).

At present there is no general agreement about how long a child should be free of seizures before medication can be discontinued. Recent investigations have suggested that under appropriate circumstances discontinuation after relatively short seizure-free periods (2 to 4 years) does not increase the risk of recurrent convulsions.[12-16] In our study, 11 patients experienced a minimum of 2 seizure-free years on medication and thus could be candidates for discontinuation of medication. Within this group of children, intelligence was the only variable that distinguished seizure remission from recurrence following withdrawal of therapy. Based on these results, we are currently recommending that, when a child of normal intelligence with congenital hydrocephalus has been seizure free for 3 years, strong consideration should be given to withdrawing antiepileptic drug treatment.

Other investigators[13,17] have suggested that in some children at "high risk" for seizure recurrence, withdrawal of antiepileptic drugs should be attempted, in view of the potential economic and psychosocial consequences of termination of medication as well as the possible effect of anticonvulsants on learning and behavior.[18,19] Three of the five patients in our study who suffered recurrent seizures following discontinuation of medication did so only after several years (range, 2 to 6 years) following the cessation of therapy. It seems likely that these patients and their families benefited from the medication-free periods. In all five patients, even the individuals who relapsed within 2 months after discontinuation of therapy, there was no difficulty in reestablishing seizure control. Thus our study provides limited evidence suggesting that withdrawal of antiepileptic drugs, even from children with hydrocephalus who are at high risk for seizure recurrence, may provide some benefit to the patient without substantial health risks.

Acknowledgements

We are indebted to Drs. Jean Holowach Thurston and Philip R. Dodge for their critical review of the manuscript and helpful suggestions, to Dr. Sandra J. Holmes for her assistance in statistical analysis, and to Ms. Debby O'Leary for preparation of the manuscript.

—by Michael J. Noetzel, MD, and Jeffrey N. Blake, BA

References

1. Pampiglione G, Lawrence KM. Electroencephalic and clinicopathological observations in hydrocephalic children. *Arch Dis Child* 1962; 37:491-499.

2. Hosking GP. Fits in hydrocephalic children. *Arch Dis Child* 1974; 49:633-635.

3. Varfis G, Berney J, Beaumanoir A. Electroclinical follow-up of shunted hydrocephalic children. *Childs Brain* 1977; 3:129-139.

4. Lorber J, Sillanpaa M, Greenwood N. Convulsions in children with hydrocephalus. *Z Kinderchir* 1978; 25:346-351.

5. Blaauw G. Hydrocephalus and epilepsy. *Z Kinderchir* 1978; 25:341-345.

6. Stellman GR, Bannister CM, Hillier V. The incidence of seizure disorder in children with acquired and congenital hydrocephalus. *Z Kinderchir* 1986; 41(suppl I):38-41.

7. Faillace WJ, Canady AI. Cerebrospinal fluid shunt malfunction signaled by new or recurrent seizures. *Childs Nerv Syst* 1990; 6:37-40.

8. Noetzel MJ, Blake JN. Prognosis for seizure control and remission in children with myelomeningocele. *Dev Med Child Neurol* 1991; 33:803-810.

9. Noetzel MJ, Marsh JL, Palkes H, Gado M. Hydrocephalus and mental retardation in craniosynostosis. *J Pediatr* 1985; 107:885-892.

10. Fishman MA, Palkes HS. The validity of psychometric testing in children with congenital malformations of the central nervous system. *Dev Med Child Neurol* 1974; 16:180-185.

11. SAS Institute Inc. SAS/STAT guide for personal computers version 6.03 edition. Cary, NC: SAS Institute, 1987.

12. Holowach J, Thurston DL, O'Leary J. Prognosis of childhood epilepsy: follow-up study of 148 cases in which therapy had been suspended after prolonged anticonvulsant control. *N Engl J Med* 1972; 286:169-174.

13. Emerson R, D'Souza BJ, Vining EP, Holden KR, Mellits ED, Freeman JM. Stopping medication in children with epilepsy: predictors of outcome. *N Engl J Med* 1981; 304:1125-1129.

14. Holowach Thurston J, Thurston DL, Hixon BB, Keller AJ. Prognosis in childhood epilepsy: additional follow-up of 148 children 15 to 23 years after withdrawal of anticonvulsant therapy. *N Engl J Med* 1982; 306:831-836.

15. Shinnar A, Vining EPG, Mellits ED, et al. Discontinuing antiepileptic medication in children with epilepsy after two years without seizures: a prospective study. *N Engl J Med* 1985; 313:976-980.

16. Matricardi M, Brinciotti M, Benedetti P. Outcome after discontinuation of antiepileptic drug therapy in children with epilepsy. *Epilepsia* 1989; 30:582-589.

17. Gordon N. Duration of treatment for childhood epilepsy. *Dev Med Child Neurol* 1982; 24:81-88.

18. Bourgeois BF, Prensky AL, Palkes HS, Talent BK, Busch SG. Intelligence in epilepsy: a prospective study in children. *Ann Neurol* 1983; 14:438-444.

19. Trimble M. Anticonvulsant drugs, behavior, and cognitive abilities. In: Essman WB, Valzelli L, eds. *Current developments in psychopharmacology*, vol 6. New York: Spectrum, 1981:65-91.

Chapter 10

Third Ventriculostomy

What Is Third Ventriculostomy?

Third ventriculostomy is a procedure in which a tiny (one millimeter) perforation is made in the wall of the third ventricle, thus allowing movement of cerebrospinal fluid out of the blocked ventricle and into the interpeduncular cistern. This procedure is an "intracranial CSF diversion," a process whereby cerebrospinal fluid within the ventricle is diverted elsewhere in an attempt to relieve pressure. The objective of this procedure is to reduce pressure on the brain from excess fluid in the ventricle without using a shunt. The ultimate goal is to remove or render unnecessary the shunt. Unlike shunts, which can require numerous revisions, third ventriculostomy is a one-time procedure.

Ventriculostomies are made possible by the development of a technique called neuroendoscopy, or simply endoscopy. Neuroendoscopy involves passing a tiny catheter (roughly the size of a strand of spaghetti) through brain tissue. A minuscule camera, light and other tools are then slid through the catheter. The camera projects images of the brain fissures and formations onto a monitor located next to the operating table, allowing the surgeon to view the inside of the brain before and during surgery.

Typically, the surgeon places the endoscopic catheter through a small hole drilled in the skull. In people who already have a shunt,

---

From the Winter 1996 issue of the Hydrocephalus Association *Newsletter*; reprinted with permission.

the surgeon may be able to use the original hole made when the shunt catheter was first placed. In contrast to shunt surgeries where removal of part of the skull exposes a large portion of brain, ventriculostomy requires only a tiny hole.

Though third ventriculostomies were performed as early as 1922, inadequate instruments and technology prevented the technique from achieving popularity. The advent of shunt systems in the 1960s replaced the ventriculostomy as the most common method of treating hydrocephalus.

Even today, however, we are well aware that despite the advances in shunt technology and surgical technique, there are many cases in which shunts are inadequate. Extracranial shunts are subject to complications such as blockage, infection and overdrainage, necessitating surgical revisions of the shunt. For this reason, in selected cases, a growing number of neurosurgeons are recommending the third ventriculostomy in place of shunting.

Although in the best case scenario, third ventriculostomy can produce the much-desired result of treating hydrocephalus without a shunt, doctors caution that this procedure is not appropriate for everyone.

With new technologies, such as magnetic resonance imaging (MRI) and endoscopic guidance, the risks of ventriculostomy, including severe bleeding, have been minimized and the technique has become more accepted. The sophisticated imaging of the MRI allows doctors to see the stenosed aqueduct and the absence of flow void phenomenon, while neuroendoscopic procedures offer unprecedented intraventricular views. According to pediatric neurosurgeon Harold Rekate, Chairman of the Pediatric Section of the American Association of Neurological Surgeons, "miniaturization of instruments and improved imaging technology are allowing us to go places in the brain we have never gone before."

How Is Success Defined?

Doctors categorize as "successful" patients who have clinical evidence of normal ICP (intracranial pressure) and structural evidence of improved cortical mantle. If previously shunted, the shunt has to be either removed or proved to be nonfunctional.

Results are determined by assessing clinical signs, head circumference, and fontanelle tension, as well as by MRI. It is important to note that in some cases, ventricles may remain large despite signs of clinical normalization.

Currently published statistics of "success" may not tell the whole story, cautions Dr. Sainte-Rose of Paris, France, in a recent article on "Third Ventriculostomy." Because CSF reabsorption pathways require some time to accommodate the increased amounts of CSF following the ventriculostomy, it may not be possible to determine success for some time after the operation. Post-operation evaluations of success may in fact be understated because of this delay.

Doctors classify as "improvement" cases in which there was significant, immediate reversal of intracranial hypertensive symptoms, slowing of head growth, or an apparently successful outcome that proved to be short-lived.

"Failure" concerns cases in which patients had no change in their clinical progress or structural studies, or needed a shunt within six months of the procedure.

Significantly, 38% of the patients in one recent study remained shunt dependent. The doctors attribute this to the inability of arachnoid villi to absorb the excess CSF or, alternatively, to a block at the incisure preventing the movement of CSF.

While achieving shunt independence is a critical element of "success," the procedure can also serve to improve the way the shunt functions, even if the shunt is not eliminated altogether. For instance, if a patient still requires a shunt, malfunctions are less likely to be life-threatening.

Dr. Robert F. C. Jones of Paddington, Australia, describes the case of a female patient who benefited from third ventriculostomy even though she remained shunt dependent in his article, "Neuroendoscopic Third Ventriculostomy." Before the procedure, she would be unconscious a few hours after her shunt blocked. Now, she simply complains of a headache when her shunt blocks—and the shunt can be revised the next day.

Who Is a Candidate?

Recent studies indicate that the two factors most responsible for successful ventriculostomies are:

1. previous shunt

2. noncommunicating hydrocephalus (obstructed ventricular pathways).

Doctors hypothesize that shunts may allow subarachnoid space to develop, thus making more room for the procedure, while the presence of a functioning shunt may also buy time while the patient develops absorption abilities.

Successful procedures have been performed on babies, as well as elderly patients, indicating that age does not seem to be a factor.

Speaking at a recent meeting of the American Association of Neurological Surgeons, Marion L Walker, M.D., President of the American Society of Pediatric Neurosurgeons, recommended the procedure mainly for children and young adults with a diagnosis of aqueductal stenosis. Aqueductal stenosis, the most common cause of congenital hydrocephalus, is obstruction of the long narrow passageway between the third and fourth ventricle, causing fluid to accumulate upstream from the obstruction.

The primary criteria for successful ventriculostomy appears to be:

- noncommunication—obstruction of the cerebrospinal fluid pathways within the ventricles
- ventricular width of 7 mm or more
- no structural anomalies
- no previous radiation treatment
- *people with certain brain malformations or hemorrhaging are usually not eligible*

What are the Potential Complications?

The primary complications are fever and bleeding. The use of a cold light source and a monopolar coagulation in the confined volume of the third ventricle can increase the temperature of the CSF to high levels, which in turn can cause a fever. Attempts to perforate insufficiently thin ventricular floors can cause bleeding, as can damage to ventricular walls.

Conclusion

Although in the best case scenario, third ventriculostomy can produce the much-desired result of treating hydrocephalus without a shunt, doctors caution that this procedure is not appropriate for everyone. Though the procedure is becoming more common, it is still fairly rare and only a limited number of doctors are skilled in the technique. For those who meet the criteria, ventriculostomy is a promising procedure that may offer freedom from shunt dependency.

References

"Neuroendoscopic Third Ventriculostomy,"** Robert F. C. Jones, M.D., Charles Teo, M.D., Warwick A. Stening, M.D., Bernard C.T. Kwok, M.D.

"Third Ventriculostomy,"** Christian Sainte-Rose. M.D.

Harold Rekate, M.D., Chairman, Section on Pediatric Neurological Surgery of the American Association of Neurological Surgeons

Marion L. Walker, M.D., President, American Society of Pediatric Neurosurgeons

Note

**The two articles referenced above are available in the Hydrocephalus Association Resource Guide, #'s 247 and 256. For information on how to order these articles, or for a copy of The Guide, contact the Association.

The conference tape "New Technologies in the Treatment of Hydrocephalus" discusses Third Ventriculostomy in detail.

Hydrocephalus Association
870 Market Street #955
San Francisco, CA 94102
Telephone: (415) 732-7040
Fax: (415) 732-7044

—by Rachel Fudge

Chapter 11

The Variable Pressure Programmable Valve

A New System for the Management of Hydrocephalus

Fifteen U.S. medical centers are testing a programmable variable pressure valve used in shunt systems to manage hydrocephalus.

The valve, currently in clinical trials, provides clinicians with the flexibility to incrementally adjust resistance to the flow of CSF—a feature which allows each valve to be titrated to fit the unique physiological needs of the individual patients. Flow resistance, measured in millimeters of water can be increased or decreased by units of 10 mm with a range of 20-300 mm. "The valve will open and drain CSF when CSF pressure reaches the selected pressure level. A low pressure setting, for example, would mean more frequent opening and more CSF drainage," explains Mark Luciano, MD, PhD, Head of Pediatric Neurosurgery at the Cleveland Clinic.

The adjustable feature is particularly important for patients whose acceptable range of CSF flow (drainage) is narrowly defined. "Some patients have a small window of tolerance to the rate of CSF flow. This valve is designed to allow for the small variations which could never be accomplished before," says Luciano.

From *Hydrocephalus News and Notes*, Winter 1995; by Ann Marie Liakos, Executive Director of the Hydrocephalus Research Foundation and The National Hydrocephalus Foundation, 1670 Green Oak Circle, Lawrenceville, Georgia 30243; and Mark G. Luciano, MD, PhD, Head of the Pediatric Neurosurgery Section, Cleveland Clinic Children's Hospital, 9500 Euclid Avenue (S/80), Cleveland, Ohio 44195; reprinted with permission.

Congenital Disorders Sourcebook

Although some patients respond well to the traditionally available low, medium or high-pressure fixed flow systems, the symptoms of others are not relieved even in the presence of a functioning device. In other words, some patients require a rate of drainage greater or less than allowed by the design limits of traditionally available systems.

Programmable variable pressure valve technology is promising for these patients—in fact, it may mean that patients who would otherwise have required surgical intervention may avoid that kind of invasive procedure. Adjustment of the programmable system is performed through a non-invasive procedure using a magnetic field.

Follow-up for patients who receive the variable pressure programmable valve is effectively the same as follow-up for patients who have received other conventional devices with one primary difference: plain skull x-rays are also taken of patients with the programmable system. These x-rays record pictures of the valve itself and provide clinicians with confirming information about the resistance setting.

"The immediate benefit of this valve," says Luciano, "could be to reduce the number of times a valve needs to be changed surgically to adjust drainage pressure, and to reduce the incidence of problems of over-drainage such as subdural hematomas. The ability to adjust valve pressure may also allow, however, a tailoring of valve drainage to each individual patient which may allow an optimization of symptomatic relief and function. It is important to add, however, that this valve is still under investigation. Its equivalence or added benefits as compared to other systems is yet to be proven."

Currently use of this valve in the U.S. is limited to investigational centers as part of a clinical trial.

The term "clinical trial" which is unfamiliar to many people, describes an investigational or experimental treatment available to patients participating in research. Treatments or therapies, developed on the basis of scientific theory and observation, are offered through clinical trials after having been tested in laboratory settings, and having shown promise in the laboratory environment.

Several events must take place between the laboratory observation and the actual trials. In the case of hydrocephalus shunt valves, a shunt manufacturer agrees to produce the experimental valves in quantities sufficient to meet the needs of participating patients. A treatment protocol must also be written defining the goals of the study; it must describe the profiles of the patients who may participate, and a protocol for patient follow-up and evaluation must be established.

The Variable Pressure Programmable Valve

All participating patients must meet the same criteria for entry, receive the same treatment, and be evaluated in the same way. Very often these studies involve two groups: an experimental group and a control group. The experimental device is evaluated alongside conventional treatments with random assignment of patients to receive either device. All of these factors help researchers measure the effectiveness of the new valve objectively.

The goal of the trials investigating the valve is to collect sufficient data about the valve to gain FDA permission for general use and distribution. Two pathways are currently available for approval. The "510(k) Pathway Premarket Notification" requires evidence demonstrating that the new valve is equivalent in performance to existing, marketed systems. By contrast, the "Premarket Approval" pathway requires that the valve be proven safe and effective through controlled clinical trials.

As with any clinical trial, the results of this study await completion of patient enrollment and final analysis. A thorough review is necessary to evaluate the potential benefits and problems with such a device, although the preliminary results are promising.

For More Information

For updates on the status of the project or for information about the quarterly newsletter *Hydrocephalus News and Notes* contact:

The Hydrocephalus Research Foundation
1670 Green Oak Circle
Lawrenceville, GA 30243
(770) 995-9570
(770) 995- 8982 fax
e-mail to Ann_Liakos@atlmug.org

Chapter 12

Prenatal Onset Hydrocephalus: Fetal Diagnosis

As an investigator, one of the most frustrating situations one can encounter is being asked for information vital to clinical and/or personal decisions, and not being able to provide it because the necessary research has simply not been done. Such is the case with hydrocephalus diagnosed *in utero*. While advancements in diagnostic imaging, primarily ultrasound, have enabled clinicians to suspect hydrocephalus as early as 15 weeks gestation, correct identification and accurate prognosis are still extremely difficult to obtain and predict.

That this dilemma persists is evident historically in the literature. In the mid-1980's, in response to the marvels of ultrasound, investigators rushed to define the "new" abnormalities that could be visualized (reviewed in Bannister and Tew). Even then, the major conclusions were that the causes of the hydrocephalus were very heterogeneous and prognosis was uncertain (Harrod, et al. 1984). More than twenty years later, these issues are still being debated (Mori, et al. 1995; Guiffre et al. 1995). As Carys Bannister and Brian Tew state so well in their excellent book and enigmatic way (Bannister and Tew, 1991), only a great deal more experimental and clinical research will bring us closer to accurate diagnoses, proper treatments, and improved outcomes.

From *Hydrocephalus News and Notes*, Summer 1996; by J. Pat McAllister, II, PhD, Director of Neurosurgical Research, Department of Neurosurgery (S/80). The Cleveland Clinic Foundation, 9500 Euclid Avenue, Cleveland, Ohio 44195; reprinted with permission.

And yet, while we recognize the limits of current knowledge, and the need for more research, we must also acknowledge that much has been learned about fetal diagnosis, thanks to ultrasound. Probably the most important message for the family facing this situation is that an accurate diagnosis cannot be made before the 20th week of gestation (Bannister and Tew, 1991). Normal ventricles and choroid plexus can be observed as early as the 10th week of gestation, and most major brain structures are recognizable by 16 weeks; however, up to the 20th week of gestation, even normal ventricles are large because of the growth of the surrounding brain (cerebral cortex), has not caught up to the growth of the lateral ventricles. Furthermore, the choroid plexus, which produces cerebrospinal fluid, is larger than usual and fills the lateral ventricles. It is not until after the 20th week of gestation, when the cortical mantle has begun to thicken, that the true size of the lateral ventricles can be judged accurately. These changing patterns in development, as well as the fact that occasionally fetal-onset hydrocephalus can "resolve" on its own, have prompted clinicians to follow the course of the disorder with repeat ultrasounds every 1 to 2 weeks to determine if hydrocephalus is progressing or has become arrested.

If hydrocephalus is diagnosed properly, the agonizing decisions of treatment must be addressed, and this is where information on prognosis is lacking. In Japan a great deal of research is being conducted on hydrocephalus. Koreaki Mori, a leading Japanese investigator, has attempted to shed new light on the issue of prognosis. In a superb study of 1450 cases, Mori and colleagues have defined 7 classifications of hydrocephalus that were associated with neurologic deficit: 1) early fetal hydrocephalus; 2) overt neonatal hydrocephalus; 3) hydrocephalus associated with severe brain malformations such as hydranencephaly, holoprosencephaly, and lissencephaly; 4) hydrocephalus associated with severe brain damage; 5) hydrocephalus associated with epilepsy; 6) hydrocephalus shunted late after detection; and 7) hydrocephalus complicated by a shunting operation.

While not all of these classifications involve prenatal onset, the conclusions of this study are very profound: "The postnatal functional outcome was significantly poor in fetal hydrocephalus diagnosed in early gestation." This disappointing prognosis is even more devastating when the possibility a recurrence ranges from negligible to 25% (Harrod, et al. 1984).

Once fetal hydrocephalus is diagnosed accurately, treatment decisions become problematic because options are very limited. Nonintervention until term is possible, but dramatically increases the risk of permanent neurologic deficits. Intra-uterine intervention may seem like the most appropriate approach, but it is fraught with difficulties. Several experimental (Edwards et al. 1984) and clinical (Manning et al. 1986) models have tested the procedure of *in utero* shunting with ventriculo-amniotic shunts. In theory, this procedure could be carried out in fetuses between 20 and 25 weeks of gestation. In a small study of 44 fetal cases of aqueductal stenosis (n=32), communicating hydrocephalus (n=2), Dandy-Walker malformation (n=1), and hydrocephalus due to multiple causes (n=9), Manning et al. (1986) attempted ventriculo-amniotic shunting. Ten fetuses died during treatment or within three months of birth because of technical difficulties with shunt insertions, preterm delivery, infection, or abnormalities of the central nervous system, heart, lungs or gastrointestinal tract. Of the survivors followed by up to 2 years, 12 (35%) of the 34 were normal for their age, 4 (12%) had mild neurologic deficits, and 18 (53%) had severe deficits. These data demonstrate why this type of procedure is not performed at present.

A third alternative, early delivery followed immediately by ventricular shunting, is feasible. At 32-33 weeks of gestation, the lungs have matured sufficiently to support independent breathing of the prematurely-delivered infant. Nevertheless, this approach involves a delay of about 12 weeks, during which a considerable amount of damage may occur to the developing brain.

The dilemma that this situation presents is frustrating to all involved. We now have some of the research tools required to explore new treatments, and given the resources, should begin to make progress in this important area.

Selected References

Bannister, CM, and Tew, B. Current Concepts in Spina Bifida and Hydrocephalus. *Clinic in Developmental Medicine*. No. 122. New York: Cambridge University. 1991.

Edwards, MSB; Harrison, MR; Halks-Miller, M; Nakayama, DK; Berger, MS; Glick, PL; Chinn, DH. Kaolin-induced congenital hydrocephalus *in utero* in fetal lambs and rhesus monkeys. *Journal of Neurosurgery*. 60: 115-122. 1984.

Guiffre, R; Pastores, FS; DeSanto, S. Connatal (fetal) hydrocephalus: an acquired pathology? *Childs Nervous System*. 11: 97-101. 1995.

Harrod, MJ; Friedman, JM; Santos-Ramos, R; Rutledge, J; Weinberg, A. Etiologic heterogeneity of fetal hydrocephalus diagnosed by ultrasound. *American Journal of Obstetrics and Gynecology*. 150: 38-40. 1984.

Manning, FA; Harrison, MR; Rodeck, C; and members of the International Fetal Medicine and Surgical Society. Catheter shunts for fetal hydronephrosis and hydrocephalus. Report of the International Fetal Surgery Registry. *New England Journal of Medicine*. 315: 336-340.

Mori, K; Shimada, J; Kurisaka, M; Sato, K; Watanabe, K Classification of hydrocephalus and outcome of treatment. *Brain Development*. 17: 338-348. 1995.

For More Information

For more information about hydrocephalus research, contact:

The Hydrocephalus Research Foundation
1670 Green Oak Circle
Lawrenceville, GA 30243
(770) 995-9570
(770) 995- 8982 fax
e-mail to Ann_Liakos@atlmug.org

Chapter 13

Pregnancy and Maternal Hydrocephalus Survey

Nancy Bradley, a shunt-dependent mother in her early 30s, has developed a database designed to collect information about pregnancy and maternal hydrocephalus.

Working with different support groups, Bradley has obtained relevant references. A paper by M. D. Cusimano summarizes the known cases in the medical literature. In this reference, there are 17 cases. All mothers and babies had favorable outcomes; however, 25% of mothers with VA (ventriculoatrial) and 46% of mothers with VP (ventriculoperitoneal) shunts had shunt obstructions during the pregnancies.

A second reference by J. B. Landwehr summarizes the results of 25 pregnancies and yields significantly different results than the paper published by Cusimano. Pregnancy outcomes were two elective abortions, five miscarriages, two preterm vaginal deliveries, one midforceps rotation, two primary low transverse caesareans, two repeat low transverse caesareans, and eleven spontaneous vaginal deliveries. No patient received prophylactic antibiotics during labor and vaginal delivery because of the shunt. There were no related shunt complications.

To make more data available on the effects of pregnancy on shunted women, Bradley started a computerized database. Since its inception in May of 1994, the database has grown considerably and now includes participants from the United States, Canada, and England.

From *Hydrocephalus News and Notes*, Summer 1996; by Nancy Bradley, The Maternal Shunt Dependency Database, Project Coordinator, 8403 Boyne Street, Downey, California 90242; reprinted with permission.

To date, twenty-five shunted mothers have responded to Bradley's questionnaire; twenty-one with VP shunts, three with VA shunts, and one with a ventriculopleural shunt. Ten women have given birth twice, one has given birth three times, and one has given birth four times.

Two respondents reported having both spina bifida and hydrocephalus and two mothers reported having Dandy-Walker and hydrocephalus.

The questionnaire is divided into two sections, requesting both maternal and pregnancy information. In part 1, the mothers were asked their age, medical history and type of shunt (VA, VP). In part 2, the respondents were asked about their shunt's performance during the pregnancy, the delivery and the postpartum period. Several questions were asked about the type of delivery, use of forceps or suction, use of anesthesia, position of the baby, and any noted birth defects.

There are no discernable trends relating the four cases involving shunt malfunction during pregnancy. In two of the four cases, the surgery was postponed until after delivery. One mother reported "feeling" her shunt was failing near the end of her pregnancy. Her doctor chose to deliver the baby by cesarean section. The lower end of her shunt was changed 8 weeks after delivery. One year later, her shunt obstructed due to scar tissue from the cesarean that had formed around the lower end of her shunt. The entire shunt was revised and rerouted at that time.

Three mothers reported experiencing "stabbing" pains at the lower end of their VP shunts throughout their pregnancies.

One respondent with a VP shunt reported that she had a severe headache during delivery. It subsided after delivery, and did not result in a revision.

There were no shunt infections reported as a result of shunt surgery during pregnancy or delivery by cesarean section. The reasons doctors chose to deliver by cesarean section varied significantly. Five caesareans were performed because the babies were in a breech position (2 of these babies had birth defects). External breech version (a turning procedure) was discussed with one mother who felt the abdominal pressure used in the procedure might harm her VP shunt and decided against trying. One cesarean was performed because the baby turned on his side during labor. Another mother's labor failed to progress after 26 hours resulting in a cesarean delivery. Her second baby was also delivered by cesarean section. In still another case, a respondent reported that her doctor felt it was better for the shunt if she had both of her deliveries by cesarean section.

Pregnancy and Maternal Hydrocephalus Survey

Table 13.1. Summary of Results (updated August 1996)

Total Number of Respondents 25
Number of Pregnancies 48

Reported Miscarriages 6 (12%)
Tubal Pregnancies 2 (4%)
Elective Abortion 2 (4%)
Live Births 38 (79%)
Pre-Term Live Births 1 (2%)

Shunt Malfunctions
Prior to Delivery 4 (10%)
During Delivery 0 (0%)
After Delivery 3 (8%)
No Malfunction 31 (79%)

Maternal Fatalities 0 (0%)
Birth Defects 4 (10%)
Babies with Hydrocephalus 1 (2.5%)
Number of C-Sections 15 (38%)
Average Weight of Babies .... 7 lbs 15 oz

One mother had an appendectomy 15 weeks into her pregnancy without shunt complications. She experienced premature labor from 30 gestational weeks until her baby's full term delivery.

After delivery, two women observed that they had pressure headaches while breastfeeding. Eight mothers noticed no headaches while breast-feeding.

Two women with VP shunts reported that their shunts had disconnected, slipped into their pelvises, and wrapped around their reproductive organs. Neither was pregnant at the time this happened. One woman went on to have three pregnancies. The other had a hysterectomy as a result of the damage done by the shunt to her reproductive organs.

Nine women took seizure medication during pregnancy. Two women were prescribed Tegretol, and six women reported taking phenobarbital, and one woman was prescribed Dilantin. One of the mothers on 90-180 mg of Phenobarbital reported a large weight gain (45 lbs), and the development of latent diabetes. Her doctor felt that

Table 13.2. Post Delivery Shunt Related Complications (updated August 1996)

Type of Delivery	Malfunctions
Cesarean: 15 cases	7% (1 malfunction)
Vaginal: 23 cases	9% (2 malfunctions)

Type of Anesthesia	Malfunctions
Epidural: 15 cases	0%
General: 5 cases	20% (1 malfunction)
Spinal: 2 cases	0%
None: 16 cases	9% (2 malfunctions)

Delivery Aids	Malfunctions
Forceps: 3 cases	0%
Suction: 3 cases	0%
Pressure: 2 cases	50%
None: 11 cases	9%

Type of Shunt	Malfunctions
VP: 35 cases	8% (3 malfunctions)
VA: 2 cases	0%
V-Lung: 1 case	0%

Antibiotics	Malfunctions
Yes: 13 cases	0%
No: 25 cases	12% (3 cases)

the Phenobarbital had contributed to her weight gain. One mother with spina bifida, hydrocephalus and seizures reported that her daughter also suffers from seizures.

The four reported birth defects were hydronephrosis (water on the kidney) with neurofibromatosis, spina bifida with hydrocephalus, Vaters syndrome, and Trisomy-13.

A supplementary questionnaire has been sent to previous respondents asking additional questions about their pregnancies.

Bradley hopes that this information is useful to women with hydrocephalus and their doctors. She would also like to thank all of the women who have contributed to this database.

Pregnancy and Maternal Hydrocephalus Survey

Women interested in participating, please contact:

Nancy Bradley
8403 Boyne Street
Downey, CA 90242
(310) 869-3689

References

Cusimano, MD, et al., Management of Pregnant Women with Cerebrospinal Fluid Shunts, *Pediatric Neurosurgery* 1991-1992;17:10-13.

Landwehr, JB, Jr., et al., Maternal Neurosurgical Shunts and Pregnancy Outcome, *Obstetrics-Gynecology*, 1994, January, 83(1):134-137.

For More Information

To receive future updates on the Pregnancy and Maternal Hydrocephalus Survey as they become available or for information about receiving *Hydrocephalus Notes and News*, contact:

The Hydrocephalus Research Foundation
1670 Green Oak Circle
Lawrenceville, GA 30243
(770) 995-9570 phone
(770) 995-8982 fax
e-mail to: Ann_Liakos@atlmug.org

Part Three

Cerebral Palsy

Chapter 14

Cerebral Palsy: Hope through Research

Introduction

In the 1860s, an English surgeon named William Little wrote the first medical descriptions of a puzzling disorder that struck children in the first years of life, causing stiff, spastic muscles in their legs and, to a lesser degree, their arms. These children had difficulty grasping objects, crawling, and walking. They did not get better as they grew up nor did they become worse. Their condition, which was called Little's disease for many years, is now known as *spastic diplegia*. It is just one of several disorders that affect control of movement and are grouped together under the term cerebral palsy.

Because it seemed that many of these children were born following complicated deliveries, Little suggested their condition resulted from a lack of oxygen during birth. This oxygen shortage damaged sensitive brain tissues controlling movement, he proposed. But in 1897, the famous physician Sigmund Freud disagreed. Noting that children with cerebral palsy often had other problems such as mental retardation, visual disturbances, and seizures, Freud suggested that the disorder might sometimes have roots earlier in life, during the brain's development in the womb. "Difficult birth, in certain cases" he wrote, "is merely a symptom of deeper effects that influence the development of the fetus."

National Institute of Neurological Disorders and Stroke (NINDS), NIH Pub. No. 93-159, September 1993.

Despite Freud's observation, the belief that birth complications cause most cases of cerebral palsy was widespread among physicians, families, and even medical researchers until very recently. In the 1980s, however, scientists analyzed extensive data from a government study of more than 35,000 births and were surprised to discover that such complications account for only a fraction of cases—probably less than 10 percent. In most cases of cerebral palsy, no cause could be found. These findings from the National Institute of Neurological Disorders and Stroke (NINDS) perinatal study have profoundly altered medical theories about cerebral palsy and have spurred today's researchers to explore alternative causes.

At the same time, biomedical research has also led to significant changes in understanding, diagnosing, and treating persons with cerebral palsy. Identification of infants with cerebral palsy very early in life gives youngsters the best opportunity for developing to their full capacity. Biomedical research has led to improved diagnostic techniques—such as advanced brain imaging and modern gait analysis—that are making this easier. Certain conditions known to cause cerebral palsy, such as *rubella* (German measles) and *jaundice*, can now be prevented or treated. Physical, psychological, and behavioral therapy that assist with such skills as movement and speech and foster social and emotional development can help children who have cerebral palsy to achieve and succeed. Medications, surgery, and braces can often improve nerve and muscle coordination, help treat associated medical problems, and either prevent or correct deformities.

Much of the research to improve medical understanding of cerebral palsy has been supported by the NINDS, one of the Federal Government's National Institutes of Health. The NINDS is America's leading supporter of biomedical research into cerebral palsy and other neurological disorders. Through this publication the NINDS hopes to help the more than 4,500 American babies and infants diagnosed each year, their families, and others concerned about cerebral palsy benefit from these research results.

What Is Cerebral Palsy?

Cerebral palsy is an umbrella-like term used to describe a group of chronic disorders impairing control of movement that appear in the first few years of life and generally do not worsen over time. The term *cerebral* refers to the brain's two halves, or hemispheres, and *palsy* describes any disorder that impairs control of body movement. Thus, these disorders are not caused by problems in the muscles or nerves. Instead, faulty development or damage to motor areas in the brain disrupts the brain's ability to adequately control movement and posture.

Symptoms of cerebral palsy lie along a spectrum of varying severity. An individual with cerebral palsy may have difficulty with fine motor tasks, such as writing or cutting with scissors; experience trouble with maintaining balance and walking; or be affected by involuntary movements, such as uncontrollable writhing motion of the hands or drooling. The symptoms differ from one person to the next, and may even change over time in the individual. Some people with cerebral palsy are also affected by other medical disorders, including seizures or mental impairment. Contrary to common belief, however, cerebral palsy does not always cause profound handicap. While a child with severe cerebral palsy might be unable to walk and need extensive, lifelong care, a child with mild cerebral palsy might only be slightly awkward and require no special assistance. Cerebral palsy is not contagious nor is it usually inherited from one generation to the next. At this time, it cannot be cured, although scientific research continues to seek improved treatments and methods of prevention.

How Many People Have This Disorder?

The United Cerebral Palsy Associations estimate that more than 500,000 Americans have cerebral palsy. Despite advances in preventing and treating certain causes of cerebral palsy, the number of children and adults it affects has remained essentially unchanged or perhaps risen slightly over the past 30 years. This is partly because more critically premature and frail infants are surviving through improved intensive care. Unfortunately, many of these infants have developmental problems of the nervous system or suffer neurological damage. Research is under way to improve care for these infants, as in ongoing studies of technology to alleviate troubled breathing and trials of drugs to prevent bleeding in the brain before or soon after birth.

What Are the Different Forms?

Spastic diplegia, the disorder first described by Dr. Little in the 1860s, is only one of several disorders called cerebral palsy. Today doctors classify cerebral palsy into four broad categories—spastic, athetoid, ataxic, and mixed forms—according to the type of movement disturbance.

Figure 14.1. The four key forms of spastic cerebral palsy. Doctors name them by combining the terms plegia *(meaning paralyzed) or* paresis *(weak) with a Latin description of the affected limbs. (Source: Paul Wiegmann, medical illustrator)*

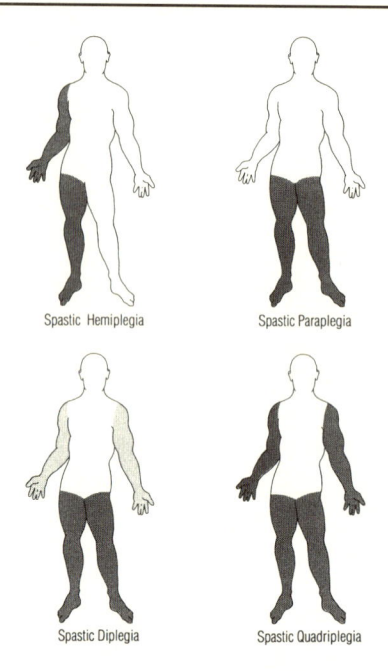

Spastic Hemiplegia

Spastic Paraplegia

Spastic Diplegia

Spastic Quadriplegia

Spastic cerebral palsy. In this form of cerebral palsy, which affects 70 to 80 percent of patients, the muscles are stiffly and permanently contracted. Doctors will often describe which type of spastic cerebral palsy a patient has based on which limbs are affected. The names given to these types combine a Latin description of affected limbs with the term *plegia* or *paresis*, meaning paralyzed or weak. The four commonly diagnosed types of spastic cerebral palsy are shown in the figure above.

When both legs are affected by spasticity, they may turn in and cross at the knees. This abnormal leg posture, called scissoring, can interfere with walking.

Individuals with spastic hemiparesis may also experience *hemiparetic tremors*, in which uncontrollable shaking affects the limbs on one side of the body. If these tremors are severe, they can seriously impair movement.

Athetoid, or dyskinetic, cerebral palsy. This form of cerebral palsy is characterized by uncontrolled, slow, writhing movements. These abnormal movements usually affect the hands, feet, arms, or legs and, in some cases, the muscles of the face and tongue, causing grimacing or drooling. The movements often increase during periods of emotional stress and disappear during sleep. Patients may also have problems coordinating the muscle movements needed for speech, a condition known as *dysarthria*. Athetoid cerebral palsy affects about 10 to 20 percent of patients.

Ataxic cerebral palsy. This rare form affects balance and coordination. Affected persons may walk unsteadily with a wide-based gait, placing their feet unusually far apart, and experience difficulty when attempting quick or precise movements, such as writing or buttoning a shirt. They may also have intention tremor. In this form of tremor, beginning a voluntary movement, such as reaching for a book, causes a trembling that affects the body part being used. The tremor worsens as the individual gets nearer to the desired object. The ataxic form affects an estimated 5 to 10 percent of cerebral palsy patients.

Mixed forms. It is common for patients to have symptoms of more than one form of cerebral palsy mentioned above. The most common combination includes spasticity and athetoid movements but other combinations are possible.

What Other Medical Disorders Are Associated with Cerebral Palsy?

Many individuals who have cerebral palsy have no associated medical disorders. However, disorders that involve the brain and impair its motor function can also cause seizures and impair an individual's intellectual development, attentiveness to the outside world, activity and behavior, and vision and hearing. Medical disorders associated with cerebral palsy include:

Mental impairment. About one-third of children who have cerebral palsy are mildly intellectually impaired, one-third are moderately or severely impaired, and the remaining third are intellectually normal. Mental impairment is more commonly seen in children with spastic quadriplegia.

Seizures or epilepsy. As many as half of all children with cerebral palsy have seizures. During a seizure, the normal, orderly pattern of electrical activity in the brain is disrupted by uncontrolled bursts of electricity. When seizures recur without a direct trigger, such as fever, the condition is called epilepsy. In the person who has cerebral palsy and epilepsy, this disruption may be spread throughout the brain and cause varied symptoms all over the body—as in tonic-clonic seizures—or may be confined to just one part of the brain and cause more specific symptoms—as in partial seizures.

Tonic-clonic seizures generally cause patients to cry out and are followed by loss of consciousness, twitching of both legs and arms, convulsive body movements, and loss of bladder control.

Partial seizures are classified as simple or complex. In simple partial seizures, the individual has localized symptoms, such as muscle twitches, numbness, or tingling. In complex partial seizures, the individual may hallucinate, stagger, perform automatic and purposeless movements, or experience impaired consciousness or confusion.

Growth problems. A syndrome called *failure to thrive* is common in children with moderate-to-severe cerebral palsy, especially those with spastic quadriparesis. Failure to thrive is a general term physicians use to describe children who seem to lag behind in growth and development despite having enough food. In babies, this lag usually takes the form of too little weight gain; in young children, it can appear as abnormal shortness; in teenagers, it may appear as a combination of shortness and lack of sexual development. Failure to thrive probably has several causes, including, in particular, poor nutrition and damage to the brain centers controlling growth and development.

In addition, the muscles and limbs affected by cerebral palsy tend to be smaller than normal. This is especially noticeable in some patients with spastic hemiplegia, because limbs on the affected side of the body may not grow as quickly or as large as those on the more normal side. This condition usually affects the hand and foot most severely. Since the involved foot in hemiplegia is often smaller than the unaffected foot even among patients who walk, this size difference is probably not due to lack of use. Scientists believe the problem is more likely to result from disruption of the complex process responsible for normal body growth.

Impaired vision or hearing. A large number of children with cerebral palsy have *strabismus*, a condition in which the eyes are not aligned because of differences in the left and right eye muscles. In an adult, this condition causes double vision. In children, however, the brain often adapts to the condition by ignoring signals from one of the misaligned eyes. Untreated, this can lead to very poor vision in one eye and can interfere with certain visual skills, such as judging distance. In some cases, physicians may recommend surgery to correct strabismus.

Children with hemiparesis may have *hemianopia*, which is defective vision or blindness that impairs the normal field of vision. For example, when hemianopia affects the right field of vision, a child looking straight ahead might have perfect vision except on the far right. In homonymous hemianopia, the impairment affects the same part of the visual field of both eyes.

Impaired hearing is also more frequent among those with cerebral palsy than in the general population.

Abnormal sensation and perception. Some children with cerebral palsy have impaired ability to feel simple sensations like touch and pain. They may also have *stereognosia*, or difficulty perceiving and identifying objects using the sense of touch. A child with stereognosia, for example, would have trouble identifying a hard ball, sponge, or other object placed in his hand without looking at the object.

What Causes Cerebral Palsy?

Cerebral palsy is not one disease with a single cause, like chicken pox or measles. It is a group of disorders that are related but have different causes. When physicians try to uncover the cause of cerebral palsy in an individual child, they look at the form of cerebral palsy, the mother's and child's medical history, and onset of the disorder.

About 10 to 20 percent of children who have cerebral palsy acquire the disorder after birth. Acquired cerebral palsy results from brain damage in the first few months or years of life and often follows brain infections, such as bacterial meningitis or viral encephalitis, or results from head injury—most often from a motor vehicle accident, a fall, or child abuse.

Congenital cerebral palsy, on the other hand, is present at birth, although it may not be detected for several months. In most cases, the cause of congenital cerebral palsy is unknown. Thanks to research, however, scientists have pinpointed some specific events during pregnancy or around the time of birth that can damage motor centers in the developing brain. Some of these causes of congenital cerebral palsy include:

Infections during pregnancy. German measles, or rubella, is caused by a virus that can infect pregnant women and, therefore, the fetus in the uterus, to cause damage to the developing nervous system. Other infections that can cause brain injury in the developing fetus include cytomegalovirus and toxoplasmosis.

Jaundice in the infant. *Bile pigments*, compounds that are normally found in small amounts in the bloodstream, are produced when blood cells are destroyed. When many blood cells are destroyed in a short time, as in the condition called Rh incompatibility (see below), the yellow-colored pigments can build up and cause jaundice. Severe, untreated jaundice can damage brain cells.

Perinatal asphyxia. During labor and delivery, a shortage of oxygen in the blood, reduced brain blood flow, or both can impair the supply of oxygen to the newborn's brain, causing the condition known as perinatal asphyxia. When asphyxia is severe enough to put the newborn at risk for long-term brain damage, it immediately causes problems with brain function (as in moderate-to-severe hypoxic-ischemic encephalopathy). Asphyxia this severe is very uncommon, is always linked to dysfunction of other body organs, and is often accompanied by seizures.

In the past, physicians and scientists attributed most cases of cerebral palsy to asphyxia or other complications during birth if they could not identify another cause. However, extensive research by NINDS scientists and others has shown that very few babies who experience asphyxia during birth develop encephalopathy after birth. Research also shows that most babies who experience asphyxia do not grow up to have cerebral palsy or other neurological disorders. In fact, current evidence suggests that cerebral palsy is associated with asphyxia and other birth complications in no more than 10 percent of cases.

Rh incompatibility. In this blood condition, the mother's body produces immune cells called antibodies that destroy the fetus's blood cells, leading to a form of jaundice in the newborn.

Stroke/intracranial hemorrhage. Bleeding in the brain (intracranial hemorrhage) has several causes—including broken blood vessels in the brain, clogged blood vessels, or abnormal blood cells—and is one form of stroke. Newborn respiratory distress, a breathing disorder that is particularly common in premature infants, is one cause. Although strokes are better known for their effects on older adults, they can also occur in the fetus during pregnancy or the newborn around the time of birth, damaging brain tissue and causing neurological problems. Ongoing research is testing potential treatments that may one day help prevent stroke in fetuses and newborns.

What Are the Risk Factors?

Research scientists have examined thousands of expectant mothers, followed them through childbirth, and monitored their children's early neurological development. As a result, they have uncovered certain characteristics, called risk factors, that increase the possibility that a child will later be diagnosed with cerebral palsy:

Breech presentation. Babies with cerebral palsy are more likely to present feet first, instead of head first, at the beginning of labor.

Complicated labor and delivery. Vascular or respiratory problems of the baby during labor and delivery may sometimes be the first sign that a baby has suffered brain damage or that a baby's brain has not developed normally during the pregnancy. Such complications can cause permanent brain damage.

Inborn malformations outside the nervous system. Babies with physical birth defects—including faulty formation of the spinal bones, hernia (a protrusion of organs through an abnormal opening inside the body) in the groin area, or an abnormally small jaw bone—are at an increased risk for cerebral palsy.

Low Apgar score. The *Apgar score* (named for anesthesiologist Virginia Apgar) is a numbered rating that reflects a newborn's condition. To determine an Apgar score, doctors periodically check the baby's heart rate, breathing, muscle tone, reflexes, and skin color in the first minutes after birth. They then assign points; the higher the score, the more normal the baby's condition. A low score at 10-20 minutes after delivery is often considered an important sign of potential problems.

Low birthweight and premature birth. The risk of cerebral palsy is higher among babies who weigh less than 2500 grams (5 lbs., 7 ½ oz.) at birth and among babies who are born less than 37 weeks into pregnancy. This risk increases as birthweight falls.

Multiple births. Twins, triplets, and other multiple births are linked to an increased risk of cerebral palsy.

Nervous system malformations. Some babies born with cerebral palsy have visible signs of nervous system malformation, such as an abnormally small head (microcephaly). This suggests that problems occurred in the development of the nervous system while the baby was in the womb.

Maternal bleeding or severe proteinuria late in pregnancy. Vaginal bleeding during the sixth to ninth months of pregnancy and severe proteinuria (the presence of excess proteins in the urine) are linked to a higher risk of having a baby with cerebral palsy.

Maternal hyperthyroidism, mental retardation, or seizures. Mothers with any of these conditions are slightly more likely to have a child with cerebral palsy.

Seizures in the newborn. An infant who has seizures faces a higher risk of being diagnosed, later in childhood, with cerebral palsy.

Knowing these warning signs helps doctors keep a close eye on children who face a higher risk for long-term problems in the nervous system. However, parents should not become too alarmed if their child has one or more of these factors. Most such children do not have and do not develop cerebral palsy.

Can Cerebral Palsy Be Prevented?

Several of the causes of cerebral palsy that have been identified through research are preventable or treatable:

- **Head injury** can be prevented by regular use of child safety seats when driving in a car and helmets during bicycle rides, and elimination of child abuse. In addition, common sense measures around the household—like close supervision during bathing and keeping poisons out of reach—can reduce the risk of accidental injury.

- **Jaundice** of newborn infants can be treated with phototherapy. In phototherapy, babies are exposed to special blue lights that break down bile pigments, preventing them from building up and threatening the brain. In the few cases in which this treatment is not enough, physicians can correct the condition with a special form of blood transfusion.

- **Rh incompatibility** is easily identified by a simple blood test routinely performed on expectant mothers and, if indicated, expectant fathers. This incompatibility in blood types does not usually cause problems during a woman's first pregnancy, since the mother's body generally does not produce the unwanted antibodies until after delivery. In most cases, a special serum given after each childbirth can prevent the unwanted production of antibodies. In unusual cases, such as when a pregnant woman develops the antibodies during her first pregnancy or antibody production is not prevented, doctors can help minimize problems by closely watching the developing baby and, when needed, performing a transfusion to the baby while in the womb or an exchange transfusion (in which a large volume of the baby's blood is removed and replaced) after birth.

- **Rubella**, or German measles, can be prevented if women are vaccinated against this disease *before* becoming pregnant.

In addition, it is always good to work toward a healthy pregnancy through regular prenatal care and good nutrition and by eliminating smoking, alcohol consumption, and drug abuse. Despite the best efforts of parents and physicians, however, children will still be born with cerebral palsy. Since in most cases the cause of cerebral palsy is unknown, little can currently be done to prevent it. As investigators learn more about the causes of cerebral palsy through basic and clinical research, doctors and parents will be better equipped to help prevent this disorder.

What Are the Early Signs?

Early signs of cerebral palsy usually appear before 3 years of age, and parents are often the first to suspect that their infant is not developing motor skills normally. Infants with cerebral palsy are frequently slow to reach developmental milestones, such as learning to roll over, sit, crawl, smile, or walk. This is sometimes called developmental delay.

Some affected children have abnormal muscle tone. Decreased muscle tone is called *hypotonia*; the baby may seem flaccid and relaxed, even floppy. Increased muscle tone is called *hypertonia*, and the baby may seem stiff or rigid. In some cases, the baby has an early period of hypotonia that progresses to hypertonia after the first 2 to 3 months of life. Affected children may also have unusual posture or favor one side of their body.

Parents who are concerned about their baby's development for any reason should contact their physician, who can help distinguish normal variation in development from a developmental disorder.

How Is Cerebral Palsy Diagnosed?

Doctors diagnose cerebral palsy by testing an infant's motor skills and looking carefully at the infant's medical history. In addition to checking for those symptoms described above—slow development, abnormal muscle tone, and unusual posture—a physician also tests the infant's reflexes and looks for early development of hand preference.

Reflexes are movements that the body makes automatically in response to a specific cue. For example, if a newborn baby is held on its back and tilted so the legs are above its head, the baby will automatically extend its arms in a gesture, called the Moro reflex, that looks like an embrace. Babies normally lose this reflex after they reach 6 months, but those with cerebral palsy may retain it for abnormally long periods. This is just one of several reflexes that a physician can check.

Doctors can also look for hand preference—a tendency to use either the right or left hand more often. When the doctor holds an object in front and to the side of the infant, an infant with hand preference will use the favored hand to reach for the object, even when it is held closer to the opposite hand. During the first 12 months of life, babies do not usually show hand preference. But infants with spastic hemiplegia, in particular, may develop a preference much earlier, since the hand on the unaffected side of their body is stronger and more useful.

The next step in diagnosing cerebral palsy is to rule out other disorders that can cause movement problems. Most important, doctors must determine that the child's condition is not getting worse. Although its symptoms may change over time, cerebral palsy by definition is not progressive. If a child is continuously losing motor skills, the problem is probably due to other causes—including genetic diseases, muscle diseases, disorders of metabolism, or tumors in the nervous system. The child's medical history, special diagnostic tests, and, in some cases, repeated check-ups can help confirm that other disorders are not the cause.

The doctor may also order specialized tests to learn more about the possible cause of cerebral palsy. One such test is *computed tomography*, or CT, a sophisticated imaging technique that uses X rays and a computer to create an anatomical picture of the brain's tissues and structures. A CT scan may reveal brain areas that are underdeveloped, abnormal cysts (sacs that are often filled with liquid) in the brain, or other physical problems. With the information from CT scans, doctors may be better equipped to judge the long-term outlook for an affected child.

Magnetic resonance imaging, or MRI, is a relatively new brain imaging technique that is rapidly gaining widespread use for identifying brain disorders. This technique uses a magnetic field and radio waves, rather than X rays. MRI gives better pictures of structures or abnormal areas located near bone than CT.

Figure 14.2. Like a scar that records an old injury to the skin, the large cyst (arrows) seen in this MRI scan reflects earlier damage or faulty development in the brain. (Source: Dr. Laura Ment, Yale University School of Medicine)

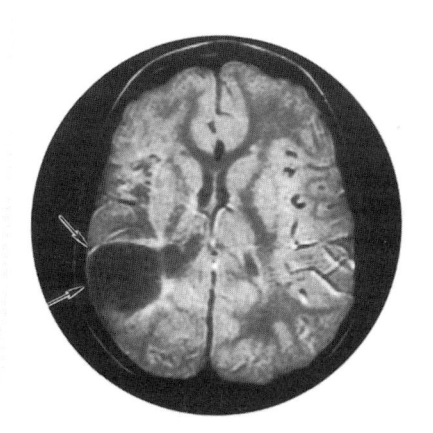

A third test that can expose problems in brain tissues is *ultrasonography*. This technique bounces sound waves off the brain and uses the pattern of echoes to form a picture, or sonogram, of its structures. Ultrasonography can be used in infants before the bones of the skull harden and close. Although it is less precise than CT and MRI scanning, this technique can detect cysts and structures in the brain, is less expensive, and does not require long periods of immobility.

Finally, physicians may want to look for other conditions that are linked to cerebral palsy, including seizure disorders, mental impairment, and vision or hearing problems.

When the doctor suspects a seizure disorder, an *electroencephalogram*, or EEG, may be ordered. An EEG uses special patches called electrodes placed on the scalp to record the natural electrical currents inside the brain. This recording can help the doctor see telltale patterns in the brain's electrical activity that suggest a seizure disorder.

Figure 14.3. Sharp peaks and valleys on this EEG tracing reveal bursts of abnormal electrical activity in the brain during seizures in a 2-year-old child. (Source: Dr. Susumu Sato, NINDS)

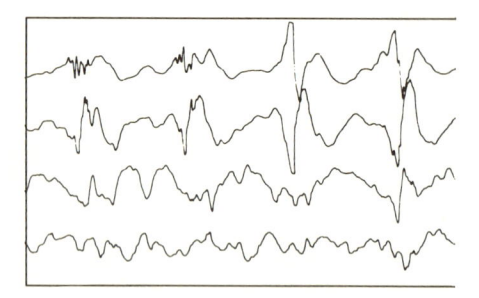

Intelligence tests are often used to determine if a child with cerebral palsy is mentally impaired. Sometimes, however, a child's intelligence may be underestimated because problems with movement, sensation, or speech due to cerebral palsy make it difficult for him or her to perform well on these tests.

If problems with vision are suspected, the doctor may refer the patient to an ophthalmologist for examination; if hearing impairment seems likely, an otologist may be called in.

Identifying these accompanying conditions is important and is becoming more accurate as ongoing research yields advances that make diagnosis easier. Many of these conditions can then be addressed through specific treatments, improving the long-term outlook for those with cerebral palsy.

How Is Cerebral Palsy Managed?

Cerebral palsy can not be cured, but treatment can often improve a child's capabilities. In fact, progress due to medical research now means that many patients can enjoy near-normal lives if their neurological problems are properly managed. There is no standard therapy that works for all patients. Instead, the physician must work with a team of health care professionals first to identify a child's unique needs and impairments and then to create an individual treatment plan that addresses them.

Some approaches that can be included in this plan are drugs to control seizures and muscle spasms, special braces to compensate for muscle imbalance, surgery, mechanical aids to help overcome impairments, counseling for emotional and psychological needs, and physical, occupational, speech, and behavioral therapy. In general, the earlier treatment begins, the better chance a child has of overcoming developmental disabilities or learning new ways to accomplish difficult tasks.

The members of the treatment team for a child with cerebral palsy should be knowledgeable professionals with a wide range of specialties. A typical treatment team might include:

- *a physician*, such as a pediatrician, a pediatric neurologist, or a pediatric physiatrist, trained to help developmentally disabled children. This physician, often the leader of the treatment team, works to synthesize the professional advice of all team members into a comprehensive treatment plan, implements treatments, and follows the patient's progress over a number of years.

- *an orthopedist*, a surgeon who specializes in treating the bones, muscles, tendons, and other parts of the body's skeletal system. An orthopedist might be called on to predict, diagnose, or treat muscle problems associated with cerebral palsy.

- *a physical therapist*, who designs and implements special exercise programs to improve movement and strength.

- *an occupational therapist*, who can help patients learn skills for day-to-day living, school, and work.

- *a speech and language pathologist*, who specializes in diagnosing and treating communication problems.

- *a social worker*, who can help patients and their families locate community assistance and education programs.

- *a psychologist*, who helps patients and their families cope with the special stresses and demands of cerebral palsy. In some cases, psychologists may also oversee therapy to modify unhelpful or destructive behaviors or habits.

- *an educator*, who may play an especially important role when mental impairment or learning disabilities present a challenge to education.

Individuals who have cerebral palsy and their family or caregivers are also key members of the treatment team, and they should be intimately involved in all steps of planning, making decisions, and applying treatments. Studies have shown that family support and personal determination are two of the most important predictors of which individuals who have cerebral palsy will achieve long-term goals.

Too often, however, physicians and parents may focus primarily on an individual symptom—especially the inability to walk. While mastering specific skills is an important focus of treatment on a day-to-day basis, the ultimate goal is to help individuals grow to adulthood and have maximum independence in society. In the words of one physician, "After all, the real point of walking is to get from point A to point B. Even if a child needs a wheelchair, what's important is that they're able to achieve this goal."

What Specific Treatments Are Available?

Physical, Behavioral, and Other Therapies

Therapy—whether for movement, speech, or practical tasks—is a cornerstone of cerebral palsy treatment. The skills a 2-year-old needs to explore the world are very different from those that a child needs in the classroom or a young adult needs to become independent. Cerebral palsy therapy should be tailored to reflect these changing demands.

Physical therapy. Physical therapy usually begins in the first few years of life, soon after the diagnosis is made. Physical therapy programs use specific sets of exercises to work toward two important goals: preventing the weakening or deterioration of muscles that can follow lack of use (called disuse atrophy) and avoiding *contracture*, in which muscles become fixed in a rigid, abnormal position.

Contracture is one of the most common and serious complications of cerebral palsy. A contracture is a chronic shortening of a muscle due to abnormal tone and weakness associated with cerebral palsy. A muscle contracture limits movement of a bony joint, such as the elbow, and can disrupt balance and cause loss of previous motor abilities. Physical therapy alone, or in combination with special braces (sometimes called *orthotic devices*), works to prevent this complication by stretching spastic muscles. For example, if a child has spastic hamstrings (tendons located behind the knee), the therapist and parents should encourage the child to sit with the legs extended to stretch them.

Cerebral Palsy: Hope through Research

A third goal of some physical therapy programs is to improve the child's motor development. A widespread program of physical therapy that works toward this goal is the Bobath technique, named for a husband and wife team who pioneered this approach in England. This program is based on the idea that the primitive reflexes retained by many children with cerebral palsy present major roadblocks to learning voluntary control. A therapist using the Bobath technique tries to counteract these reflexes by positioning the child in an opposing movement. So, for example, if a child with cerebral palsy normally keeps his arm flexed, the therapist would repeatedly extend it.

A second such approach to physical therapy is "patterning," which is based on the principle that motor skills should be taught in more or less the same sequence that they develop normally. In this controversial approach, the therapist guides the child with movement problems along the path of normal motor development. For example, the child is first taught elementary movements like pulling himself to a standing position and crawling before he is taught to walk—regardless of his age. Some experts and organizations, including the American Academy of Pediatrics, have expressed strong reservations about the patterning approach, because studies have not documented its value.

Physical therapy is usually just one element of an infant development program that also includes efforts to provide a varied and stimulating environment. Like all children, the child with cerebral palsy needs new experiences and interactions with the world around him in order to learn. Stimulation programs can bring this valuable experience to the child who is physically unable to explore.

As the child with cerebral palsy approaches school age, the emphasis of therapy shifts away from early motor development. Efforts now focus on preparing the child for the classroom, helping the child master activities of daily living, and maximizing the child's ability to communicate.

Physical therapy can now help the child with cerebral palsy prepare for the classroom by improving his or her ability to sit, move independently or in a wheelchair, or perform precise tasks, such as writing. In **occupational therapy**, the therapist works with the child to develop such skills as feeding, dressing, or using the bathroom. This can help reduce demands on caregivers and boost self-reliance and self-esteem. For the many children who have difficulty communicating, **speech therapy** works to identify specific difficulties and overcome them through a program of exercises. For example, if a child has difficulty saying words that begin with "b," the therapist may suggest daily practice with a list of "b" words, increasing their difficulty as each list is mastered. Speech therapy can also work to help the child learn to use special communication devices, such as a computer with voice synthesizers.

Behavioral therapy. Behavioral therapy provides yet another avenue to increase a child's abilities. This therapy, which uses psychological theory and techniques, can complement physical, speech, or occupational therapy. For example, behavioral therapy might include hiding a toy inside a box to reward a child for learning to reach into the box with his weaker hand. Likewise, a child learning to say his "b" words might be given a balloon for mastering the word. In other cases, therapists may try to discourage unhelpful or destructive behaviors, such as hair-pulling or biting, by selectively presenting a child with rewards and praise during other, more positive activities.

As a child with cerebral palsy grows older, the need for and types of therapy and other support services will continue to change. Continuing physical therapy addresses movement problems and is supplemented by vocational training, recreation and leisure programs, and special education when necessary. Counseling for emotional and psychological challenges may be needed at any age, but is often most critical during adolescence. Depending on their physical and intellectual abilities, adults may need attendant care, living accommodations, transportation, or employment opportunities.

Regardless of the patient's age and which forms of therapy are used, treatment does not end when the patient leaves the office or treatment center. In fact, most of the work is often done at home. The therapist functions as a coach, providing parents and patients with the strategy and drills that can help improve performance at home, at school, and in the world. As research continues, doctors and parents can expect new forms of therapy and better information about which forms of therapy are most effective for individuals with cerebral palsy.

Drug Therapy

Physicians usually prescribe drugs for those who have seizures associated with cerebral palsy, and these medications are very effective in preventing seizures in many patients. In general, the drugs given to individual patients are chosen based on the type of seizures, since no one drug controls all types. However, different people with the same type of seizure may do better on different drugs, and some individuals may need a combination of two or more drugs to achieve good seizure control.

Drugs are also sometimes used to control spasticity, particularly following surgery. The three medications that are used most often are diazepam, which acts as a general relaxant of the brain and body; baclofen, which blocks signals sent from the spinal cord to contract the muscles; and dantrolene, which interferes with the process of muscle contraction. Given by mouth, these drugs can reduce spasticity for short periods, but their value for long-term control of spasticity has not been clearly demonstrated. They may also trigger significant side effects, such as drowsiness, and their long-term effects on the developing nervous system are largely unknown. One possible solution to avoid such side effects may lie in current research to explore new routes for delivering these drugs.

Patients with athetoid cerebral palsy may sometimes be given drugs that help reduce abnormal movements. Most often, the prescribed drug belongs to a group of chemicals called anticholinergics that work by reducing the activity of acetylcholine. Acetylcholine is a chemical messenger that helps some brain cells communicate and that triggers muscle contraction. Anticholinergic drugs include trihexyphenidyl, benztropine, and procyclidine hydrochloride.

Occasionally, physicians may use alcohol "washes"—or injections of alcohol into a muscle—to reduce spasticity for a short period. This technique is most often used when physicians want to correct a developing contracture. Injecting alcohol into a muscle that is too short weakens the muscle for several weeks and gives physicians time to work on lengthening the muscle through bracing, therapy, or casts. In some cases, if the contracture is detected early enough, this technique may avert the need for surgery. In addition, a number of experimental drug therapies are under investigation.

Surgery

Surgery is often recommended when contractures are severe enough to cause movement problems. In the operating room, surgeons can lengthen muscles and tendons that are proportionately too short. First, however, they must determine the exact muscles at fault, since lengthening the wrong muscle could make the problem worse.

Finding problem muscles that need correction can be a difficult task. To walk two strides with a normal gait, it takes more than 30 major muscles working at exactly the right time and exactly the right force. A problem in any one muscle can cause abnormal gait. Furthermore, the natural adjustments the body makes to compensate for muscle problems can be misleading. A new tool that enables doctors to spot gait abnormalities, pinpoint problem muscles, and separate real problems from compensation is called *gait analysis*. Gait analysis combines cameras that record the patient while walking, computers that analyze each portion of the patient's gait, force plates that detect when feet touch the ground, and a special recording technique that detects muscle activity (known as *electromyography*). Using these data, doctors are better equipped to intervene and correct significant problems. They can also use gait analysis to check surgical results.

Figure 14.4. In gait analysis, video cameras, sensitive force plates on the floor, and a computer help tease apart the hundreds of individual movements needed to take a single stride. This process can help physicians spot and treat problems with specific muscles and tendons in cerebral palsy. (Source: Paul Wiegmann, medical illustrator)

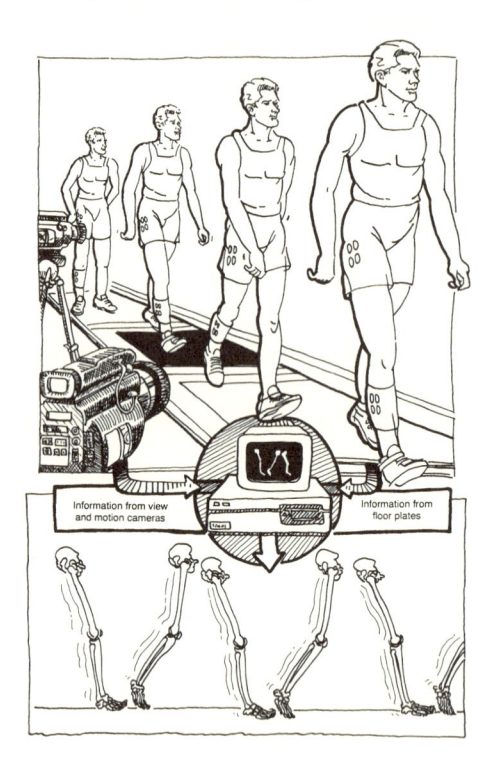

Because lengthening a muscle makes it weaker, surgery for contractures is usually followed by months of recovery. For this reason, doctors try to fix all of the affected muscles at once when it is possible or, if more than one surgical procedure is unavoidable, they may try to schedule operations close together.

A second surgical technique, known as *selective dorsal root rhizotomy*, aims to reduce spasticity in the legs by reducing the amount of stimulation that reaches leg muscles via nerves. In the procedure, doctors try to locate and selectively sever some of the overactivated nerve fibers that control leg muscle tone. Although there is scientific controversy over how selective this technique actually is, recent research results suggest it can reduce spasticity in some patients, particularly those who have spastic diplegia. Ongoing research is evaluating this surgery's effectiveness.

Experimental surgical techniques include chronic cerebellar stimulation and stereotaxic thalamotomy. In chronic cerebellar stimulation, electrodes are implanted on the surface of the cerebellum—the part of the brain responsible for coordinating movement—and are used to stimulate certain cerebellar nerves. While it was hoped that this technique would decrease spasticity and improve motor function, results of this invasive procedure have been mixed. Some studies have reported improvements in spasticity and function, others have not.

Stereotaxic thalamotomy involves precise cutting of parts of the thalamus, which serves as the brain's relay station for messages from the muscles and sensory organs. This has been shown effective only for reducing hemiparetic tremors (see Glossary at end of chapter).

Mechanical Aids

Whether they are as humble as Velcro shoes or as advanced as computerized communication devices, special machines and gadgets in the home, school, and workplace can help the child or adult with cerebral palsy overcome limitations.

The computer is probably the most dramatic example of a new device that can make a difference in the lives of those with cerebral palsy. For example, a child who is unable to speak or write but can make head movements may be able to learn to control a computer using a special light pointer that attaches to a headband. Equipped with a computer and voice synthesizer, this child could communicate with others. In other cases, technology has led to new versions of old devices, such as the traditional wheelchair and its modern offspring that runs on electricity.

What Other Major Problems Are Associated with Cerebral Palsy?

A common complication is **incontinence**, caused by faulty control over the muscles that keep the bladder closed. Incontinence can take the form of bed-wetting (also known as enuresis), uncontrolled urination during physical activities (or stress incontinence), or slow leaking of urine from the bladder. Possible medical treatments for incontinence include special exercises, biofeedback, prescription drugs, surgery, or surgically implanted devices to replace or aid muscles. Specially designed undergarments are also available.

Poor control of the muscles of the throat, mouth, and tongue sometimes leads to **drooling**. Drooling can cause severe skin irritation and, because it is socially unacceptable, can lead to further isolation of affected children from their peers. Although numerous treatments for drooling have been tested over the years, there is no one treatment that always helps. Drugs called anticholinergics can reduce the flow of saliva but may cause significant side effects, such as mouth dryness and poor digestion. Surgery, while sometimes effective, carries the risk of complications, including worsening of swallowing problems. Some patients benefit from a technique called biofeedback that can tell them when they are drooling or having difficulty controlling muscles that close the mouth. This kind of therapy is most likely to work if the patient has a mental age of more than 2 or 3 years, is motivated to control drooling, and understands that drooling is not socially acceptable.

Difficulty with eating and swallowing—also triggered by motor problems in the mouth—can cause **poor nutrition**. Poor nutrition, in turn, may make the individual more vulnerable to infections and cause or aggravate "failure to thrive"—a lag in growth and development that is common among those with cerebral palsy. When eating is difficult, a therapist trained to address swallowing problems can help by instituting special diets and teaching new feeding techniques. In severe cases of swallowing problems and malnutrition, physicians may recommend tube feeding, in which a tube delivers food and nutrients down the throat and into the stomach, or *gastrostomy*, in which a surgical opening allows a tube to be placed directly into the stomach.

What Research Is Being Done?

Investigators from many arenas of medicine and health are using their expertise to help improve treatment and prevention of cerebral palsy. Much of their work is supported through the National Institute of Neurological Disorders and Stroke (NINDS), the National Institute of Child Health and Human Development, other agencies within the Federal Government, nonprofit groups such as the United Cerebral Palsy Research and Educational Foundation, and private institutions.

Cerebral Palsy: Hope through Research

The ultimate hope for overcoming cerebral palsy lies with prevention. In order to prevent cerebral palsy, however, scientists must first understand the complex process of normal brain development and what can make this process go awry.

Between early pregnancy and the first months of life, one cell divides to form first a handful of cells, and then hundreds, millions, and, eventually, billions of cells. Some of these cells specialize to become brain cells. These brain cells specialize into different types and migrate to their appropriate site in the brain. They send out branches to form crucial connections with other brain cells. Ultimately, the most complex entity known to us is created: a human brain with its billions of interconnected neurons.

Mounting evidence is pointing investigators toward this intricate process in the womb for clues about cerebral palsy. For example, a group of researchers has recently observed that more than one-third of children who have cerebral palsy also have missing enamel on certain teeth. This tooth defect can be traced to problems in the early months of fetal development, suggesting that a disruption at this period in development might be linked both to this tooth defect and to cerebral palsy.

As a result of this and other research, many scientists now believe that a significant number of children develop cerebral palsy because of mishaps early in brain development. They are examining how brain cells specialize, how they know where to migrate, how they form the right connections—and they are looking for preventable factors that can disrupt this process before or after birth.

Scientists are also scrutinizing other events—such as bleeding in the brain, seizures, and breathing and circulation problems—that threaten the brain of the newborn baby. Through this research, they hope to learn how these hazards can damage the newborn's brain and to develop new methods for prevention.

Some newborn infants, for example, have life-threatening problems with breathing and blood circulation. A recently introduced treatment to help these infants is extracorporeal membrane oxygenation (ECMO), in which blood is routed from the patient to a special machine that takes over the lungs' task of removing carbon dioxide and adding oxygen. Although this technique can dramatically help many such infants, some scientists have observed that a substantial fraction of treated children later experience long-term neurological problems, including developmental delay and cerebral palsy. Investigators are studying infants through pregnancy, delivery, birth, and infancy, and are tracking those who undergo this treatment. By observing them at all stages of development, scientists can learn whether their problems developed before birth, result from the same breathing problems that made them candidates for the treatment, or spring from errors in the treatment itself. Once this is determined, they may be able to correct any existing problems or develop new treatment methods to prevent brain damage.

Other scientists are exploring how brain insults like hypoxic-ischemic encephalopathy (brain damage from a shortage of oxygen or blood flow), bleeding in the brain, and seizures can cause the abnormal release of brain chemicals and trigger brain damage. For example, research has shown that bleeding in the brain unleashes dangerously high amounts of a brain chemical called glutamate. While glutamate is normally used in the brain for communication, too much glutamate overstimulates the brain's cells and causes a cycle of destruction. Scientists are now looking closely at glutamate to detect how its release harms brain tissue and spreads the damage from stroke. By learning how such brain chemicals that normally help us function can hurt the brain, scientists may be equipped to develop new drugs that block their harmful effects.

In related research, some investigators are already conducting studies to learn if certain drugs can help prevent neonatal stroke. Several of these drugs seem promising because they appear to reduce the excess production of potentially dangerous chemicals in the brain and may help control brain blood flow and volume. Earlier research has linked sudden changes in blood flow and volume to stroke in the newborn.

Low birthweight itself is also the subject of extensive research. In spite of improvements in health care for some pregnant women, the incidence of low birth-weight babies born each year in the United States remains at about 7½ percent. Some scientists currently investigating this serious health problem are working to understand how infections, hormonal problems, and genetic factors may increase a woman's chances of giving birth prematurely. They are also conducting more applied research that could yield: 1) new drugs that can safely delay labor, 2) new devices to further improve medical care for premature infants, and 3) new insight into how smoking and alcohol consumption can disrupt fetal development.

While this research offers hope for preventing cerebral palsy in the future, ongoing research to improve treatment brightens the outlook for those who must face the challenges of cerebral palsy today. An important thrust of such research is the evaluation of treatments already in use so that physicians and parents have the information they need to choose the best therapy. A good example of this effort is an ongoing NINDS-supported study that promises to yield new information about which patients are most likely to benefit from selective dorsal root rhizotomy, a recently introduced surgery that is becoming increasingly in demand for reduction of spasticity.

Similarly, although physical therapy programs are a popular and widespread approach to managing cerebral palsy, little scientific evidence exists to help physicians, other health professionals, and parents determine how well physical therapy works or to choose the best approach among many. Current research on cerebral palsy aims to provide this information through careful studies that compare the abilities of children who have had physical and other therapy with those who have not.

As part of this effort, scientists are working to create new measures to judge the effectiveness of treatment, as in ongoing research to precisely identify the specific brain areas responsible for movement. Using such techniques as magnetic pulses, researchers can locate brain areas that control specific actions, such as raising an arm or lifting a leg, and construct detailed maps. By comparing charts made before and after therapy among children who have cerebral palsy, researchers may gain new insights into how therapy affects the brain's organization and new data about its effectiveness.

Investigators are also working to develop new drugs—and new ways of using existing drugs—to help relieve cerebral palsy's symptoms. In one such set of studies, early research results suggest that doctors may improve the effectiveness of the anti-spasticity drug called baclofen by giving the drug through spinal injections, rather than by mouth. In addition, scientists are also exploring the use of tiny implanted pumps that deliver a constant supply of anti-spasticity drugs into the fluid around the spinal cord, in the hope of improving these drugs' effectiveness and reducing side effects, such as drowsiness.

Other experimental drug development efforts are exploring the use of minute amounts of the familiar toxin called botulinum. Ingested in large amounts, this toxin is responsible for botulism poisoning, in which the body's muscles become paralyzed. Injected in tiny amounts into specific muscles, however, this toxin has shown early promise in reducing local spasticity.

A large research effort is also directed at producing more effective, nontoxic drugs to control seizures. Through its Antiepileptic Drug Development Program, the NINDS screens new compounds developed by industrial and university laboratories around the world for toxicity and anticonvulsant activity and coordinates clinical studies of efficacy and safety. To date, this program has screened more than 13,000 compounds and, as a result, five new antiepileptic drugs—carbamazepine, clonazepam, valproate, clorazepate, and felbamate—have been approved for marketing. A new project within the program is exploring how the structure of a given antiseizure medication relates to its effectiveness. If successful, this project may enable scientists to design better antiseizure medications more quickly and cheaply.

As researchers continue to explore new treatments for cerebral palsy and to expand our knowledge of brain development, we can expect significant medical advances to prevent cerebral palsy and many other disorders that strike in early life.

Glossary

Apgar score—a numbered score doctors use to assess a baby's physical state at the time of birth.

asphyxia—interference with oxygen delivery to the brain and other vital organs.

bile pigments—yellow-colored substances produced by the human body as a byproduct of digestion and red blood cell destruction.

cerebral—relating to the two hemispheres of the human brain.

computed tomography (CT)—an imaging technique that uses X rays and a computer to create a picture of the brain's tissues and structures.

congenital—present at birth.

contracture—chronic shortening of a muscle that limits movement of a bony joint, such as the knee.

dysarthria—problems with speaking caused by difficulty moving or coordinating the muscles needed for speech.

electroencephalogram (EEG)—a technique for recording the pattern of electrical currents inside the brain.

Cerebral Palsy: Hope through Research

electromyography—a special recording technique that detects muscle activity.

failure to thrive—a condition characterized by lag in physical growth and development.

gait analysis—a technique that uses camera recording, force plates, electromyography, and computer analysis to objectively measure an individual's pattern of walking.

gastrostomy—a surgical procedure to create an artificial opening in the stomach.

hemianopia—defective vision or blindness that impairs half of the normal field of vision.

hemiparetic tremors—uncontrollable shaking affecting the limbs on the spastic side of the body in those who have spastic hemiplegia.

hypertonia—increased tone.

hypotonia—decreased tone.

hypoxic-ischemic encephalopathy—brain damage caused by poor blood flow or insufficient oxygen supply to the brain.

jaundice—a blood disorder caused by the abnormal buildup of bile pigments in the bloodstream.

magnetic resonance imaging (MRI)—an imaging technique which uses radio waves, magnetic fields, and computer analysis to create a picture of body tissues and structures.

orthotic devices—special devices, such as splints or braces, used to treat problems of the muscles, ligaments, or bones.

palsy—paralysis, or problems in the control of voluntary movement.

paresis or plegia—weakness or paralysis. In cerebral palsy, these terms are typically combined with another phrase that describes the distribution of paralysis and weakness, e.g., paraparesis.

reflexes—movements that the body makes automatically in response to a specific cue.

Rh incompatibility—a blood condition in which antibodies in a pregnant woman's blood can attack fetal blood cells, impairing the fetus's supply of oxygen.

rubella—also known as German measles, rubella is a viral infection that can damage the nervous system in the developing fetus.

selective dorsal root rhizotomy—a surgical procedure in which selected nerve fibers are severed to reduce spasticity in the legs.

spastic diplegia—a form of cerebral palsy in which both arms and both legs are affected, the legs being more severely affected.

spastic hemiplegia (or hemiparesis)-a form of cerebral palsy in which spasticity affects the arm and leg on one side of the body.

spastic paraplegia (or paraparesis)—a form of cerebral palsy in which spasticity affects both legs, but the arms are relatively or completely spared.

spastic quadriplegia (or quadriparesis)—a form of cerebral palsy in which all four limbs are affected equally.

stereognosia—difficulty perceiving and identifying objects using the sense of touch.

strabismus—misalignment of the eyes.

ultrasonography—a technique that bounces sound waves off of tissues and structures and uses the pattern of echoes to form an image, called a sonogram.

Where Can I Find More Information?

The NINDS is the Federal Government's leading supporter of biomedical research on brain and nervous system disorders, including cerebral palsy. The NINDS conducts research in its own laboratories at the National Institutes of Health in Bethesda, MD, and supports research at institutions worldwide. The Institute also sponsors an active public information program. Other NINDS publications that may be of interest to those concerned about cerebral palsy include "Epilepsy: Hope Through Research" and "The Dystonias."

For more information contact:

NIH Neurological Institute
PO Box 5801
Bethesda, MD 20824
(301) 496-5751
(800) 352-9424

—by Frances Taylor,
Office of Scientific and Health Reports, NINDS

Chapter 15

Cerebral Palsy: Statistics and Risk Factors

Cerebral Palsy: Contributing Risk Factors and Causes

Cerebral palsy is a term used to describe a chronic condition affecting body and/or limb movement and the control of muscle tone and coordination. It is caused by damage to one or more specific areas of the brain during periods of brain development; there is usually no damage to the sensory or motor nerves controlling the muscles. The brain damage is not progressive; however, the characteristics of disabilities resulting from brain damage often change over time.

In examining the contributing factors that influence the occurrence of cerebral palsy and the specific causes of cerebral palsy, five (5) time periods need to be considered:

1. Preconception (parental background)
2. First trimester of pregnancy (0 to 3 months)
3. Second trimester of pregnancy (3+ to 6 months)
4. Third trimester of pregnancy (6+ to 9 months)
5. Perinatal period and infancy (first 2 years post natal)

At a "critical time," either a single factor or a combination of factors can contribute to or can cause damage to the developing brain.

This chapter compiles information from three *Research Fact Sheets* produced by the United Cerebral Palsy Research and Educational Foundation: "Cerebral Palsy: Contributing Risk Factors and Causes," © 1995; "Statistics," © 1994; and "Recurrence of Birth Defects," © 1994; all documents are reprinted with permission.

All factors have not yet been identified. However, a large number are known, and their most influential times of occurrence are being identified.

These factors and the times when they are most likely to have an impact on the developing brain, are listed below.

1. Preconception (Parental Background)

- Biological aging (parent or parents over age 35)
- Biological immaturity (very young parent or parents)
- Environmental toxins
- Genetic background and genetic disorders
- Malnutrition
- Metabolic disorders
- Radiation damage

2. First Trimester of Pregnancy (0 to 3 Months)

Early:

- Endocrine: thyroid function; progesterone insufficiency
- Nutrition: malnutrition; vitamin deficiencies; amino acid intolerance
- Toxins: alcohol; drugs; poisons; smoking

Late:

- Endocrine: thyroid function; progesterone insufficiency
- Maternal disease: thyrotoxicosis; genetic disorders
- Nutrition: malnutrition; amino acid intolerance

3. Second Trimester of Pregnancy (3+ to 6 Months)

Early:

- Infection: CM virus; rubella; toxoplasma; HIV; syphilis; chicken pox; subclinical uterine infection

Late:

- Placental pathology: vascular occlusion; fetal malnutrition; chronic hypoxia; growth factor deficiencies

Cerebral Palsy: Statistics and Risk Factors

4. Third Trimester of Pregnancy (6+ to 9 Months)

Early:

- **Prematurity and low birth weight**
- Blood factors: Rh incompatibility; jaundice
- Cytokines: neurological tissue destruction
- Inflammation and infection: chorioamnionitis

Late:

- **Prematurity and low birth weight**
- Hypoxia: placental insufficiency; perinatal hypoxia
- Infection: listeria; meningitis; streptococcus group B; septicemia; chorioamnionitis

5. Perinatal Period and Infancy (First 2 Years Post Natal)

- Endocrine: hypoglycemia; hypothyroidism
- Hypoxia: perinatal hypoxia; respiratory distress syndrome
- Infection: meningitis; encephalitis
- Multiple births: death of a twin or triplet
- Stroke: hemorrhagic or embolic stroke
- Trauma: abuse; accidents

Statistics

A recent publication in an international research journal, *Developmental Medicine and Child Neurology*, (1994, 36: Pg. 473-483) reported on a study of persons with cerebral palsy in southwest Germany and western Sweden:

In children of *normal* birth weight who have disabilities associated with cerebral palsy,

- about 80% of the disabilities were due to factors occurring before birth; and
- about 20% were due to factors occurring around the birth or immediate post-birth periods (first four weeks of life);

In children of *low birth weight* who developed disabilities associated with cerebral palsy,

- the occurrence is about 0.7 per 1000 live births; and
- there is still uncertainty as to when the brain damage occurred:

  1. did the brain damage occur during embryonic development and because of modern neo-natal care, the infant survived?
  2. did the brain damage occur during or after birth to infants with a "vulnerable" brain?

Spasticity of one or more limbs is the most common disability now associated with new cases of cerebral palsy. There appears to be a predominantly pre-natal cause of limb spasticity in normal birth weight infants; there appears to be a predominantly peri-natal and neo-natal cause of limb spasticity in low birth weight infants.

The study also reports that the number of people with disabilities due to cerebral palsy in the populations they studied is 2.0-2.5 per thousand people (the same as is reported in the U.S.) Cerebral palsy is the second most common neurological impairment in childhood; mental retardation is the first.

Comments

This study reinforces similar findings from studies in the U.S. It helps focus attention on when brain damage associated with cerebral palsy occurs, risk factors that endanger the infant and the most common disabilities resulting from cerebral palsy. Because of the increasing survival of low birth weight infants and the resulting increases in the probability of brain damage, the UCP Research & Educational Foundation is targeting the causes of low birth weight and prematurity as a research priority.

Recurrence of Birth Defects

Cerebral palsy is generally not included in the broad category called "birth defects"; instead cerebral palsy is usually referred to as a "developmental disorder." Typical examples of birth defects are: clubfoot; cleft lip; or a cardiac anatomical defect. However, studies of birth defects also tell us a great deal about forces that influence the developing brain. Therefore, studies of birth defects are of importance to scientists studying developmental brain disorders such as cerebral palsy.

A recent study on birth defects published in *The New England Journal of Medicine* (Lie RT, et al. A Population-Based Study of the

Cerebral Palsy: Statistics and Risk Factors

Risk of Recurrence of Birth Defects; *NEJM* 330:1-6, July 7, 1994) is of interest. The study was done in Norway which has a national health care system and an excellent medical registry that documents birth defects. The study was based on the records of the first and second infants delivered by nearly 400,000 women from 1967 through 1989.

Certain birth defects are known to recur in families. For the nearly 9,200 women whose first infant had a birth defect, the study determined the risk for the second infant having a similar or dissimilar birth defect.

The results were:

- among first infants born to the 400,000 women, 2.5% had a birth defect;

- the mothers of affected first infants were 2.4 times more likely than other women to have a second infant with a birth defect;

- the increased risk was due primarily to an increased risk of the *same* defect occurring in the second infant:

- there was only a slightly increased risk of a *different* defect in the second infant;

- if the women lived in the same municipality during both pregnancies, there was a substantial increase in the risk of having a second infant with the same defect. This risk was decreased when women moved to another municipality after the birth of their first infant with a birth defect;

- thus, a change in environment removed the increased risk of a second child being born with a birth defect.

Comments

Birth defects can be due to: genetic factors; environmental factors; or as now more frequently recognized, genetic susceptibility to environmental factors. The above study documents the importance of environmental factors in the occurrence of repeated birth defects and that changes in the external environment in which a mother lives or works can strongly influence the occurrence of birth defects. The study did not address what the specific environmental factors were, but lays the foundation for new studies to identify these.

Cerebral palsy is not usually included in the category "birth defects." It is important to recognize that there is no evidence that a change in the environment in which a mother lives or works has any effect on the occurrence of cerebral palsy. However developmental disorders such as cerebral palsy have a number of factors in common with birth defects, particularly internal environmental factors influencing the developing brain. Since cerebral palsy rarely "runs in families," genetic causes are not believed at this time to play a primary role in its occurrence; however, a genetic factor could influence the developing brain's susceptibility to other factors such as an intra-uterine infection.

If there is no genetic disorder influencing brain development and, if the intrauterine environment is appropriate, the newborn infant should have a fully functioning brain. Since 75-85% of cases of cerebral palsy now occurring in the U.S.A. are believed to be due to events before birth, the role of the intra-uterine environment in the prevention of cerebral palsy is a critical issue.

The "environment" in which the fetus is developing *in utero* is clearly very important. What "things" in that environment adversely affect brain development, how they got there, how they can be prevented from being there, and how to eliminate them are among the important research issues that the Foundation's program is addressing. Some of the intra-uterine environmental factors being studied include the effects on the developing brain of abnormalities in the functioning of the placenta; infection of the fetus; infection of the mother; metabolic and endocrine disorders of the mother; influence of maternal use of cigarettes, alcohol, and drugs; and influence of environmental "pollutants" such as high levels of radiation.

For More Information

For more information about cerebral palsy, contact:

United Cerebral Palsy Research and Educational Foundation
1660 L Street, NW
Suite 700
Washington, DC 20036
1-800-USA-5UCP
(202) 776- 0406
TDD (202) 973-7197
FAX (202) 776-0414

Chapter 16

Treating Muscle Spasticity in Cerebral Palsy

BOTOX™

BOTOX™ is the commercial name given to a preparation made from *Clostridium botulinum*, a bacterium that causes a serious form of food poisoning. The food poisoning blocks the transmission of the nerve impulse from a nerve to a muscle, causing muscle weakness or paralysis.

The effect of BOTOX™ is to relieve muscle spasm, generally within three days after its injection into a spastic muscle. The effects of each injection lasts approximately three months; sometimes it may be as long as six months before another injection of BOTOX™ is needed. It is suggested that once severe muscle spasms have been relieved, physical therapy may be more effective in building muscle strength and coordination.

Studies of BOTOX™'s usefulness in treating muscle spasms in humans were begun in 1973. Since then, BOTOX™ has been studied for treating a variety of conditions involving inappropriate muscle activity. When injected into specific places in selected muscles,

---

This chapter compiles information from six *Research Fact Sheets* produced by the United Cerebral Palsy Research and Educational Foundation: "BOTOX™," © 1993; "BOTOX™ Update," © 1995; "Baclofen and the Baclofen Pump," © 1994; "Update: Baclofen and the Baclofen Pump," © 1995; "Selective Dorsal Rhizotomy: A Neurosurgical Approach to Muscle Spasticity," © 1994; and "The Use of Electrical Stimulation of Spastic Muscles," ©1994; all documents are reprinted with permission.

BOTOX™ has been found useful in treating muscle spasms affecting vision (*strabismus* and *blepharospasm*). It has also been found useful in treating long term spasticity in neck muscles as well as in treating spasticity in the throat muscles affecting speech. A number of persons with these disorders have been followed for several years, and there have been few reports of side effects. Most difficulties appear to be relatively mild and of short duration. The use of BOTOX™ for specific disorders of eye and facial muscles has been approved by the U.S. Government Food and Drug Administration.

Because of the above, it has been proposed that BOTOX™ may be useful for relieving muscle spasticity In persons with *cerebral palsy*. Allergan which produces BOTOX™, is conducting a clinical trial of its effectiveness in selected medical centers around the country. The clinical trial is in its final phases, and information about the effectiveness of BOTOX™ in treating muscle spasticity associated with cerebral palsy should be available by mid-1994.

BOTOX™ Update

In November 1993, a Foundation Research Fact Sheet discussed the status of BOTOX™ in the treatment of the muscle spasticity associated with cerebral palsy.

In summary of the November 1993 Fact Sheet: BOTOX™ is used to relieve muscle spasm by blocking the transmission of the nerve impulse to a muscle, causing the muscle to be weakened or paralyzed. It is administered by fine needle injection into one or more spastic muscles, usually taking effect within three days and often lasting three to six months. The relief of spasticity by BOTOX™ injections is usually followed by an organized program of physical therapy. BOTOX™ has been approved by the U.S. Food and Drug Administration for use in specific disorders of the eye and of facial and neck muscles. It is available to physicians through pharmacies. BOTOX™ has been undergoing evaluation for relieving the muscle spasticity in the extremities that is associated with cerebral palsy. Readers are referred to the November 1993 Foundation Research Fact Sheet for additional background information (see section above).

A number of clinical trials of BOTOX™ for use in relieving limb spasticity in persons with cerebral palsy have now been completed. The data have been submitted to the U.S. Food and Drug Administration (FDA) for approval of its use for this purpose. As of now, the FDA review has not been completed.

Treating Muscle Spasticity in Cerebral Palsy

At the 1995 Annual Meeting of the American Academy of Cerebral Palsy and Developmental Medicine, a number of research papers were presented on the clinical evaluation of BOTOX™. In general, the results reported were favorable. There were reports of meaningful improvements in limb positioning and of some improvement in gait of selected patients; other patients had minimal results. The persons most likely to benefit were young people, with no tendon contractures and who do not have significant spasticity of muscles in the thigh.

Comment

The final story on the use of BOTOX™ is not yet available. Hopefully, the information submitted to the FDA and the evaluation of those data will be made available in the near future. In the interim, physicians are continuing to explore the use of BOTOX™ in muscle spasticity due to cerebral palsy. Some physicians suggest that a trial of BOTOX™ is a reasonable way to evaluate what effects selective dorsal rhizotomy may have on spasticity and on gait. However, we must remember that the basic problem is lack of muscle coordination, not muscle disease. An improvement in limb positioning may be the reason for the benefit in gait. Additional information about the use and availability of BOTOX™ can be obtained by writing to:

BOTOX™
Allergan, Inc.
2525 Dupont Drive
Irvine, CA 92715

Baclofen and the Baclofen Pump

Persons with cerebral palsy often experience muscle spasticity that limits their mobility. Clinical approaches to the control of spasticity include drug therapy, surgery and/or physical therapy.

Drug therapies for the treatment of spasticity have had limited clinical success. New drug therapies are under study, as are new methods of using older therapies. One such new method is the use of baclofen administered by means of a pump implanted under the skin of the abdomen.

Baclofen is a muscle relaxant and antispasmodic that works by inhibiting the nervous system. Its precise mechanism of action is unknown although it is thought to inhibit the transmission of impulses between nerve cells. Since it is a nervous system inhibitor, it can affect the action of nerve cells in the brain and cause confusion, drowsiness, dizziness, and difficulties with gait and balance. In high doses, it is reported to have caused problems with breathing and with heart and kidney function.

Baclofen has been used clinically for the relief of muscle spasticity in the limbs, through its action of inhibiting nerve cell transmission in the spinal cord. It is reported that baclofen is of value in diminishing muscle spasticity in persons with injury to the spinal cord and diseases of the spinal cord. **However, its usefulness in muscle spasticity associated with cerebral palsy has not been established; also, it is not recommended for use in children under 12 years of age.**

One reason for the adverse side effects associated with baclofen is a result of its oral administration. In order to act on the nerve cells in the spinal cord, baclofen first enters the fluid surrounding the spinal cord (the cerebral spinal fluid) and then the spinal cord. When taken by mouth and in order to obtain therapeutic levels in the cerebrospinal fluid, relatively large amounts of the drug are needed. However, in high oral doses, the drug also enters the cerebrospinal fluid surrounding the brain and affects brain function, causing lethargy and difficulties with balance. In order to offset the effects of high oral doses, a technique has been developed that uses a pump about the size of a hockey puck. The pump is implanted under the skin of the abdomen, and a tube from the pump is placed into the fluid chamber surrounding the spinal cord. The pump has a reservoir in which baclofen is stored. The pump is programmed to discharge specified amounts of baclofen into the cerebrospinal fluid at a predetermined rate. This method of delivery can more precisely control how much of the drug is administered and where the drug is introduced into the cerebrospinal fluid.

Update: Baclofen and the Baclofen Pump

In April 1994, a Research Foundation Fact Sheet described the status of information about the use of a drug to reduce muscle spasticity—baclofen—and its administration by a pump implanted under the skin (see section above). Baclofen decreases the excitability of nerve cells in the spinal cord and is being used to diminish spasticity in the lower limbs in persons with spinal cord injury and disease of the spinal cord, The pump is used as a method of administering controlled

Treating Muscle Spasticity in Cerebral Palsy

amounts of the drug by a tube from the pump to the spinal fluid in the space which surrounds the spinal cord. The usefulness of baclofen for the treatment of muscle spasticity associated with cerebral palsy has not been established and is under study. Also, the usefulness and safety of the pump and tube for delivering baclofen into the spinal fluid is under study. Thus, the usefulness and role of baclofen delivered by pump into the spinal fluid is undergoing clinical evaluation.

The Research Foundation has been informed by Medtronic Neurological (manufacturer of the pump) that the U.S. Food and Drug Administration (FDA) has approved a treatment protocol (a "treatment IND") to study the use of baclofen (Lioresal®) being delivered to the spinal fluid in the treatment of spasticity of cerebral origin: this includes severe spasticity related to cerebral palsy and to head injury.

The treatment protocol approved by the FDA allows this therapy to be used at this time under investigative conditions. Persons with cerebral palsy wishing to participate in one of the clinical trials must receive treatment at a medical center that is enrolled in the Medtronic clinical study. Several medical centers are participating in the study evaluating this therapy.

In the consideration of this therapy for cerebral palsy, there are several issues that need to be addressed:

- Is the drug administered in this way effective in the treatment of spasticity associated with cerebral palsy?

- What are the side-effects of the use of the drug administered in this way?

- What are the benefits, complications and dangers of the use of the implanted pump and the delivery system to the spinal fluid?

- What is the role of other therapies usually given in conjunction with baclofen (e.g., physiotherapy)?

Selective Dorsal Rhizotomy: A Neurosurgical Approach to Muscle Spasticity

A number of pediatric neurological surgeons are utilizing a surgical procedure to diminish spasticity (increased muscle tone) in children with cerebral palsy. The goals of the procedure are improvement in walking, increase in range of motion, and better body positioning;

this latter for non-ambulatory persons requiring assistance with hygiene for body care.

The surgical procedure is done in the lower back region, principally to diminish tone in spastic muscles of the lower limbs. It involves identifying sensory nerve fibers just dorsal (posterior) to the spinal cord and then selectively cutting those nerve fibers (rhizotomy)—"selective dorsal rhizotomy." The nerve fibers selected for cutting during surgery are those which when stimulated electrically are reported to generate unusual electrical activity. After part of its nerve supply is cut, the muscle usually has less tone (is less spastic) and may show temporary or permanent weakness. The surgery is always followed by other clinical procedures, often a program of intensive physical therapy for periods of three to six months.

Surgeons who use this procedure find it important that an expert team use specified criteria to evaluate any child being considered for surgical treatment of spasticity. The presurgical evaluation team is usually multi-disciplinary and uses a combination of clinical, laboratory and behavioral guidelines for evaluating the child. It generally requires assurances of the parent or other caregiver to adhere to the program of follow-up therapy. The presence of muscle-tendon contractures, a history of previous surgery, and/or hip displacement are considered by some physicians as contraindications to rhizotomy, particularly if the purpose of rhizotomy is to improve function such as walking.

A number of side effects of the procedure have been reported. One side effect is sensory loss, numbness or uncomfortable sensations in limb areas which the cut nerve supplied; however, these usually disappear. Another reported side effect is hip dislocation in children who had previous problems in hip alignment. Also, there are some reports of difficulty in bladder and/or bowel control after surgery. An important post-operative problem is patient discouragement, usually due to the length and intensity of the follow-up program of physical therapy.

Several "case series" have been published by individual pediatric neurosurgeons and physical medicine specialists on their clinical experience in using selective dorsal rhizotomy. There have also been a number of medical symposia in which these case series have been discussed. Most series report a decrease in muscle tone; however, there are mixed reports about the long term effects of selective dorsal rhizotomy on function. Some specialists report that if the patient is selected properly and follow-up therapy is adequate, the clinical results in their patients are good; other specialists report that limited clinical improvement in their patients does not justify the risks or complications of the surgery.

Controversial issues include: What is the biological rationale explaining why the procedure should be clinically useful? What are the characteristics of the person for whom the procedure should be used (age, contractures, previous therapy, neuromuscular laboratory findings, etc.)? Is there a meaningful and long term diminution in spasticity after surgery? Does the diminution in spasticity provide for improved function such as ambulation? What are the respective contributions to improvement of function of the surgical procedure and of the intensive follow-up care?

The majority of articles published about selective rhizotomy indicate its effectiveness in reducing muscle tone. However, there is still debate as to whether the long term benefits of the procedure justify the risks, cost, and expenditure of family resources. **At this time, the available data indicate that selective dorsal rhizotomys decreases muscle tone (spasticity); however, there are inadequate data to support or reject the usefulness of selective rhizotomy to improve long term function in patients with disabilities due to cerebral palsy.**

Some investigators are evaluating the usefulness of this procedure in controlled clinical trials of their patients. However, proper evaluation will probably require a larger number of persons participating in a trial than can be enrolled in any single institution. The UCP Research & Educational Foundation has urged the pediatric neurosurgical community to undertake a national cooperative study to evaluate the role and place of this neurosurgical procedure. Until an adequate controlled clinical trial is done, we won't know if selective dorsal rhizotomy is useful in the treatment of persons with disability due to spasticity associated with cerebral palsy.

The Use of Electrical Stimulation of Spastic Muscles

The use of electrical stimulation in the treatment of muscle spasticity and tendon contracture associated with cerebral palsy has been used by a number of clinicians over many years. The desired effects of electrical stimulation were increased muscle strength and greater mobility of restricted joint motion; both, important to increased function. The results of clinical use have been varied and often difficult to evaluate. This is particularly true about the long term effects of electrical stimulation.

In a recent article in the journal *Developmental Medicine and Child Neurology* (Hazelwood, ME et al. *DMCN*; August 1994, 36/8; Pgs 661-673), a group of clinician-investigators did a carefully designed study of the use of electrical stimulation in the treatment of one sided muscle spasticity (hemiplegia) associated with cerebral palsy. The muscles tested were those responsible for dorso-flexion of the ankle (the upward movement of the foot on the leg).

The authors report that "electrical stimulation can be effective as a home-based therapy for the reduction of contracture (tendon shortening) in children with cerebral palsy." They suggest that electrical stimulation may be most helpful in preventing additional contracture. They also report an increase in the range of passive (involuntary) movement of the ankle. However, functional analysis of gait showed no evidence of significant improvement.

Comment

The effects of electrical stimulation appear to be limited and temporary. It is usually used intermittently as one part of a broader treatment program. It appears to be most useful at times of rapid body growth or of increasing contracture of tendons. Although electrical stimulation can contribute to an increase in range of motion, there is little indication that when used alone it provides for improvement in function.

For More Information

For more information about muscle spasticity in cerebral palsy, contact:

United Cerebral Palsy Research and Educational Foundation
1660 L Street, NW
Suite 700
Washington, DC 20036
1-800-USA-5UCP
(202) 776-0406
TDD (202) 973-7197
FAX (202) 776-0414

Chapter 17

Surgical Treatment of Drooling

The September 1995 issue of the journal *Developmental Medicine and Child Neurology* included a report of an Australian study on the "Long Term Outcome of Saliva-control Surgery" by K. Webb et al. (Vol. 37/ No.9, Pgs. 755-762). The following summarizes and comments on some of the highlights of that report.

When present, drooling is a difficult problem in persons with developmental brain disorders. Drooling is normal in infancy but usually subsides around 18 months of age. Persistence beyond four years of age is not considered normal (Crysdale 1989). It is generally accepted that drooling occurs because of a defect in the oral or voluntary phase of swallowing, resulting in an overflow of secretions which builds up in the front of the mouth (Shott et al. 1989).

Any treatment which reduces the amount of drooling must also consider the several important functions of saliva; these include lubrication of the material being swallowed, the digestion of starch, oral hygiene and dental protection. It is important that the benefits of therapy outweigh its disadvantages, particularly for the long run.

Treatments proposed for saliva control and drooling include behavioral conditioning, oromotor training, drug therapy and several types of surgical procedures. Behavioral and oromotor training have been reported to give modest improvement but usually, these procedures do not provide long term beneficial results. Drug therapies are generally directed at decreasing the amount of saliva and usually result

---

Research Fact Sheet, United Cerebral Palsy Research and Educational Foundation, © January 1996; reprinted with permission.

in an unacceptable dry mouth with resultant swallowing difficulties and poor oral hygiene.

There are a number of surgical procedures which have been used for the treatment of drooling; most have not been found to be satisfactory. The recent study describes the results of a surgical procedure which involves the redirection of flow from some salivary ducts (the submandibular ducts) and closing of one salivary duct (a parotid duct). Unfortunately, there was only a superficially favorable outcome. The authors report that a significant proportion of persons or their caregivers did not find the surgery helpful, generally because they found the complications unacceptable.

Comment

At this time there is no single acceptable treatment for drooling. A combination of approaches is usually necessary and benefits of therapy need to be considered in respect to complications. The fundamental issue is we don't really understand the neurological and neuromuscular mechanisms responsible for drooling. Until we do, it will continue to be "hit and miss". Drooling is one of the research areas identified for Research Foundation support. So far, we have had very few research grant requests.

For More Information

For more information about drooling in cerebral palsy contact:

United Cerebral Palsy Research and Educational Foundation
1660 L Street, NW
Suite 700
Washington, DC 20036
1-800-USA-5UCP
(202) 776-0406
TDD (202) 973-7197
FAX (202) 776-0414

Chapter 18

Current Research Initiatives in Cerebral Palsy

How Does the Brain Heal?

Cerebral palsy is caused by injury to the developing brain. The brain injury in cerebral palsy can occur during fetal development (prenatal), during labor, delivery and shortly thereafter (perinatal), or during the first two years of infant life (post natal). There are a broad spectrum of causes, individually or in combination, that can bring about damage to the developing brain. The damage can occur in one small area of the brain, in a large area of the brain, or in several areas of the brain; it can damage nerve cells, the nerve cell fibers (axons) that conduct messages, or both. To be called cerebral palsy, the injury must result primarily in a defect in motor control (control of muscle coordination) with resulting problems in muscle strength and muscle movement. It is important to emphasize that the problem of impaired motor control in cerebral palsy is not due to an inherent problem in the muscle or to the peripheral nerves connecting the central nervous system (brain; spinal cord) to the muscle; the defect is in the brain and its effect on the peripheral nerves which control the muscles.

This chapter compiles information from four *Research Fact Sheets* produced by the United Cerebral Palsy Research and Educational Foundation: "How Does the Brain Heal?" © 1996; "The Role of the Placenta in Cerebral Palsy," © 1995; "Protection of the Developing Brain of Very Low Birth Weight Infants," © 1995; and "Cerebral Palsy Associated with Low levels of Thyroid in Premature Infants," © 1996; all documents reprinted with permission.

Most clinical treatments used to diminish or remove the disability caused by cerebral palsy focus on the dysfunction of peripheral nerve or muscle; these clinical treatments generally include drugs, surgery, rehabilitation or assistive technology. They address the result of brain damage, not the damaged brain. These interventions have had wide variations in their success, dependent usually on the specific type and degree of the disability; on the reliability of the therapy; on the skill of the therapist; and on the dedication of the person with the disability and his/her caregiver to the program of intervention. Important studies are in progress and are being developed to study the usefulness of these interventions (outcomes research) and to improve on them (clinical and engineering research).

Although interventions to influence the effects of cerebral palsy are essential at this time in order to improve the quality of life of persons with disabilities, a fundamental issue still is: can we "repair" the injured brain? Also, if it is repaired, will the disabilities be lessened or eliminated?

The brain's control of movement involves the integrated activity of several brain processes; these include: sensory perception (e.g., touch, vision); memory storage and retrieval; gross motor control (e.g., arm movement): and fine motor control (e.g., finger skills). It is also influenced by the several other processes occurring concurrently in the brain but not directly concerned with control of movement (e.g., control of breathing). In addition, we must remember that the brain changes over time (e.g., learning), and these changes interact with the brain's pattern of response to the previous damage. Thus, changing the damaged area can also change other brain processes; when the existing balance is changed and overall brain function also changes—but usually very little.

Despite all these "ifs," "ands," and "buts," research is providing us with information about how we might help to change the injured brain and restore motor function. Excellent examples of the success of this approach—more properly, the partial success—is in Parkinson's Disease and several forms of epilepsy.

What are the research strategies being pursued to help restore function in the injured brain?

Sprouting. When nerve cells die and the nerve fibers they send to other cells (nerve or muscle) also die, adjacent healthy nerve cells send their fibers into the damaged area and make new connections:

Current Research Initiatives in Cerebral Palsy

thus, new pathways are established by which adjacent brain areas can take over functions of the damaged area. This is one of the brain's repair processes which occurs spontaneously following a stroke. The problems are how to encourage sprouting when it doesn't occur spontaneously; how to make the connections work (become functional) and not just "be there"; and how to make the function an appropriate (useful) one and not an "abnormal" one (e.g., a muscle spasm). This is a very active area of research, particularly in animal models. The results are very promising, but as yet practical only in humans in very special situations; this does not yet include cerebral palsy. However, if we could identify the brain damage very early (*in utero*? in the neonatal nursery?), it may be possible to influence sprouting and assist the brain in making functional new connections.

Regeneration. Very often when a nerve cell is injured but not killed, its connecting fibers die; the nerve cell's connection to other cells are lost. This is the usual event in spinal cord trauma. However, the body of the nerve cell can recover and grow new fibers; the fibers are "regenerated." Like sprouting, this is a normal reaction to injury and is believed to occur spontaneously; for example, in peripheral nerve injury. However, in the central nervous system, the process that guided the growing nerve fiber to make the proper connections is active only in specific stages of fetal development; after birth, the guidance mechanism is thought not to be available in the brain. Why? Can we reactivate the guidance mechanism? Can we provide substitutes for it? Also, as in sprouting, the growing fiber needs to become activated after the connection is made in order to control its target. This functional connection occurs regularly when nerves in the peripheral nervous system are injured, but poorly when nerve cells in the central nervous system (brain and spinal cord) are injured. There have been very good results in assisting the guidance mechanism in experimental animal models, particularly following spinal cord injury; the results in the brain are still unsatisfactory. Thus, this method of restoring function in the brain of a person with cerebral palsy is still a goal yet to be achieved.

Tissue Implants. The use of nerve tissue implants in the damaged brain or spinal cord has received a lot of public attention in recent years; this is particularly true because of its reported success in humans with Parkinson's Disease. In Parkinson's Disease, tissue implants work because the disorder is due primarily to the death of a localized area of the brain that produces a chemical, dopamine. If embryonic brain cells that produce dopamine are implanted in the damaged area, they become mature cells that produce dopamine and relieve many of the disease's symptoms. This is a form of chemical replacement therapy, like taking insulin. However, in cerebral palsy, there is no evidence that the motor control problem is due to a loss of a brain chemical. Thus it seems highly unlikely that the strategy of tissue implantation is applicable to cerebral palsy.

However, there is a variation of this that may be more applicable. In spinal cord injury (more like cerebral palsy than Parkinson's Disease), nerve cell implants have served to support the growth of nerve cell fibers into the area of injury. The implant appears to provide the growing nerve cell fibers (sprouting; regeneration) with a favorable environment in which to grow, probably because of the implant's production of nerve growth factors essential to cell growth and health. However, a major problem still exists: growth to where? As in sprouting and regeneration, will the nerve cell fibers know where to go?

Electronic Implants. There have been some remarkable successes under experimental conditions in both animals and humans in which implanted electronic devices have been used to substitute for damaged nerve cells. One such example is the cochlear implant which is now being used commonly to stimulate the inner ear of persons with profound hearing loss and send interpretable sound to the brain. Similar types of experiments have been done in attempts to restore vision in people who are blind; this latter is at a very early stage of development. However, both of these depend on stimulating organs outside the brain (ear; eye) which in turn sends messages to the brain. As yet similar success for electronic stimulation of the brain to produce purposeful muscle movement has not been reported. The brain can be stimulated electrically and a muscle (generally a group of muscles) made to contract. However, being able to provide a program of electronic stimuli to the brain which results in purposeful movement (e.g., finger control) is a goal yet to be achieved.

Learning. No discussion of strategies for restoring brain function would be complete without discussion of learning. We don't really know how the brain "learns." What is memory? How is it stored? How is it retrieved? But we do know that learning stimulates brain activity; that brain cells respond to stimulation; and that brain cell stimulation is very important both in brain development and in brain repair.

Current Research Initiatives in Cerebral Palsy

For example, the brain is regularly stimulated by muscle activity. The muscles tell the brain that they have contracted. In brain repair, these incoming stimuli from muscle can excite existing pathways in the brain which are already there, but are not used—or rarely used—to perform a function. Stimuli arising in muscle probably encourage the invasion of nerve cell fibers from adjacent brain cells into areas of cell death (encouraging sprouting), and support the growth of new fibers from recovering cells (supporting regeneration). We also know that stimulated target tissues (e.g., muscle) send out chemical messages to growing nerve cell fibers inviting them to become connected. The controlled stimulation of muscle not only helps maintain its viability, but also encourages its reconnection to peripheral nerves. Is the same true for reconnecting nerve cells in the brain? Can the person learn to use other parts of the brain to perform a motor task? Evidence indicates the answer may be yes.

Comment

The above is a very generalized overview of research and research strategies addressing the repair of injured brain. Fortunately, the developing and young brain are very responsive to change and probably to repair. Practical results in brain healing are still to be achieved, particularly in developmental brain injury like cerebral palsy. However, the best scientists in the world are addressing these issues, and our Foundation is doing everything we can to help them. Will we get there? We will—but we can't predict when! Our Foundation's motto says it all: "Hope Through Research."

The Role of the Placenta in Cerebral Palsy

There is a growing body of evidence that a lack of sufficient oxygen to the infant during the birth period (the perinatal period) is not the major reason for the brain damage usually found in cerebral palsy; this is particularly true if the infant is full term (40 weeks) and of normal birth weight (5.5 lbs. or more). Studies indicate that less than 15% of cerebral palsy is attributable to insufficient oxygen at birth. It is believed that prenatal factors are the major reasons for developmental brain damage.

Attention has been drawn to a number of prenatal factors that influence fetal growth and development at different times in intrauterine life. These prenatal factors are being identified and their influence studied as contributors to the damage of the developing brain resulting in cerebral palsy (see September 1995 Fact Sheet on Risk Factors and Causes). One contributor of importance is malfunction and/or pathology of the placenta, The placenta serves two major purposes:

- A selective filter between the circulation of the mother and the fetus; and
- A site for the storage, production and timely release of substances necessary for the growth and development of the fetus.

If these placental functions are seriously impaired, fetal growth and development are believed to be threatened, particularly brain development.

There are four major factors recognized at this time as causes of placental malfunction:

- poor placental structure and/or placement in the uterus
- infection of the placenta
- genetic and metabolic disorders of the mother
- inadequate blood supply to the placenta

In order to investigate the relationship of placental malfunction and the later development of cerebral palsy, studies will probably require the storing of placentas delivered at the time of birth of infants who are recognized to be at risk; of developing cerebral palsy (e.g., multiple births; poor muscle tone; respiratory distress; very low birth weight).

These infants can be followed and those who develop cerebral palsy identified. Following development of cerebral palsy, the stored placentas associated with the birth of these children can be examined anatomically, microscopically and biochemically. These findings can be compared to those from a sample of stored placentas from infants who did not develop cerebral palsy. The differences will provide the leads necessary to explore the role of the placenta in the development of cerebral palsy.

Because of this research area's potential importance, the Foundation is stimulating needed research on the role of placental damage and/or malfunction in the development of cerebral palsy.

Protection of the Developing Brain of Very Low Birth Weight Infants

Very low birth weight (3.3 lbs. or less) is an important risk factor for damage to the infant's developing brain. Nationally, 45,000 infants are born each year with a birth weight of 3.3 lbs or less. Of these 85% survive. Of the survivors, 5-15% develop cerebral palsy. Thus, measures to protect the brain of the infant born with a very low birth weight can be of significance in reducing the occurrence of cerebral palsy. The Foundation has designated as areas of priority: research to prevent low birth weight and prematurity; and the development of methods to protect the low birth weight infant's brain.

A recent article in the journal *Pediatrics* [Nelson, K.B., Grether, J.K., "Can magnesium sulfate reduce the risk of cerebral palsy in very low birth weight infants?" *Pediatrics* 1995, 95 (2)] presents information which may have significance for the protection of the brain of infants born with very low birth weights.

The authors report on the use of magnesium sulfate, sometimes given to mothers shortly before delivery as a treatment for premature labor and/or toxemia brought on by pregnancy. Children with birth weights of less than 3.3 lbs and with moderate to severe disabilities due to cerebral palsy were compared to children of similar very low birth weights who did not develop these disabilities. The authors report that in women who gave birth to very low birth weight babies, there was a significant decrease in the occurrence of moderate to severe cerebral palsy when magnesium sulfate was administered to the mother prior to delivery. The marked reduction in the rate of occurrence of cerebral palsy was seen regardless of the medical reason for early delivery. They suggest that magnesium is protective to the very low birth weight infant's brain.

This study is based on an analysis of previous records (a "retrospective" study) by a scientist in the National Institute of Neurological Disorders and Stroke working with a scientist in the California Birth Defects Monitoring Program, the latter an organization receiving research grant support from our Foundation. However exciting the results of the study, they must be interpreted with caution. Retrospective studies rarely "prove" anything; they usually serve to develop an idea which is then tested in a "prospective" study of new cases in a controlled clinical trial done under exacting conditions. The Foundation is working with the authors of the study to develop and initiate the needed clinical trial to test the hypothesis that the use of magnesium sulfate before early delivery may help in protecting the brain of very low birth weight infants.

In conclusion, at this time the results of the study reported in *Pediatrics* are exciting and provocative, but not conclusive. With the Foundation's assistance, they will be put to the test.

Cerebral Palsy Associated with Low Levels of Thyroid Hormone in Premature Infants

Two articles in the March 28, 1996 issue of the *New England Journal of Medicine* ("The Relation of Transient Hypothyroxinemia in Preterm Infants to Neurologic Development at Two Years of Age;" Reuss M.L. et al. "Prematurity-Associated Neurologic and Developmental Abnormalities and Neonatal Thyroid Function," Vulsma, T. and Kok, J.H.) explore the relationship of a temporary low level of thyroid hormone in premature infants in the first week of life and the occurrence of severe cerebral palsy and/or mental retardation.

One article is the report of a research study supported by the National Institutes of Health (NIH), the government's medical research agency; the other is an editorial review of the research area by international experts.

The articles point out that thyroxin (thyroid hormone) is necessary for brain development and crosses the placenta from mother to fetus. When the infant is born, its own mechanism becomes active for the production and adjustment of necessary levels of thyroxin. However, it takes time for the premature infant to take over this function; the more premature the infant, the lower the level of thyroxin available to it, particularly in the first few weeks after birth. Most infants are finally able to make the adjustment, thus the low level of thyroxin available is usually a temporary phenomenon—but one that occurs at a critical time in brain development.

In the past, several studies have shown that low levels of thyroxin are present in infants who are mentally retarded. The present study shows that the same is true with those who have severe cerebral palsy.

Comment

Temporary low levels of thyroxin in the premature infant can be associated with the occurrence of severe cerebral palsy.

Does this temporary low level of thyroxin cause brain damage? Or are both due to some other factor influencing the occurrence of both?

Current Research Initiatives in Cerebral Palsy

We don't know. Should all premature infants be tested shortly after birth for thyroxin levels? Probably. Will treating premature infants who have low levels of thyroxin help prevent cerebral palsy? We don't know, but a clinical trial would tell us.

The present study is important in that it identifies several specific research questions that can and need to be answered. The Research Foundation is working with the NIH to get the answers.

For More Information

For more information on cerebral palsy and on-going research initiatives contact:

United Cerebral Palsy Research and Educational Foundation
1660 L Street, NW
Suite 700
Washington, DC 20036
1-800-USA-5UCP
(202) 776-0406
TDD (202) 973-7197
FAX (202) 776-0414

Chapter 19

Magnesium Linked to Lower Incidence of Cerebral Palsy

A new study shows that very low birth weight babies have a lower incidence of cerebral palsy (CP) when their mothers are treated with magnesium sulfate soon before giving birth. The findings come from a study sponsored by the California Birth Defects Monitoring Program (CBDMP) and the National Institute of Neurological Disorders and Stroke (NINDS) and reported in the February 1995 issue of *Pediatrics* (Karin B. Nelson, M.D.; Judith K. Grether, Ph.D. "Can Magnesium Sulfate Reduce the Risk of Cerebral Palsy in Very Low Birth Weight Infants?" *Pediatrics*, February, 1995, Vol. 95, Number 2, p. 263.)

The study compared a group of 42 very low birth weight children who had moderate or severe congenital CP to a control group of 75 very low birth weight children without the disability. Three of the 42 mothers of children with CP and 29 of the 75 mothers of children in the control group received magnesium sulfate during pregnancy. The researchers concluded that magnesium sulfate seems to have a protective effect against CP in very low birth weight infants.

The investigators caution however that more research will be required to establish a definitive relationship between the drug and prevention of the disorder. The current study results are based on observations of a group of children born in four northern California counties.

"This intriguing finding means that use of a simple medication could significantly decrease the incidence of cerebral palsy and prevent

---

National Institute of Neurological Disorders and Stroke (NINDS), February 8, 1995.

lifelong disability and suffering for thousands of Americans," said Zach W. Hall, Ph.D., director of NINDS.

CP is a serious disorder that causes problems in movement control in more than half a million Americans at an estimated cost of $5 billion a year. Many people with CP suffer additional neurological disabilities, including mental retardation and epilepsy. More than 25 percent of all CP occurs in very low birth weight babies, defined as those born weighing less than 1500 grams, or 3.3 pounds. There are approximately 52,000 very low birth weight babies born each year. Of these, one in 20 who survives infancy has CP.

"Although medicine has made striking advances in allowing more preterm babies to survive, some of these children face grievous, lifelong disabilities. We hope the findings from our study will help prevent cerebral palsy in some of these vulnerable infants," said Karin B. Nelson, M.D., acting chief of the NINDS neuroepidemiology branch and lead author of the paper. She added that very low birth weight babies are 100 times more likely to have disabling CP than infants of the most common birth weight (3000-3500 grams).

Magnesium sulfate, an inexpensive natural chemical, is commonly used in the United States by obstetricians to prevent preterm labor or to treat preeclampsia, high blood pressure brought on by pregnancy. The drug, which is usually delivered intravenously in the hospital, is considered relatively safe when given under medical supervision.

The beneficial effect of the magnesium sulfate seen in this study was similar whether the mothers received the drug to prevent convulsions associated with preeclampsia, or for preterm labor. The investigators also found that magnesium sulfate appeared to confer a protective effect against CP whether or not the mothers received other drugs to stop preterm labor or to enhance fetal lung maturation in premature infants.

Dr. Nelson and co-author Judith K. Grether, Ph.D., of the CBDMP, have not yet compiled data on the exact dosages of magnesium sulfate administered or on the time of treatment relative to the time of birth. This information is important since it takes 2 to 3 hours for magnesium sulfate to reach the fetus.

"Based on our work, other scientists are already looking at their data and seeing similar associations," said Dr. Grether. "If these are confirmed in clinical trials, we will be able to learn even more about the usefulness of magnesium in premature birth."

The study authors speculate that magnesium may play a role in brain development and possibly prevent cerebral hemorrhage in

Magnesium Linked to Lower Incidence of Cerebral Palsy

preterm infants. Although the precise mechanism for this effect is not known, several suggestions for effectiveness can be cited. An earlier study has shown higher survival rates in infants born weighing less than 1000 grams whose mothers were given magnesium sulfate; and in animal models magnesium has been associated with decreased brain injury after the brain has been deprived of oxygen.

Magnesium is an essential part of the diet and is found in green vegetables, beans, meat and chocolate.

The CBDMP was established by the state of California in 1982 to collect and analyze data on children with birth defects, and since that time has accumulated records on hundreds of thousands of children.

NINDS, one of the National Institutes of Health located in Bethesda, MD, is the nation's principal supporter of research on the brain and nervous system. The Institute is a lead agency for the Congressionally designated Decade of the Brain.

Part Four

Fetal Alcohol Syndrome

Chapter 20

Clinical Recognition of Fetal Alcohol Syndrome

Difficulties of Detection and Diagnosis

Verifying the diagnosis of fetal alcohol syndrome (FAS) in a specific patient is often difficult. Future diagnostic aids may include weighted checklists, laboratory and imaging studies, and psychological profiles.

Until about 20 years ago, the dangers of maternal alcohol consumption to the developing fetus were generally minimized or dismissed. Reports linking maternal alcohol use and fetal growth deficiency emerged from France in the late 1950s. Then in 1968, Lemoine and colleagues (1968) described growth deficit, mental retardation, and an unusually high rate of birth defects in 127 children born to alcoholic mothers. In addition, Ulleland (1972) found pre- and postnatal growth deficiency and developmental abnormalities in 8 of 12 children born to alcoholic mothers.

Based in part on these cases, Jones and Smith (1973) introduced the term "fetal alcohol syndrome" (FAS) to describe a pattern of abnormalities found in some children born to alcoholic women. Jones and Smith's definition was significant because it clearly delineated a clinically recognizable syndrome that was distinct from all other patterns of congenital malformation and that was seen exclusively in the off-spring of mothers who drank large amounts of alcohol during pregnancy. (FAS researchers do not always specify the amount of maternal

---

Excerpted from *Alcohol-Related Birth Defects*, National Institute on Alcohol Abuse and Alcoholism (NIAAA), NIH Pub. No. 94-3466, 1994.

drinking involved. Nonspecific phrases such as "heavy drinking" used in this article reflect the terminology of the reference cited.)

During the next few years, more than 100 patients with FAS were reported. The earliest descriptions concentrated on the most severely affected patients, in whom the syndrome was most clearly recognizable. It soon became apparent, however, that the diagnosis of FAS could encompass children with varying degrees of growth failure and mental deficiency who did not display all of the physical abnormalities originally considered essential for the diagnosis.

Most birth defect syndromes undergo expansion and redefinition of their diagnostic criteria as more cases are recognized. This refinement is useful for the identification of patients with mild or atypical symptoms. However, confirmation of the diagnosis in atypical cases may become difficult or impossible when the primary diagnostic features are relatively common nonspecific abnormalities or are occasionally found in normal individuals. This is true in FAS, as described in more detail below. Diagnosis of FAS is complicated further because the mechanisms by which alcohol causes fetal damage are still unknown. This chapter discusses the current criteria for diagnosing FAS.

Clinical Features of FAS

Jones and coworkers (1973) defined three major categories of abnormality in children with FAS:

- Slow growth both before and after birth, involving height, weight, and head circumference
- Deficient intellectual and social performance and muscular coordination
- A consistent pattern of minor structural anomalies of the face, together with more variable involvement of the limbs and heart.

With some modification, these criteria still form the basis for the clinical diagnosis of FAS. Evidence of abnormality in all three areas is enough to exclude most other birth defect syndromes, but documentation of maternal alcohol use during pregnancy is required for complete confirmation.

Growth Abnormalities

Children with FAS characteristically grow slowly during childhood, and many of the most severely affected children also experience

Clinical Recognition of Fetal Alcohol Syndrome

intrauterine growth retardation. Statural growth and weight gain are suppressed at different rates, however. In classic cases, FAS children grow taller at about 60 percent of the normal rate through early childhood, while their weight increases at about 33 percent of the normal rate. Thus, they appear unusually slender or even malnourished despite an adequate diet.

Slow growth in head circumference indicates slow brain growth, a consistent feature in infants, children, and adolescents with moderate to severe FAS. Small brain size has been confirmed at autopsy, where abnormalities of brain development also are evident. The intellectual and behavioral abnormalities in children with FAS—as well as an increased risk of seizures—are results of the effects of alcohol on the developing brain.

Physical Abnormalities

The pattern of physical abnormalities in FAS includes subtle abnormalities in the face; limitations of joint movement; and other, less frequent anomalies. Although the overall facial appearance is the single most helpful clue in the diagnosis of FAS, each specific facial abnormality represents a minor anomaly or a variant of normal and thus may escape notice unless specifically looked for by the diagnostician.

One of the most distinctive and consistent signs of FAS is found in the eyelids. Affected children often appear to have widely spaced eyes (Figure 20.1), although measurements reveal that the eyes are normally situated. This discrepancy is caused by short palpebral fissures (eye openings). That is, the distance between the inner and outer corners of each eye is shortened, making the eyes appear smaller and farther apart than normal. Measurement of palpebral fissure length is needed to confirm this observation, because a similar appearance can arise from other causes. Drooping of one or both eyelids also is seen frequently in FAS.

Slow growth in the center of the face is another hallmark of FAS. This slow growth produces a hypoplastic (underdeveloped) midface; the zone between the eyes and mouth may seem flattened or depressed, and the bridge of the nose is often low. Slow nasal growth in the outward direction, away from the plane of the face, may leave a crescent-shaped fold of skin covering the inner corner of the eye (Figure 20.1). If the nose grows slowly in length, from its attachment between the eyebrows to the tip, the nostrils often point forward as well as downward.

Congenital Disorders Sourcebook

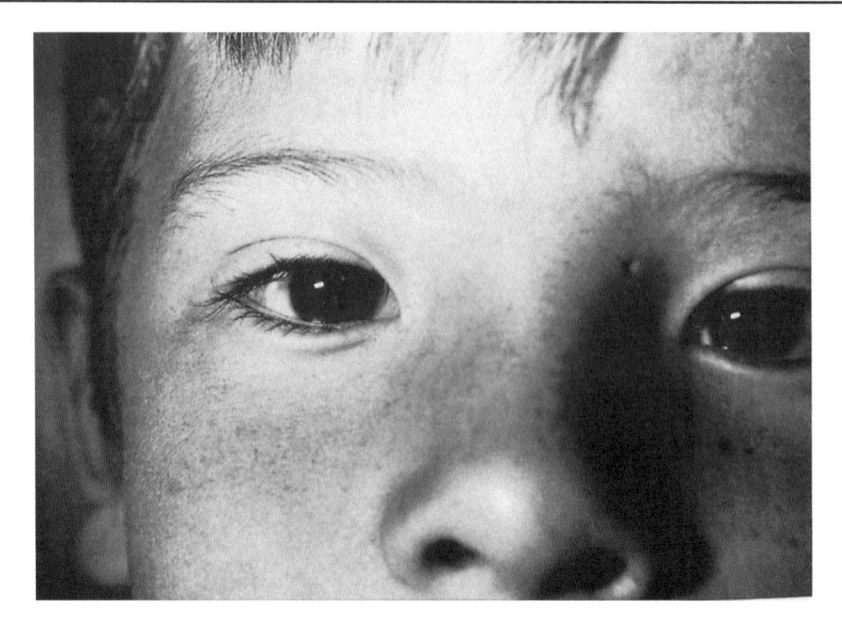

Figure 20.1. *Eyes and midface of a child with FAS, showing short eye openings and drooping eyelids. Photograph courtesy of the author.*

Another subtle but characteristic facial feature in children with FAS is found in the philtrum, the zone between the nose and the mouth. This region normally is characterized by a vertical midline groove, bordered by two vertical ridges of skin. Where the groove meets the red margin of the upper lip, an indentation usually is seen, producing a "Cupid's bow" configuration of the lip. The classic FAS face shows a long, smooth philtrum without ridges and with a smoothly arched upper lip margin (Figure 20.2).

Abnormalities of limbs and joints are less consistent features but are seen much more frequently in children with FAS than in the general population. For diagnostic purposes, the most useful such characteristics include deformities of the small joints of the hands as well as incomplete rotation at the elbow. In the hands, the typical anomalies include longitudinally oriented palmar creases; an inability to straighten a finger at one or more joints; and curving of a finger sideways, toward the middle finger (Figure 20.3).

Children with FAS also are at increased risk for many common birth defects that are not necessarily associated with alcohol. Congenital heart disease, cleft lip and palate, anomalies of the urinary tract and genitals, and spina bifida (a defect of the spinal column) occur 5

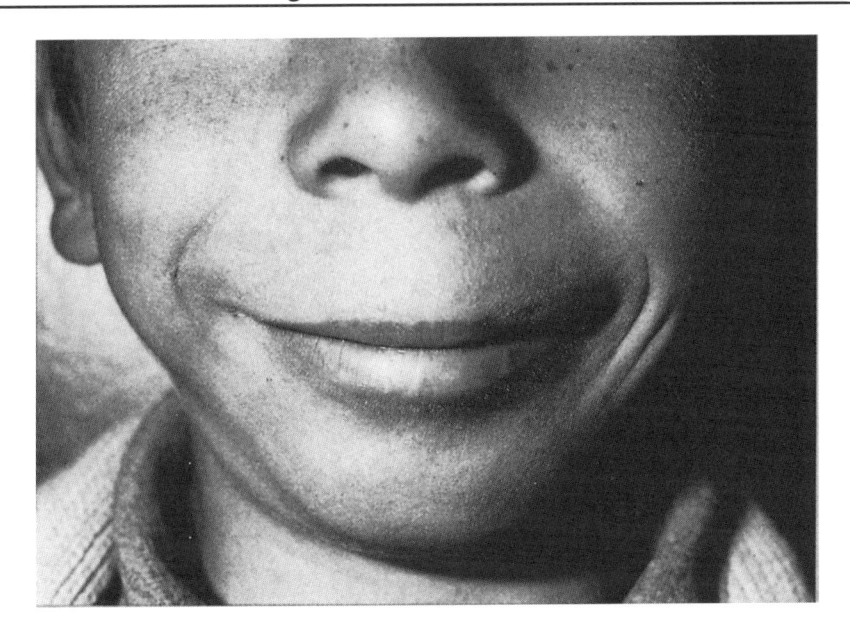

Clinical Recognition of Fetal Alcohol Syndrome

Figure 20.2. Lower face of a child with FAS, showing slightly short nose, long middle part of the upper lip without a central groove, and narrow red margin of the upper lip. Photograph courtesy of the author.

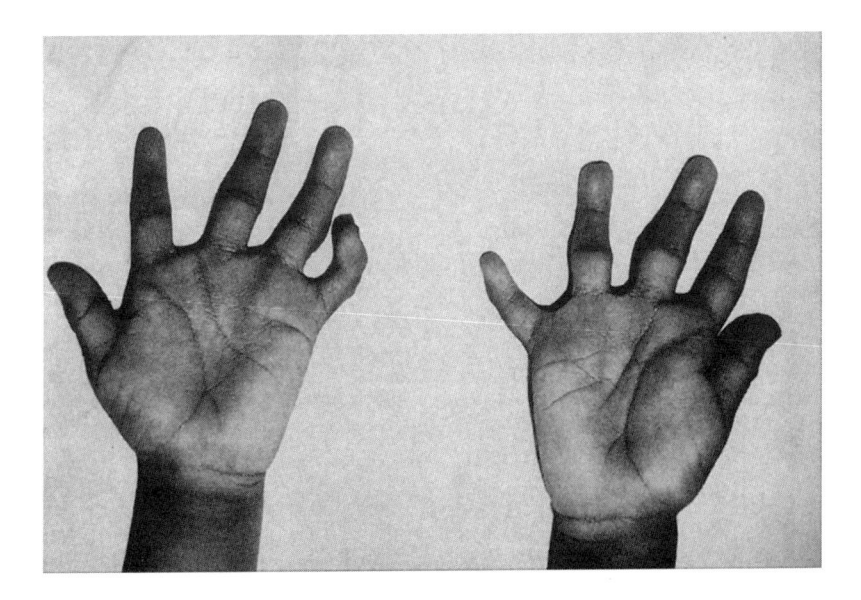

Figure 20.3. Hands of a child with FAS, showing abnormal finger joints, curved fingers, and longitudinal palmar creases. Photograph courtesy of the author.

to 60 times more often in children who were prenatally exposed to alcohol than in the general population (Abel 1990). Because none of these abnormalities is specific to FAS, they can only help to support, but not to define, the diagnosis.

Intellectual and Behavioral Abnormalities

The first reports of FAS documented delayed intellectual and behavioral development in all children studied; however, all of these children were younger than school age. Further study revealed a variety of learning and behavior problems that appeared at different ages. In infancy, feeding problems, irritability, and unpredictable patterns of sleeping and eating make the babies hard to care for and interfere with maternal bonding. During the preschool years, the children are described as affectionate but very active, "flighty" and "distractible" (Streissguth 1986). Poor fine motor coordination also becomes apparent at this age.

In the first few years of school, most children with FAS receive the diagnosis of attention-deficit hyperactivity disorder—ADHD—because of their high activity level, short attention span, and poor short-term memory (Landesman-Dwyer et al. 1981). Many need special educational help, even if their IQ falls within the normal range. (Attention-deficit hyperactivity disorder—ADHD—is a disorder of childhood characterized in general by levels of restlessness and distractibility that impair school and social functioning.)

As the FAS children grow older, their school progress is further compromised by inadequate communication skills, impulsivity, and difficulty with social interactions. Their adolescence is marked by poor judgment, trouble with abstract thinking, and limited problem-solving skills. Many affected children eventually drop out of school, and their ensuing integration into society is tenuous at best (Streissguth et al. 1991) (see the article by Streissguth in Chapter 24).

In the few studies of long-term social outcome that currently exist, anecdotal reports and case histories of adolescents and adults with FAS show a distressingly similar pattern (Dorris 1989). They have difficulty finding and holding jobs because of their unreliability; lack of social skills; and often, functional illiteracy. Establishing and maintaining lasting interpersonal relationships also is a common problem. For this reason, affected adults often lack a social support system and therefore have a higher-than-average risk of becoming involved in drug abuse and criminal behavior.

Diagnostic Pitfalls

In summary, the current criteria for the diagnosis of FAS depend on recognition of a consistent pattern of minor, often subtle physical anomalies; generalized but disproportionate growth retardation; and nonspecific developmental and behavioral aberration. Some of these characteristics change with time, and their degree of severity may vary among individuals. Confirming the diagnosis of FAS in a specific patient is often difficult, even for clinicians with considerable experience with FAS.

Underdiagnosis usually occurs when the complete pattern of abnormalities cannot be substantiated, often because of the patient's age, racial background, or familial characteristics. Clinicians also may be reluctant to make the diagnosis because they fear stigmatizing both the mother and the child (Morse et al. 1992). Overdiagnosis may result from too much emphasis on maternal drinking history, the presence of nonspecific abnormalities, or failure to recognize a different but similar congenital disorder. These problems are discussed below.

Changes in Features with Age

Recently, it has become clear that many of the critical diagnostic features of FAS change as the child grows older. The diagnosis is most difficult in newborns and adults. For example, relative mid-facial hypoplasia and a short nose with a low nasal bridge are normal features of many babies in the newborn period; however, if these features persist into the second year of life and beyond, they may be diagnostically helpful. Conversely, continued slow growth of the face and nose through adolescence compensates for earlier midfacial hypoplasia and obscures the typical facial appearance of individuals with FAS as they pass into adult life.

New information also suggests that prenatal growth retardation is found in only about 70 to 75 percent of children eventually diagnosed as having full-fledged FAS (Hymbaugh et al. 1993). The characteristic slender body build begins to change during adolescence in many affected children, especially girls, who may become moderately obese in late adolescence (Streissguth et al. 1991). Final adult height and head circumference, however, tend to remain below normal and thus have some diagnostic value at later ages.

Judgments of intellectual performance and behavior are critically dependent on the patient's age. As mentioned above, the typical learning problems and maladaptive behavior in children with FAS continue to evolve throughout childhood and into adolescence, involving far more than simple mental retardation. Therefore, any psychologically based diagnostic criteria must take into account the patient's developmental stage. For example, testing for elementary school-aged children might concentrate on measures of attention and memory, whereas that for teenagers might focus on judgment and self-regulation.

Influence of Racial and Familial Traits

Because most of the clinical features of FAS are not discrete abnormalities but fall somewhere along a continuum, it is important to consider the normal variation of features in the patient's racial group or family. For example, a moderate degree of midfacial hypoplasia is a normal characteristic in many Native American groups and should be considered when examining children from that population. Similarly, the broader lips normally seen in children of black parentage may cancel out the narrowing of the upper lip border in children with FAS. Also, the tall stature of some northern European and central African populations may compensate to a large degree for the statural growth deficiency of a child with FAS.

Similar modification of the classic FAS characteristics may be related to inheritance within a particular family. Two parents with very high IQs may have a child with FAS whose intelligence is within the normal range but well below what would be expected, based on the parents' intellect. Height growth, some facial features, and even creases on the palms may be influenced so much by heredity that the signs of FAS are obscured or mimicked.

Similarities to Other Disorders

Few birth defect syndromes resemble FAS, and they can be distinguished on examination. Nevertheless, children with a wide variety of other diagnoses have been initially suspected of having FAS. Such errors usually result when only a few features are considered, while the broader pattern goes unnoticed. Thus, a child with Cornelia de Lange syndrome (a hereditary form of mental retardation) may have slow growth, a small head, and a long philtrum, but the overall constellation of features is quite different from that of FAS. Often, a physician must correct an erroneous diagnosis of FAS given to a child who has some other disorder with vastly different implications.

Clinical Recognition of Fetal Alcohol Syndrome

Nonspecific Abnormalities

Most of the difficulties with diagnosis described above are based upon one underlying theme: none of the abnormalities found in FAS is specific to that diagnosis. Many otherwise normal children may display one or two of the common features of FAS. Isolated mental deficits or behavioral abnormalities also may occur as part of birth defect syndromes other than FAS. Slow statural growth, for example, occurs in more than 600 conditions, and small head circumference is found in about 250. Mental deficiency is a recognized component of some 700 physical deformity syndromes; it also occurs as an isolated feature in 2 to 4 percent of most populations in the absence of any abnormal physical features or history of prenatal exposure of any kind. Beyond this, some of the behavioral manifestations so frequently displayed by children with FAS can be part of a broader pattern that has recently been associated with abuse and neglect in early infancy and lack of parental bonding (Magid and McKelvey 1987).

Distribution in Various Populations

Many of the earliest case reports and epidemiologic studies of FAS involved Native American subjects, giving rise to the mistaken impression that FAS is peculiar to Native American populations. This

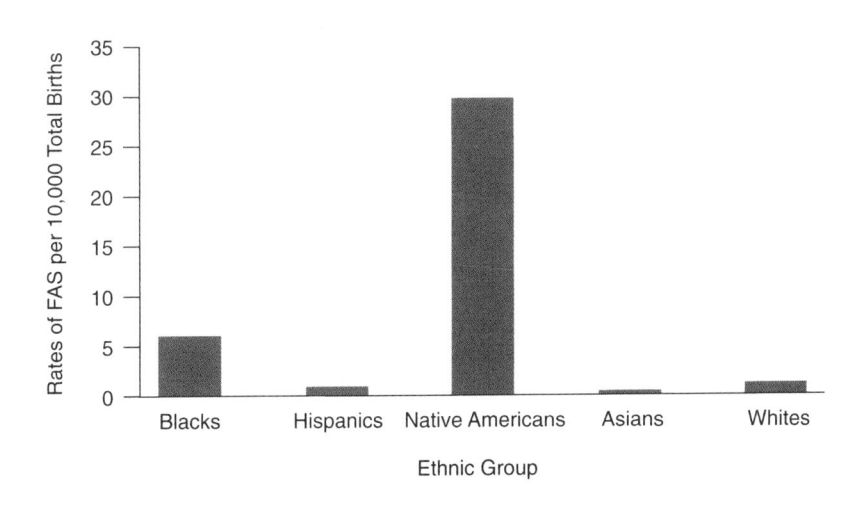

Figure 20.4. Relative frequency of FAS in newborns in the United States by ethnic group, 1981-1986. (Source: Adapted from Chávez et al. 1988.)

misconception may have led to overdiagnosis of FAS in Native American groups and perhaps to underdiagnosis in other groups. In fact, FAS has been found in every population that uses alcohol.

In the United States, epidemiologic data suggest that the rates of FAS tend to be higher in blacks and Native Americans than in whites of similar socioeconomic status and areas of residence (Abel 1990). A survey compiled by the Centers for Disease Control and Prevention (CDC) (Chávez et al. 1988) reviewed more than 4.6 million births in approximately 1,200 U.S. hospitals and showed considerable differences in occurrence of FAS among racial subgroups (Figure 20.4). The reasons for the variance among these groups remain unclear, but the figures must be interpreted with caution because of the difficulty of confirming the diagnosis of FAS in the newborn.

FAS Versus Less Specific Diagnoses

A 3-year-old girl, whose mother drank four bottles of beer a day until the middle of pregnancy, has no unusual facial features, but her weight and head circumference fall at the fifth percentile for her age, and she is hyperactive with a short attention span.

Cases such as this provide a major diagnostic dilemma. Initially, children who seemed to have several signs of FAS but not enough to confirm the diagnosis, were said to have "possible fetal alcohol effects" (Clarren and Smith 1978). This was intended as a "bookmark" rather than a diagnosis, indicating suspicion that although prenatal alcohol exposure could be responsible for the abnormalities, further proof was needed to confirm the diagnosis. Unfortunately, the word "possible" was soon dropped, and fetal alcohol effects took on a life of its own as a distinct diagnosis. Often, this judgment was based primarily on acknowledged or suspected maternal alcohol abuse during pregnancy.

In one epidemiologic study (May et al. 1983), only about one-third of babies born to mothers who drank heavily during pregnancy were found to have classic FAS, whereas almost one-half seemed to be entirely normal. Roughly 20 percent of the children were not categorized as having FAS but had some combination of mental deficit, growth delay, and maladaptive behavior. Because these abnormalities can be caused by a wide variety of environmental agents or genetic influences, it is impossible to prove that the problems in any one child were the result of prenatal alcohol exposure.

In an effort to clarify the situation, other terms were introduced, such as "alcohol-related birth defects" (Sokol and Clarren 1989). These concepts may be helpful in the epidemiologic study of large groups of children exposed prenatally to alcohol, but they have little use in the identification of FAS in a specific individual. Until a precise and unequivocal standard for diagnosis becomes available, the wisest course would be to provide a purely descriptive diagnosis for children who do not meet the criteria for FAS. Thus, the child described above could be categorized simply as alcohol exposed *in utero*, deficient in weight and head circumference, and at risk for ADHD.

Aids to Diagnosis

Weighted Checklist

Because of the difficulties in making an accurate diagnosis of FAS—especially for diagnosticians with limited experience—attempts have been made to construct checklists of distinguishing features. The first such list was produced for the U.S. Indian Health Service as part of its nationwide effort to define the extent of FAS in the Native American population. Each of 42 specific features was assigned a numeric score, or weight, based on its estimated value in confirming the diagnosis. No measures of specificity or sensitivity were provided for any of the items.

This weighted checklist proved to have considerable value in increasing appropriate referrals to diagnostic clinics but was much less effective as a diagnostic tool for clinical purposes. A newer, shorter, and more scientifically based checklist is being developed by the author and the CDC and should be ready for testing sometime in 1994.

Laboratory and Imaging Studies

No laboratory tests are available that can establish or rule out the diagnosis of FAS. However, a growing research effort is directed toward finding the underlying mechanisms that contribute to fetal alcohol damage. Scientists also are searching for genetic and biochemical characteristics associated with susceptibility to FAS. Both of these lines of research hold promise for eventual development of tests to show which mothers, babies, or pregnancies are at highest risk for adverse effects of alcohol.

During the past 3 years, several groups of investigators have been pursuing the possibility of demonstrating differences in brain structure by using special imaging techniques. Magnetic resonance imaging (MRI) and positron emission tomography (PET) already have proved useful in the diagnosis of other disorders involving brain dysfunction. MRI uses a magnetic field to produce an image of the living brain; PET uses radioactive isotopes to monitor brain metabolism. There is considerable interest in applying these technologies to the study of children with FAS.

Psychological/Behavioral Testing

As discussed earlier, the physical features of FAS are nonspecific, whereas their overall pattern is unique. Similarly, the pattern of learning and behavioral characteristics may have diagnostic value in affected children. The brain is the organ most sensitive to the prenatal damage caused by alcohol. If that damage resulted in a unique, unmistakable psychological profile, FAS could be diagnosed reliably without reliance on the variable and subtle clinical features. As yet, no such distinctive profile has been ascertained, and reliable measures of some of its components remain to be developed. If controls can be introduced for such nonspecific confounding factors as physical or emotional abuse and neglect, psychological-behavioral assessment may prove to be the long-sought "gold standard" for diagnosis of injury caused by prenatal alcohol exposure.

Summary

Since its first definition in 1973, the diagnosis of FAS has relied on the recognition of a unique pattern of structural and functional abnormalities in children with a history of exposure to alcohol before birth. The individual abnormalities are often subtle and hard to detect and mostly represent the extreme of a normal spectrum of development. For these reasons, FAS is both under- and overdiagnosed. In individual patients, it is impossible to determine with certainty whether their abnormalities were indeed caused by alcohol unless the full spectrum of FAS symptoms is present. Diagnostic aids in the form of checklists, laboratory and imaging studies, and psychological profiles may be of some assistance, but the definitive confirmatory test for intrauterine alcohol damage has not yet been developed.

—by Jon M. Aase, M.D.

Jon M. Aase, M.D., is clinical associate professor of pediatrics at the University of New Mexico, Albuquerque, New Mexico.

References

Abel, E.L. *Fetal Alcohol Syndrome.* Oradell, NJ: Medical Economics Co., Inc., 1990.

Chávez, G.F.; Cordero, J.F.; and Becerra, J.E. Leading major congenital malformations among minority groups in the United States, 1981-1986. *Morbidity and Mortality Weekly Report: CDC Surveillance Summaries* 37:17-24, 1988.

Clarren, S.K., and Smith, D.W. The fetal alcohol syndrome. *New England Journal of Medicine* 298(19):1063-1067, 1978.

Dorris, M. *The Broken Cord.* New York: Harper & Row, 1989.

Hymbaugh, K.J.; Boyle, C.A.; and Aase, J.M. "Age-Specific Differences in Physical Characteristics of Alcohol Affected Children in a Special Population Study." Poster presented at Research Society on Alcoholism, Annual Meeting, San Antonio, TX, June 1993.

Jones, K.L., and Smith, D.W. Recognition of the fetal alcohol syndrome in early infancy. *Lancet* 2:999-1001, 1973.

Jones, K.L.; Smith, D.W.; Ulleland, C.N.; and Streissguth, A.P. Pattern of malformation in offspring of chronic alcoholic mothers. *Lancet* 1:1267-1271, 1973.

Landesman-Dwyer, S.; Ragozin, A.S.; and Little, R. E. Behavioral correlates of prenatal alcohol exposure: A four-year follow-up study. *Neurobehavioral Toxicology and Teratology* 3:187-193, 1981.

Lemoine, P.; Harousseau, H.; Borteyru, J.P.; and Menuet, J.C. Les enfants de parents alcooliques: Anomalies observees a propos de 127 cas. *Ouest Medical* 21:476-482, 1968.

Magid, K., and McKelvey, C.A. *High Risk: Children Without a Conscience.* New York: Bantam Books, 1987.

May, P.A.; Hymbaugh, K.J.; Aase, J.M.; and Samet, J.M. Epidemiology of fetal alcohol syndrome among American Indians of the southwest. *Social Biology* 30(4):374-387, 1983.

Morse, B.A.; Idelson, R.K.; Sachs, W.H.; Weiner, L.; and Kaplan, L.C. Pediatricians' perspectives on fetal alcohol syndrome. *Journal of Substance Abuse* 4:187-195, 1992.

Sokol, R.J., and Clarren, S.K. Guidelines for use of terminology describing the impact of prenatal alcohol on the offspring. *Alcoholism: Clinical and Experimental Research* 13:597-598, 1989.

Streissguth A.P. The behavioral teratology of alcohol: Performance, behavioral and intellectual deficits in prenatally exposed children. In: West, J., ed. *Alcohol and Brain Development*. New York: Oxford University Press, 1986. pp. 3-44.

Streissguth, A.P.; Aase, J.M.; Clarren, S.K.; Randels, S.P.; LaDue, R.A.; and Smith, D.F. Fetal alcohol syndrome in adolescents and adults. *Journal of the American Medical Association* 265(15): 1961-1965, 1991.

Ulleland, C.N. The offspring of alcoholic mothers. *Annals of the New York Academy of Sciences* 197:167-169, 1972.

Chapter 21

Critical Periods for Prenatal Alcohol Exposure

Human Studies

Although dysmorphia, growth, and certain kinds of behavior can be studied in animal models, it is only through human clinical and epidemiologic studies that other important behaviors such as language development can be investigated. However, researchers have to be aware of the limitations of these studies, such as those that arise from the complex pattern and duration of alcohol use usually seen in pregnancy, which is discussed below. To investigate how timing affects outcome and to use statistical techniques most effectively, it would be best if information was available about alcohol exposure at different points during gestation; some fetuses would be exposed in the first trimester, others in the second, and still others in the third. It would be helpful also if levels or doses of drinking were the same so that *only* the timing of exposure was different rather than timing and amount both.

However, women who drink during pregnancy are not motivated by scientific rigor. Instead of adopting drinking patterns that range across trimesters, they are more likely to drink heavily around the time of conception, before realizing that they are pregnant, and to reduce or stop drinking later in pregnancy. Some women reduce drinking because they are aware of the potential problems; others reduce or eliminate alcohol use because of an aversion to its taste or because

---

Excerpted from *Alcohol-Related Birth Defects*, National Institute on Alcohol Abuse and Alcoholism (NIAAA), NIH Pub. No. 94-3466, 1994.

of the nausea that they feel at this time. Virtually no women begin drinking heavily only during the second or third trimesters or both. Thus, it is impossible to replicate animal results in human clinical studies. Because of these patterns of use and the likelihood that the same women will drink heavily and throughout pregnancy, there are technical difficulties in using statistics to control for *all* of the effects associated with trimester of exposure.

Another difficulty involves the administration of alcohol. Because biological measures of alcohol use such as blood and urine tests are less accurate during pregnancy due to the presence of hormones of pregnancy, it is necessary to rely on a woman's self-report for the amount and frequency of her drinking. Even when a woman is reporting her drinking as accurately as she can, such reports may be in error, particularly when they involve recall over long periods of time. Because estimates of exposure, particularly exposure during specific periods of gestation, are tentative, human research has focused not on specific days or weeks but on four broad time periods—periconception, first trimester, second trimester, and third trimester—and has asked women to estimate, usually retrospectively, their drinking during these periods. To get a feel for how accurate this information is likely to be, readers are encouraged to try to remember exactly how much they drank during a particular week 6 months ago. Typically, only abstainers and alcoholics are able to do this with any accuracy.

In contrast to most investigators, who ask women about their alcohol use only on one occasion (usually at the time they are recruited into the study), a few investigators have assessed drinking repeatedly and systematically. Day and colleagues (1989) identified women who used alcohol early in pregnancy and repeatedly interviewed them, asking about use during each trimester as well as after the birth of the baby. This method allows relatively accurate estimates of exposure by trimester and allows for the investigation of trimester effects.

Another way to examine the issue of timing of exposure is to take advantage of an experiment that results spontaneously when pregnant women are recruited into programs designed to help them stop drinking. Coles and colleagues (1985) and Larsson and colleagues (1985) have compared physical and behavioral differences in offspring of those women who stopped drinking as a result of intervention, with the offspring of those who did not stop drinking in the second trimester, to estimate the benefits of third trimester abstinence. However, it is necessary to interpret results of such studies cautiously, because it is likely that women who continue to drink despite educational and therapeutic interventions also differ in other ways from women who

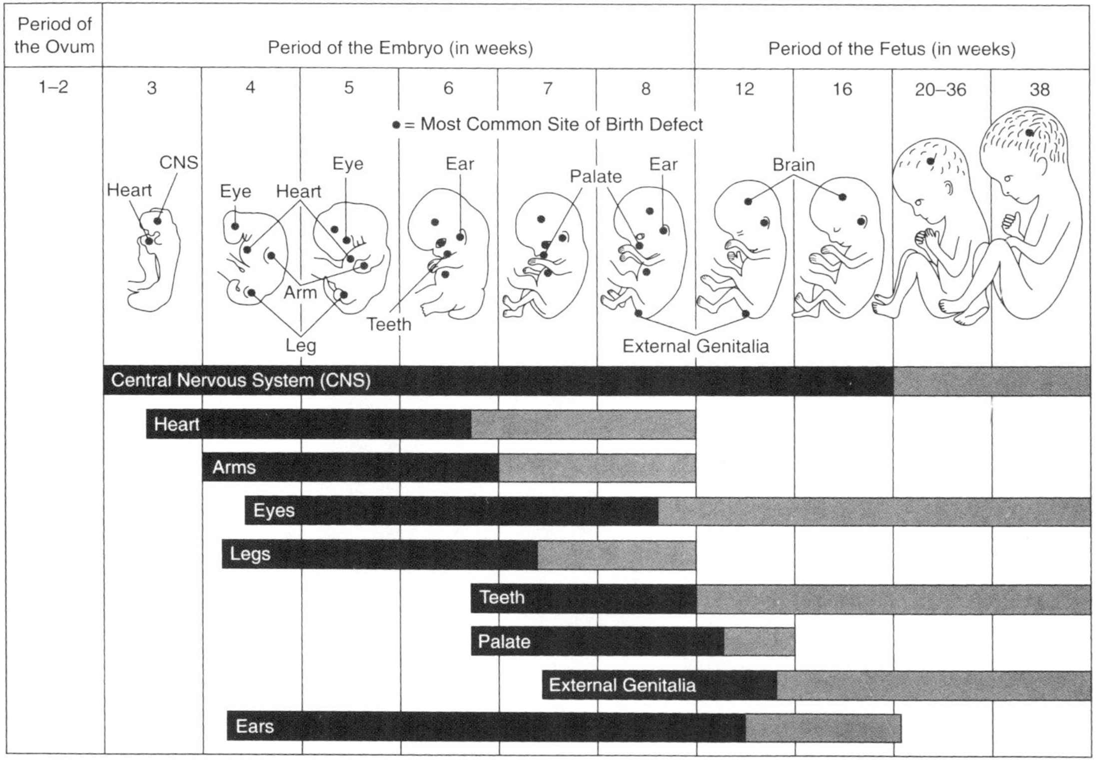

Critical Periods for Prenatal Alcohol Exposure

Figure 21.1. Vulnerability of the fetus to defects during different periods of development. The left shaded portion of the bars represents the most sensitive periods of development, during which teratogenic effects of the sites listed would result in major structural abnormalities in the child. The right shaded portion of the bars represents periods of development during which physiological defects and minor structural abnormalities would occur. (Source: Adapted from Moore 1993.)

are able to stop. For instance, those women who continue to drink also are more likely to smoke cigarettes and might be more physically addicted to alcohol than those who were able to stop. Thus, third trimester effects in the offspring of these women could stem from these differences and not only from consumption of alcohol (for more information, see Smith et al. 1986).

Timing of Alcohol Effects in Humans

Nonviability

It is probable that heavy, extremely early alcohol exposure often leads to nonviability of the fetus and spontaneous abortion. This is difficult to measure, however, because pregnancy may not have been identified and pregnancy loss may not be recognized.

Physical Anomalies (Birth Defects)

Because facial dysmorphia occurs during the embryonic period (the first 8 weeks of the first trimester), craniofacial anomalies in human subjects are probably associated with drinking during this initial stage of pregnancy. Clinical support for this period of vulnerability can be inferred from studies that examine the effects of stopping drinking during the second trimester (Coles et al. 1985), in which equivalent physical dysmorphia scores were noted in two separate groups. The first group included children whose mothers drank throughout gestation. The second group included children whose mothers stopped drinking in the second and third trimesters but drank amounts during the first trimester that were equivalent to those consumed during the first trimester by the mothers of the first group (mean amount reported for both groups was 24 drinks a week, with a range of 2 to 150 drinks a week).

In statistical studies of craniofacial anomalies in children exposed to alcohol prenatally, Ernhart and colleagues (1987) report that a relationship between these anomalies and first trimester exposure was evident. The anomalies also were related to later intellectual development in that greater dysmorphia was associated with lower IQs. In their longitudinal studies, Graham and colleagues (1988) found minor physical anomalies in alcohol-exposed children, present at birth and also at age 4 years, that were related to heavy drinking in the periconceptual period rather than at midpregnancy. Day and colleagues (1989) found that physical anomalies observed in infants were associated with reports of heavy drinking (defined in their study as at least one drink a day, or about 0.5 ounce of alcohol) in the first 2 months of pregnancy only.

Effects on Growth

Growth is usually measured by birth weight (or weight in older children), head circumference, and length (height). In contrast to the relationship observed with facial dysmorphia, effects on growth appear to be related to exposure later in pregnancy. This relationship is shown in Figure 21.2, which presents data from studies of the effect of discontinuing alcohol and other drug use by the second trimester of pregnancy on neonatal measures of growth. Drugs other than alcohol are mentioned because it cannot be proved that cigarettes and drugs such as marijuana were not used by at least some of the women in the study. (The effects of cigarettes and drug use cannot be ruled out as factors in the data presented in Figures 21.2, 21.3, and 21.4.)

These data suggest that exposure that continues throughout pregnancy produces fetal growth deficiencies that can be observed at birth. When alcohol and other drug use is discontinued by the beginning of the second trimester, children of drinkers may approach the growth of children of nondrinkers (Coles et al. 1985; Rosett et al. 1980). These findings may indicate either that the growth deficit associated with alcohol occurs in the third trimester when the fetus is known to be growing rapidly or that being alcohol-free during this time allows the previously exposed fetus to catch up on growth.

When alcohol-exposed children are studied over time, the negative effects of alcohol exposure on some aspects of growth seem to be mitigated, whereas other aspects of growth are still affected. Figure 21.3 shows the weight, height, and head circumferences of children in a longitudinal study, some of whom had a diagnosis of FAS or FAE (fetal alcohol effects), and who were reevaluated at early school age (5 to 7 years old). Notice that at this stage, although weight and height are no longer significantly lower in the alcohol-exposed groups, head circumference remains smaller among children who were exposed throughout pregnancy. These data are consistent with the results of animal studies, which found deficits in head circumference in animals exposed during the brain growth spurt (West and Goodlett 1990).

Following a larger sample (650 women) than that shown in Figure 21.3, Day and colleagues (1991) also found that as children aged, there were observable differences in growth rate that appeared to link exposure to alcohol during the second and third trimesters with the

Congenital Disorders Sourcebook

Head Circumference
(*n* = 347)

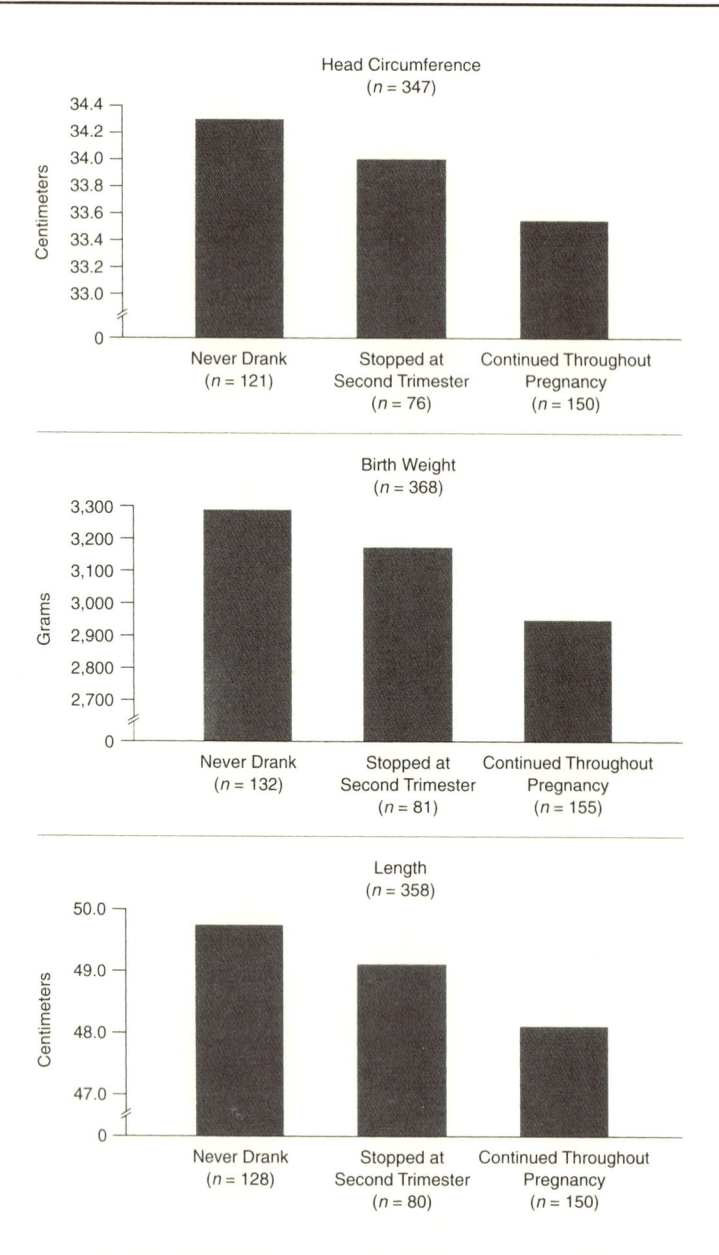

Centimeters: 34.4, 34.2, 34.0, 33.8, 33.6, 33.4, 33.2, 33.0, 0

- Never Drank (*n* = 121)
- Stopped at Second Trimester (*n* = 76)
- Continued Throughout Pregnancy (*n* = 150)

Birth Weight
(*n* = 368)

Grams: 3,300, 3,200, 3,100, 3,000, 2,900, 2,800, 2,700, 0

- Never Drank (*n* = 132)
- Stopped at Second Trimester (*n* = 81)
- Continued Throughout Pregnancy (*n* = 155)

Length
(*n* = 358)

Centimeters: 50.0, 49.0, 48.0, 47.0, 0

- Never Drank (*n* = 128)
- Stopped at Second Trimester (*n* = 80)
- Continued Throughout Pregnancy (*n* = 150)

Figure 21.2. *Effects of alcohol exposure on growth. Growth was reduced the most in children whose mothers continued to drink throughout pregnancy. Growth was not as affected in those whose mothers stopped drinking in the second trimester. These data suggest that exposure that continues throughout pregnancy produces fetal growth deficiencies that can be observed at birth. (Source: Coles et al. 1991.)*

Critical Periods for Prenatal Alcohol Exposure

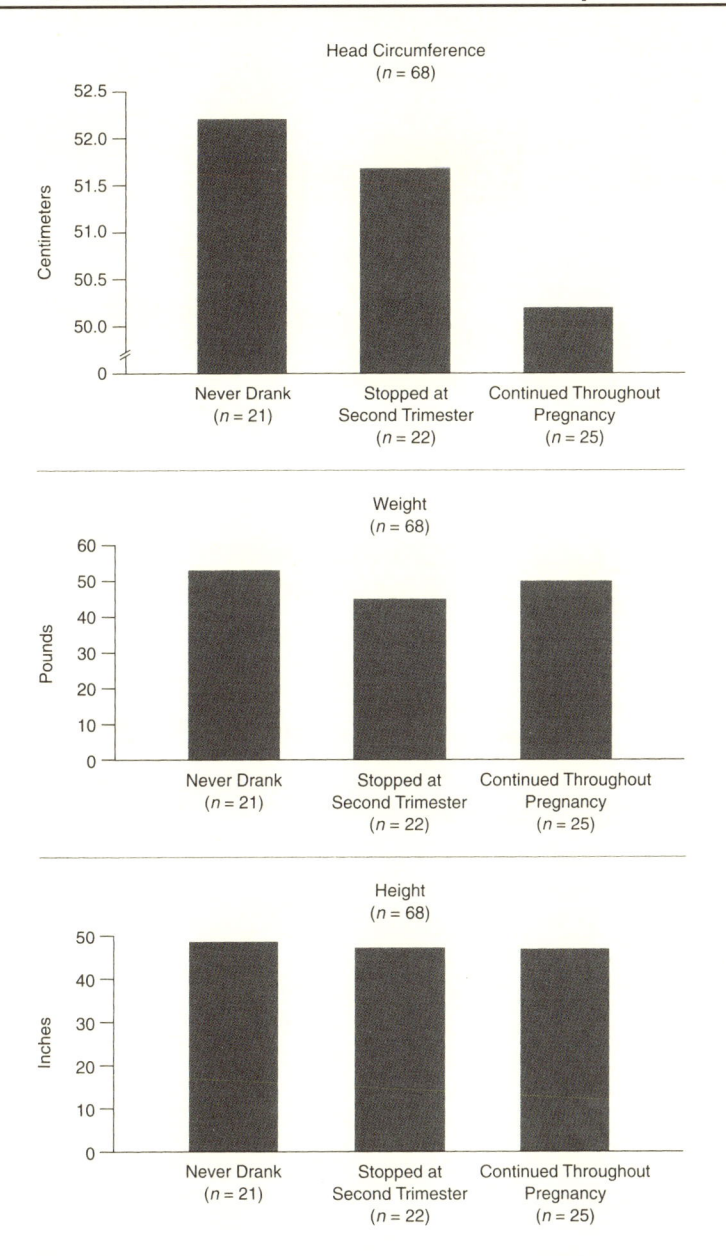

Figure 21.3. Reevaluation of growth in alcohol-exposed children at 5 to 7 years of age suggests that effects on weight and height are mitigated, whereas effects on head circumference remain. Children whose mothers drank throughout pregnancy show the greatest deficits in head circumference. (Source: Coles et al. 1991.)

effect on height and weight as well as on head circumference. In addition, due to differences in methodology from those used in the study represented in Figure 21.3, these investigators have identified an adverse effect on growth due to first trimester alcohol exposure, and, based on these data, they suggest that there may be more than one mechanism for alcohol's effects on growth.

Behavioral Effects

These effects have not been examined as closely in relation to critical periods of exposure as have facial features and growth, primarily because it is much more difficult to make such a connection. Studies of facial dysmorphia have produced a clear connection with alcohol exposure during the first trimester. However, because the relationship between specific brain sites and functions and most human and animal behaviors have not been identified (or may not exist), the same behavior may have more than one "cause." For instance, a child's poor attention may result from prenatal or traumatic brain damage, from environmental factors, or from anxiety. Therefore, observation of attention problems in alcohol-exposed children does not point to a particular period of exposure in the same way that facial dysmorphia does.

In addition, children are exposed to different amounts of alcohol at different times during their gestation, so there is a wide range of possible outcomes resulting from fetal alcohol exposure. For example, the severe central nervous system damage associated with reduced head size, or microcephaly, in some FAS children probably results from different maternal drinking patterns from those that cause the mild effects, such as lower IQ scores and alterations in behavior, found in otherwise normal children.

Despite these problems in drawing conclusions from observed behavioral effects, it is possible to tease out some relationships between particular behavioral outcomes and alcohol exposure during different periods of pregnancy. Early, heavy exposure leads to the most severe outcomes and is associated with mental retardation, sensory deficits, and motor problems. More subtle behavioral effects, such as learning disabilities and attention problems, can result from less extensive exposure. For instance, in a prospective sample (mean alcohol use by mothers before pregnancy recognition was approximately 1 drink per day, with a range of 0 to 50 drinks), Streissguth and colleagues (1989) found that reported moderate drinking (mean stated above) either before pregnancy recognition or at midpregnancy was associated

Critical Periods for Prenatal Alcohol Exposure

with relatively mild later deficits on neuropsychological tests (children scored an average of four points lower than normal on IQ tests). Early, heavier drinking (the upper limit of the range stated above) was found to result in more serious outcomes on the neuropsychological tests even in children without physical effects. In seeming contrast, Larsson and colleagues (1985) found that preschool children who were

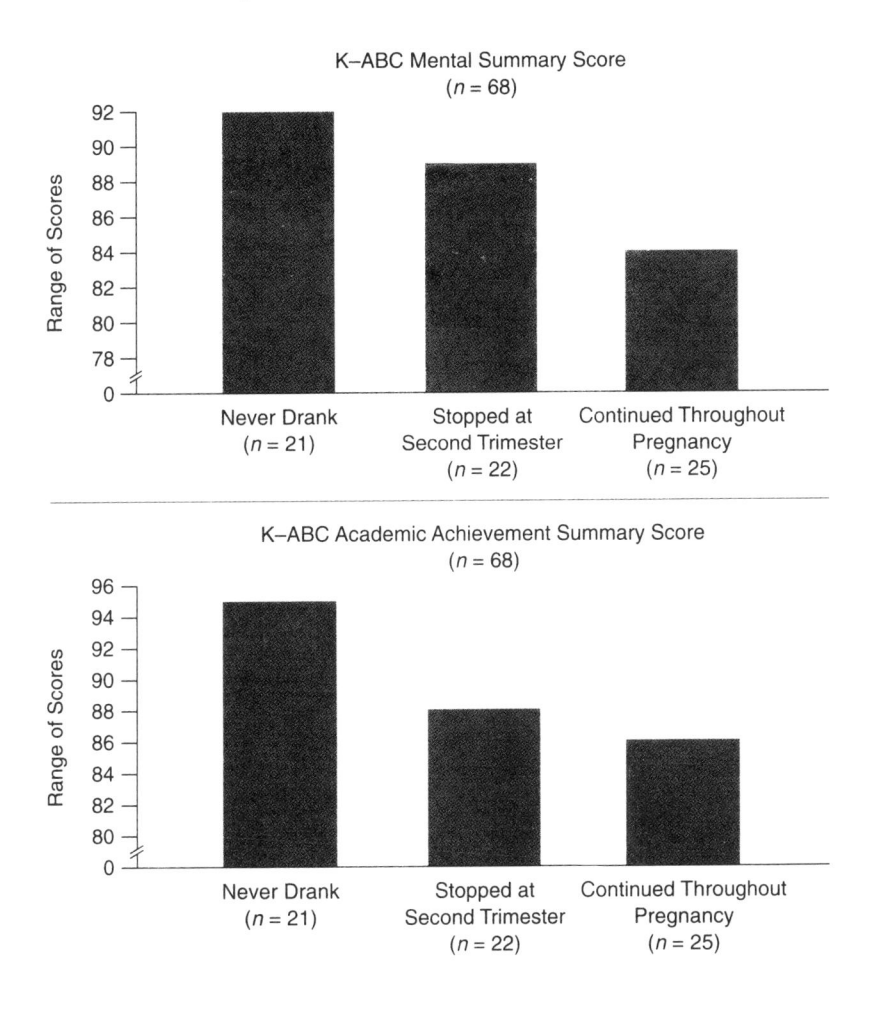

Figure 21.4. Effects on aptitude and academic achievement in alcohol-exposed children. The Kaufman Assessment Battery for Children (K-ABC) tests IQ and academic achievement for children between 2 and 12 years of age. Children whose mothers stopped drinking during the second trimester of pregnancy are less affected (i.e., have higher IQ and achievement scores) than those whose mothers drank throughout pregnancy. (Source: Coles et al. 1991.)

exposed to alcohol throughout gestation (with a range of two to nine drinks per day) were more likely to show hyperactivity, language problems, and motor deficits in comparison with those whose mothers stopped drinking by the second trimester, which implies that these effects result from later exposure.

Similar results to Larsson and colleagues' were obtained in a followup of school age children (Coles et al. 1991) that focused on cognition, attention, and behavior (Figure 21.4). In these data, alcohol exposure during any part of pregnancy appears to be associated with poorer academic achievement. Exposure during the third trimester in particular appears to be associated with lower aptitude scores, although the majority of these children cannot be classified as mentally retarded. Effects on aptitude that are associated with third trimester exposure are probably the cumulative effect of alcohol exposure throughout pregnancy. Some of the other deficits that were seen in these children exposed through the third trimester (e.g., poorer attention and sequencing and motor problems) are consistent with those seen in people with damage, such as trauma, to the hippocampus and the cerebellum (Mirsky 1987). These are the brain structures that West and Goodlett (1990) have identified as being affected by third trimester equivalent alcohol exposure in rats. Of course, because the human data results are from correlational studies, it is possible that the observed deficits stem from other factors (e.g., the child-rearing environment) rather than any specific neurological deficits that result from alcohol exposure.

Conclusions

Despite the extensive research on effects of prenatal alcohol exposure, information about timing of exposure as it relates to the fetus' vulnerability to particular effects on behaviors remains limited. Due to the nature of the developmental process, there are differences in the amount of knowledge available about specific effects of all kinds. Animal studies and epidemiologic studies strongly suggest that the facial malformation characteristic of FAS results from exposure during the first trimester and, more specifically, during the first 2 months of gestation.

However, the relationship becomes less clear in the examination of growth retardation. It appears that both early exposure (during the first 2 months of pregnancy) and exposure during the third trimester affect growth. Specifically, effects on head circumference—and, by

Critical Periods for Prenatal Alcohol Exposure

extension, brain growth—appear to be the most consistent and permanent outcomes of exposure during these two periods.

It is much more difficult to examine behavioral effects than physical anomalies, using a trimester approach, due to the nature of behavior development. Correlational studies suggest that early exposure may be more damaging to behavior than is later exposure, but some animal studies indicate that exposure in the third trimester may specifically affect the hippocampus and the cerebellum, leading to deficits in learning and motor skills. However, the many social and physical factors associated with heavy alcohol use by pregnant women as well as the difficulty in studying specific behavioral effects in children limit the interpretations. The available evidence strongly suggests that there may be specific behavioral effects of alcohol exposure during particular periods, but the limitations inherent in both animal and human studies make it difficult to be sure of these outcomes.

It also is clear from these data that although a mother's heavy alcohol use in pregnancy is potentially damaging to the fetus, her stopping use is likely to have a beneficial outcome even on many of the functions (e.g., growth and behavior) that were affected by earlier drinking. In the future, animal studies may illuminate specific brain structures and patterns of behavior that are impacted by certain patterns of alcohol exposure (West and Goodlett 1990). It may be possible to relate such findings to similar brain areas and behavior patterns in humans and thereby greatly increase understanding of these problems.

Glossary

Cerebellum: The second largest portion of the brain. It is involved in motor functions such as maintenance of posture, coordination, and balance and also may be connected with emotional development.

Correlational studies: Studies of humans that relate one behavior or interaction with the environment to observed physiological or psychological effects. Because no study of humans can eliminate other possible causes of such effects (something that can be done in controlled animal studies), only correlations can be drawn between a behavior or teratogen and an observed effect.

Hippocampus: A component of the limbic system within the brain that is involved in emotional behaviors related to survival, such as flight or fight responses. The hippocampus is associated with memory, particularly with the learning of new information and of sequentially presented information.

Neocortex: The most recently evolved portion of the cerebral cortex. The cerebral cortex (including the neocortex) covers the surface of the cerebrum (the largest portion of the brain) and is responsible for higher mental functions, general movement, perception, behavioral reactions, and the integration of these functions.

Sensory nucleus: The nucleus of termination of the sensory fibers of a peripheral nerve. The peripheral nerves carry information from the sense organs (eyes, ears, skin) to the brain. These neurons terminate in clusters of cells called nuclei. Information is then transferred from these sensory nuclei to other brain structures.

—by Claire Coles, PH.D.

Claire Coles, PH.D. is director of Clinical and Developmental Research at the Human and Behavior Genetics Laboratory of the Department of Psychiatry and is director of Psychological Services at the Marcus Development Center of the Department of Pediatrics, the Emory University School of Medicine, Atlanta, Georgia.

References

Clarren, S.K.; Astley, S.J.; and Bowden, D.M. Physical anomalies and developmental delays in nonhuman primates exposed to weekly doses of ethanol during gestation. *Teratology* 37(6):561-569, 1988.

Coles, C.D.; Smith, I.E.; Fernhoff, P.M.; and Falek, A. Neonatal neurobehavioral characteristics as correlates of maternal alcohol use during gestation. *Alcoholism: Clinical and Experimental Research* 9(5):1-7, 1985.

Coles, C.D.; Brown, R.T.; Smith, I.E.; Platzman, K.A.; Erickson, S.; and Falek, A. Effects of prenatal alcohol exposure at school age: I. Physical and cognitive development. *Neurotoxicology and Teratology* 13(4):1-11, 1991.

Day, N.L.; Jasperse, D.; Richardson, G.; Robles, N.; Sambamoorthi, U.; Scher, M.; Staffer, D.; and Cornelius, M. Prenatal exposure to alcohol: Effect on infant growth and morphological characteristics. *Pediatrics* 84(3):536-541, 1989.

Day, N.L.; Robles, N.; Richardson, G.; Geva, D.; Taylor, P.; Scher, M.; Staffer, D.; Cornelius, M.; and Goldschmidt, L. The effects of prenatal alcohol use on the growth of children at three years of age. *Alcoholism: Clinical and Experimental Research* 15(1):67-71, 1991.

Dobbing, J. The later development of the brain and its vulnerability. In: Davis, J.A., and Dobbing, J., eds. *Scientific Foundations of Paediatrics*. 2d ed. Baltimore: University Park Press, 1981. pp. 744-758.

Ernhart, C.B.; Sokol, R.J.; Martier, S.; Moron, P.; Nadler, D.; Ager, J.W.; and Wolf, A. Alcohol teratogenicity in the human: A detailed assessment of specificity, critical period, and threshold. *American Journal of Obstetrics and Gynecology* 156(1):33-39, 1987.

Fabro, S.; McLachlan, J.A.; and Dames, N.M. Chemical exposure of embryos during the preimplantation stages of pregnancy: Mortality rate and intrauterine development. *American Journal of Obstetrics and Gynecology* 148:929, 1984.

Graham, J.M.; Hanson, J.W.; Darby, B.L.; Barr, H.M.; and Streissguth, A.P. Independent dysmorphology evaluations at birth and 4 years of age for children exposed to varying amounts of alcohol in utero. *Pediatrics* 81(6):772-778, 1988.

Jones, K.L., and Smith, D.W. Recognition of fetal alcohol syndrome in early infancy. *Lancet* 2(783b): 999-1001, 1973.

Larsson, G.; Bohlin A.-B.; and Tunell, R. Prospective study of children exposed to variable amounts of alcohol in utero. *Archives of the Diseases of Children* 60:315-321, 1985.

Lemoine, P.; Harousseau, H.; Borleyru, J.P.; and Menuet, J.C. Les enfants de parents alcooliques: Anomalies observees a propos de 127 cas. [Children of alcoholic parents: Anomalies observed in 127 cases.] *Ouest Medical* 21:476-482, 1968.

Miller, M.W. Effects of prenatal exposure to ethanol on cell proliferation and neuronal migration. In: Miller, M., ed. *Development of the Central Nervous System: Effects of Alcohol and Opiates*. New York: Wiley-Liss, 1992. pp. 47-69.

Mirsky, A.F. Behavioral and psychophysiological markers of disordered attention. *Environmental Health Perspective* 74:191-199, 1987.

Moore, K.L. *The Developing Human* [1993]. © Philadelphia. W.B. Saunders Co. In: Berger, K.S. *The Developing Person*. New York: Worth Publishers, Inc., 1980. p. 121.

Rosett, H.L.; Weiner, L.; Zuckerman, B.; McKinlay, S.; and Edelin, K.C. Reduction of alcohol consumption during pregnancy with benefits to the newborn. *Alcoholism: Clinical and Experimental Research* 4:178-184, 1980.

Scialli, A.R. *A Clinical Guide to Reproductive and Developmental Toxicology*. Boca Raton, FL: CRC Press, 1992.

Smith, I.E.; Lancaster, J.S.; Moss-Wells, S.; Coles, C.D.; and Falek, A. Identifying high risk pregnant drinkers: Biological and behavioral correlates of continuous heavy drinking during pregnancy. *Journal of Studies on Alcohol* 48(4):304-309, 1986.

Streissguth, A.P.; Bookstein, F.L.; Sampson, P.D.; and Barr, H.M. Neurobehavioral effects of prenatal alcohol: Part III. PLS analyses of neuropsychologic tests. *Neurotoxicology and Teratology* 11(5):493-507, 1989.

Sulik, K.K., and Johnston, M.C. Sequence of developmental alterations following acute ethanol exposure in mice: Craniofacial features of the fetal alcohol syndrome. *American Journal of Anatomy* 166:257-269, 1983.

West, J.R., and Goodlett, C.R. Teratogenic effects of alcohol on brain development. *Annals of Medicine* 22:319-325, 1990.

Chapter 22

Effects of Paternal Exposure to Alcohol on Offspring Development

Paternal alcohol consumption may affect fetal development through a direct effect on the father's sperm or gonads. This possibility casts new light on the heritability of alcoholism in humans.

The adverse consequences of maternal alcohol intake during pregnancy on fetal outcome are well documented (for a review, see Meyer and Riley 1986). However, the possibility that paternal alcohol consumption also may induce deficits in the progeny has received relatively little attention. This is somewhat surprising, as alcoholism appears to be linked genetically with the father in humans (Merikangas 1990; Pickens et al. 1991), and studies indicate that male offspring of alcoholic fathers have behavioral problems and impaired intellectual skills as well as hormonal and nervous system anomalies (see below).

This chapter discusses the possible direct effects of paternal alcohol consumption on fetal development, distinguishing these effects from studies of the genetic heritability of alcoholism. The chapter also discusses the possibility that such paternal effects may contribute to cognitive and biochemical disturbances that may be associated with altered responses to alcohol that might lead to addiction.

For purposes of this review, alcoholism is broadly defined as the excessive and repetitive consumption of alcohol that results in significant disturbances in a person's life, such as preoccupation with drinking to the exclusion of other activities, inability to perform adequately at work, and deterioration of family or other social interactions. In

---

Excerpted from *Alcohol-Related Birth Defects*, National Institute on Alcohol Abuse and Alcoholism (NIAAA), NIH Pub. No. 94-3466, 1994.

general, the study populations discussed below meet not only these criteria but also others required for a clinical diagnosis of alcoholism.

Deficits in the Offspring of Male Alcoholics

Many studies have indicated that children of alcoholic fathers often demonstrate impaired cognitive skills and are more likely to be hyperactive than are children of nonalcoholic biological parents (Hegedus et al. 1984; Tartar et al. 1989). These studies generally adopted controls to ensure that the effects were not due to such factors as maternal drug use, socioeconomic variables, race, and psychiatric or medical disorders in the parents. These effects also were observed in children borne of alcoholic biological fathers but raised by nonalcoholic adoptive parents. (Cognition refers to intellectual functions such as information processing, learning, and memory.)

Sons of alcoholics also have abnormal electrical activity in the brain as measured by the electroencephalograph (EEG) (Begleiter and Projesz 1988; Ehlers et al. 1989; Schuckit et al. 1987*a*). Moreover, it has been shown that the sons of alcoholics, when compared with sons of nonalcoholic parents, demonstrate abnormal hormonal responses to short-term administration of alcohol (Schuckit 1988; Schuckit et al. 1987*a,b*, 1988). Hence, these data seem to suggest that genetic factors of the biological fathers that relate to their drinking behavior may have a significant effect on the intellectual and behavioral development of their offspring.

Genetic Basis for Transmission of Alcoholism

The foregoing studies generally represent attempts to identify markers for the predisposition for alcoholism. A marker can most easily be understood as a specific trait that may predict whether a person is at risk for developing a medical disorder. For example, blood tests can be used to predict the occurrence of various genetic disorders, including cystic fibrosis and Down syndrome. Researchers are attempting to identify markers that could serve as early indicators of potential susceptibility to alcoholism.

Genetic linkage studies are a more useful approach for identifying a genetic basis for alcoholism. These sophisticated molecular biological techniques attempt to establish causal links between disorders and specific genes. Using these techniques, researchers have identified genes responsible for at least some types of Alzheimer's disease, cystic fibrosis, and other genetically transmissible disorders. The discovery of an association between a medical disorder and a specific gene provides a better understanding of the mechanisms underlying the disorder and may therefore provide a basis for improved treatment.

In the case of alcoholism, genetic linkage studies have produced equivocal results. This is not surprising, as the heterogeneous nature of alcoholism is not likely to be explained by a single gene. Furthermore, the results of linkage studies depend heavily on the specific criteria used to define alcoholism in the subject population and the control populations with which they are compared. Most such studies have used widely varying sets of criteria, making comparisons between studies difficult.

Twin and Adoptee Studies

Results of twin and adoptee studies are consistent with a genetic predisposition to the development of alcoholism. These studies have demonstrated that sons borne of alcoholic biological fathers and raised by nonalcoholic fathers are at much greater risk for developing alcoholism than are sons of nonalcoholics raised by either alcoholic or nonalcoholic fathers (for reviews, see Cloninger et al. 1989; Merikangas 1990; Pickens et al. 1991). Perhaps most importantly, these studies demonstrate that the drinking history of the stepfather is irrelevant in terms of the development of alcoholism in sons borne of either alcoholic or nonalcoholic biological fathers. Sons of nonalcoholic biological fathers had the same incidence of alcoholism as in the general population, whereas sons of alcoholic biological fathers seemed to have a higher incidence of alcoholism irrespective of how they were raised.

Twin and adoptee studies are useful for establishing a familial or genetic basis for alcoholism, but they are limited in scope. Thus, it has not been possible to distinguish completely between environmental and biological factors in the development of alcoholism. Nevertheless, the studies discussed in this and previous sections suggest that there is a high incidence of alcoholism in the offspring of alcoholic fathers and that these offspring can be clearly distinguished from children of nonalcoholics in several ways.

Alcoholic Mothers and Daughters

As a result of the studies discussed above, it has been widely assumed that alcoholism is genetically transmissible only in males. These results may simply reflect the relatively low incidence of alcoholism in females compared with males (e.g., Cloninger et al. 1989). However, the diagnosis of alcoholism is being made in increasing numbers of women (Johnston et al. 1987), contradicting the earlier belief that alcoholism affects only males. (For more information on the role of genetic factors in the etiology of alcoholism of women, see Kendler, K.S.; Heath, A.C.; Neale, M.C.; Kessler, R.C.; and Eaves, L.J. Population-based twin study of alcoholism in women. *Journal of the American Medical Association* 268(14):1877-1882, 1992.) Further studies are needed to more firmly establish whether the daughters of alcoholic fathers have any higher risk for developing alcohol-related problems than daughters born of nonalcoholic parents.

In addition, not all studies have adequately considered the role of maternal alcoholism or abuse of other drugs; given the established linkage between prenatal alcohol consumption and developmental anomalies such as FAS, for example, these factors must be rigorously controlled for in such experiments. Another question that has been largely ignored is whether the mother's drinking behavior can influence alcohol consumption patterns in their offspring independently of the drinking habits of the biological fathers or stepfathers.

Studies in Animal Models

As discussed above, numerous studies clearly suggest impairments in the sons of alcoholic fathers. However, two important questions cannot be conclusively addressed in studies with humans: Are the observed deficits due to biological or to social determinants? Do these deficits represent the toxic effects of alcohol per se or the genetic transmission of specific traits? The use of an animal model permits a direct assessment of whether the paternal consumption of alcohol is a potential toxicant to the developing fetus. Although no animal model could duplicate the complex psychosocial factors that contribute to alcoholism in humans, such models can be extremely helpful in elucidating the biological aspects of alcoholism.

Teratogenic Effects of Alcohol

The initial reports of infant malformations and mortality resulting from paternal alcohol consumption in animals appeared more than 70 years ago (Stockard and Papanicolaou 1916, 1918*a,b*). These studies demonstrated profound alcohol-induced reductions in fertility, gross developmental abnormalities, and considerable levels of infant mortality. These results were initially dismissed, largely on the grounds that if these massive deficits in animals had clinical significance, they would already have been observed in humans. Another view held that as a clear-cut mechanism for these effects could not be demonstrated, the effects themselves must not exist. Moreover, several attempts to replicate these results were unsuccessful (MacDowell et al. 1926; Durham and Woods 1932).

Renewed interest in the effects of paternal drug administration emerged approximately 15 years ago as a result of studies in animal models showing that alcohol influences male sexual performance and fertility, the viability of offspring, and maturation of the fetus and newborn (for a review, see Abel 1992). These effects appeared to be qualitatively and quantitatively different from those observed in FAS. However, a few reports suggested that FAS could occur in offspring of alcoholic fathers with no evidence of heavy alcohol consumption during pregnancy by the mother (Scheiner et al. 1979; Henderson et al. 1981; Randall and Noble 1980). It remains to be resolved whether the anomalies observed in the offspring of fathers exposed to alcohol are characteristic of FAS or some other syndrome. Nevertheless, it seems clear that paternal, pregestational alcohol administration can produce adverse effects in the offspring, at least under the conditions of these early studies.

Unfortunately, methodological problems in this research have made comparisons between studies difficult and definitive conclusions nearly impossible. These problems include very limited numbers of experimental subjects; inappropriate modes of alcohol administration, causing problems with nutrition and stress; variation in the length of alcohol exposure among studies; and whether or not a drug-free interval was provided prior to mating. Moreover, some recent studies, using appropriate alcohol administration regimens and adequate control groups, failed to observe any gross anomalies characteristic of FAS such as were observed in some earlier studies.

Specific Deficits in the Offspring of Alcoholic Fathers

More recently, we and others have examined the influence of paternal alcohol consumption on offspring under well-controlled conditions in animal models (Cicero et al. 1991*b*; Wozniak et al. 1991; Abel 1989, 1992; Abel and Lee 1988; Abel and Moore 1987; Abel and Tan 1988; Berk et al. 1989).

Deficits in Puberty and Sexual Maturation. Initially, we focused on the effects of alcohol on puberty and sexual maturation, because alcoholism and alcohol use are increasing among adolescents (Johnston et al. 1987). We found that alcohol administered to prepubescent male rats significantly affected many primary indicators of puberty and sexual maturation as those rats developed. The alcohol diet was terminated when the animals were sexually mature; all reproductive hormonal indicators then quickly recovered, becoming indistinguishable from non-alcohol-fed control animals 2 to 3 weeks after termination of alcohol exposure. In contrast to these results obtained in immature rats, the effects of alcohol on reproductive hormones in the fully mature animal were transitory and of considerably lesser magnitude.

To confirm that the effects of preadolescent exposure to alcohol on reproductive hormones were fully reversible, we mated alcohol-exposed adolescent male rats, in which the effects of alcohol on reproductive hormones had apparently completely dissipated (2 to 3 weeks after termination of alcohol exposure), with drug-naive females. We examined sexual behavior, capacity to mate, and the ability to conceive healthy litters in alcohol-exposed male rats compared with controls. We also examined relatively crude indices of the development of their offspring ("alcohol-sired" rats).

Although pregnancy rates were essentially equivalent when alcohol-exposed and control animals were mated with drug-naive females, the size of the litters was modestly but significantly smaller with the alcohol-exposed males. However, in other respects, such as birth weights, ratio of males to females, mortality rates, and gross developmental features, alcohol sired offspring were identical with controls. Taken together, the results of the above experiments show that early exposure to alcohol adversely affects puberty and sexual maturation, with essentially complete recovery of reproductive function occurring within 2 to 3 weeks after alcohol withdrawal.

Offspring Effects. We more fully characterized the development of the offspring of alcohol-exposed and control animals to determine whether more subtle differences might exist. We found significant disturbances in hormonal function in adult alcohol-sired rats compared with offspring sired by normal male rats. For example, male alcohol-sired offspring had significantly lower levels of testosterone and beta-endorphin as well as lighter seminal vesicles. (Testosterone is the primary male sex hormone; beta-endorphin is a hormonelike substance in the brain, belonging to the class of endogenous peptides;

Effects of Paternal Exposure to Alcohol on Offspring

and the seminal vesicles are sperm-producing tubular structures in the testes.) We were unable to demonstrate any impairment in reproductive hormone function in female alcohol-sired offspring. However, we found that female—but not male—alcohol-sired offspring had abnormal baseline levels of certain stress-related hormones and responded differently to stress than did control female offspring.

The alcohol-sired offspring in these tests did not differ from controls in terms of body weights measured at various times during development, the appearance of various developmental landmarks, or performance on several developmental tests. However, the adult alcohol-sired males performed poorly on several spatial learning tests; other forms of learning appeared to be relatively unaffected. Female alcohol-sired offspring displayed no significant learning impairments on any test we employed.

Thus, our results indicate pronounced gender-specific hormonal function and behavioral defects in the offspring of fathers exposed to alcohol as adolescents. Perhaps of equal importance, the deficits we observed in alcohol-sired offspring appeared to be selective. We observed no differences in several hormonal systems other than those associated with reproductive hormones and stress nor were there differences on a variety of behavioral tests other than those relying on spatial learning. This selectivity might account for previous reports in which no gross developmental anomalies were observed to result from paternal alcohol exposure.

In addition, these results are highly consistent with the observations in humans, in that offspring of alcoholic fathers, as opposed to offspring suffering from FAS, are not grossly malformed or impaired but have pronounced selective intellectual and functional deficits. Thus, our animal model may prove to be useful for examining deficits derived from paternal alcohol exposure in offspring of human alcoholics.

We are unaware of any reports examining the effects of paternal drug administration using an experimental design similar to the one we used in our studies. However, several researchers have reported that exposure of fully mature male rats to environmental toxicants and drugs, including alcohol, can lead to numerous behavioral, biochemical, and hormonal disturbances in their offspring (for reviews, see Cohen 1986; Joffe and Soyka 1982; Narod et al. 1988). For example, Abel (1989, 1992) found that alcohol administration to male rodents adversely affects the hormonal and cognitive status of the offspring.

Although many studies have reported deficits in alcohol-sired offspring, earlier researchers studied only adult animals and used extremely high doses of toxicants or drugs. Moreover, alcohol exposure continued through conception, and the appearance or functional activity of the sperm was often grossly altered. Many of these studies do not permit a distinction between the chronic effects of alcohol and its acute toxicity with respect to reproductive hormonal function.

In our ongoing studies, we have shown that a period of moderate exposure of the father to alcohol during sexual maturation, followed by a drug-free period sufficient to restore normal hormonal status, resulted in the abnormal development of both male and female offspring. Thus, our results presumably do not reflect the acute effects of alcohol or the consequences of withdrawal but rather some residual effect of early exposure to alcohol during development of the future father. Consequently, the experimental design used in our studies may be useful for examining the possible consequences of heavy alcohol use by human male adolescents on the development of the offspring they bear later as adults.

Mechanisms of Paternal-Alcohol Effects on Offspring

The mechanisms underlying the deficits observed in alcohol-sired animal offspring are not easily explained. It is, however, clear that the results observed in our studies are due exclusively to paternal alcohol exposure, because they cannot reasonably be ascribed to the female. Specifically, the females were drug naive and matched to control animals in terms of their previous capacity to deliver and nurture healthy litters. Moreover, their offspring developed normally with no evidence of fetal mortality, and post mortem evaluation revealed no clinically significant problems in the females that could account for any of the observed effects.

There are three possible mechanisms for the effect of paternal alcohol consumption on the offspring. First, alcohol may directly affect the characteristics and properties of sperm, perhaps by causing mutations in the sperm's genetic material. Second, sperm may be "selected" in some way such that only a specific population is functionally intact following prolonged exposure to alcohol. Third, alcohol consumption might alter the chemical composition of semen so as to influence the activity of ejaculated sperm.

In this connection, several recent studies have shown that various drugs, including alcohol, may induce subtle mutations in sperm (Obe et al. 1986; Narod et al. 1988), and long-term alcohol exposure may result in gross abnormalities in the appearance and motility of sperm (for a review, see Abel 1992). In addition, it has been demonstrated

Effects of Paternal Exposure to Alcohol on Offspring

that drugs and toxicants accumulate in semen (e.g., Yazigi et al. 1991), and some drugs, such as cocaine, may bind to the sperm surface (Yazigi et al. 1991).

These data suggest that drugs may either impair sperm directly, thereby influencing the development of offspring, or be transported to the ovum via the seminal fluid by physically binding to sperm. Alternatively, alcohol might alter the biochemical and nutritional composition of the seminal fluid, which is necessary for the survival of sperm and to ensure successful conception. If the latter is true, then it can be postulated that the embryo may be exposed to high levels of a toxicant or that seminal substances necessary for facilitating and maintaining the embryo are altered during the earliest stages of development, adversely affecting normal maturation. These possibilities are pure conjecture, as a causal link with birth defects has not been established.

It may be significant that endogenous opioids are synthesized in the testes. Endogenous opioids are morphinelike substances, best known as chemical messengers in the brain. Their functions are not clearly understood, but they generally involve modulation of hormonal systems. Endogenous opioids carry out their functions by binding to specific receptor proteins embedded in the surfaces of cells, thereby ultimately causing chemical changes to occur within those cells. Receptors for endogenous opioids have been found to occur in certain testicular cells and on the surface of sperm.

Therefore, these substances may play a significant role in modulating the production of sex hormones and sperm in the testicles. Although the effects of alcohol on testicular endogenous opioid function are unknown, both short- and long-term alcohol use significantly affect endogenous opioid systems in the brain and other organs.

Alcohol and morphine have similar effects on puberty and sexual maturation (Cicero et al. 1991a), and the results of breeding animals exposed to morphine during adolescence with drug-naive females were similar to those observed in animals exposed to alcohol. For example, morphine-sired male offspring had lower serum testosterone and other hormone levels, lower weights of the seminal vesicles, and heavier adrenal glands. (The adrenal glands, located above the kidneys, produce hormones that help regulate various metabolic functions and the response to stress.) Female morphine-derived adult offspring had significantly higher levels of adrenal stress-related hormones in the blood.

Moreover, Friedler and associates (Friedler 1985; Friedler and Cicero 1988) have demonstrated cognitive deficits in the offspring of morphine-exposed males mated with drug-naive females, similar in some respects to those observed in the offspring of alcohol-exposed males. These similarities between two commonly used drugs, alcohol and opiates, raise several interesting questions, such as whether these drugs act through a common pathway and whether other drugs likely to be used during adolescence would produce similar effects.

Conclusions

Alcohol consumption by male rats appears to have long-lasting effects on their ability to produce normal progeny. Studies suggest that alcohol itself may be a direct toxicant to sperm, inducing subtle yet marked deficits in the offspring of alcohol-exposed fathers. If true, this will require a reassessment of the numerous studies in humans examining the heritability of specific traits predisposing the offspring to alcoholism. Specifically, it has been assumed that the sons of alcoholics inherit some genetic trait that predisposes them to alcoholism, but few investigators have considered the possibility that these deficits could be due to alcohol's being a direct gonadal toxicant or teratogenic agent.

Results relative to the paternal effects of alcohol on progeny are still in a very early stage of development. A concerted effort must be made to replicate these findings and to address other important issues, such as: How much alcohol must fathers drink to produce deficits in their offspring? Are the effects observed in the offspring of alcohol-exposed fathers transmitted from one generation to the next? Can these effects be reversed by long-term abstinence of the father prior to conception?

Whereas the paternal effects of alcohol on both male and female offspring appear to be pronounced, no studies as yet suggest that any of the deficits observed in animal models are causally related to the development of alcoholism. Studies are needed to determine whether the observed cognitive and biochemical disturbances are associated with altered responses to alcohol that might lead to addiction. Such studies would also help determine whether animal models are appropriate for examining the causal factors and heritability of alcoholism in humans.

—*by Theodore J. Cicero, Ph.D.*

Theodore J. Cicero, Ph.D., is professor of neuropharmacology in the Department of Psychiatry, Washington University School of Medicine, St. Louis, Missouri.

This work was supported by grants AA07144 and AA07466 from the National Institute on Alcohol Abuse and Alcoholism and by Research Scientist Award DA00095 and grant DA03833 from the National Institute on Drug Abuse.

References

Abel, E.L. Paternal and maternal alcohol consumption: Effects on offspring in two strains of rats. *Alcoholism: Clinical and Experimental Research* 13:533-541, 1989.

Abel, E.L. Paternal exposure to alcohol. In: Sonderegger, T.B., ed. *Perinatal Substance Abuse: Research Findings and Clinical Implications*. Baltimore: Johns Hopkins University Press, 1992. pp. 132-162.

Abel, E.L., and Lee, J.A. Paternal alcohol exposure affects offspring behavior but not body or organ weights in mice. *Alcoholism: Clinical and Experimental Research* 12:349-355, 1988.

Abel, E.L., and Moore, C. Effects of paternal alcohol consumption in mice. *Alcoholism: Clinical and Experimental Research* 11:533-535, 1987.

Abel, E.L., and Tan, S.E. Effects of paternal alcohol consumption on pregnancy outcome in rats. *Neurotoxicology and Teratology* 19:187-192, 1988.

Begleiter, H., and Projesz, B. Potential biological markers in individuals at high risk for developing alcoholism. *Alcoholism: Clinical and Experimental Research* 12:488-493, 1988.

Berk, R.S.; Montgomery, I.N.; Hazlett. L.D.; and Abel, E.L. Paternal alcohol consumption: Effect on ocular response and serum antibody response to *Pseudomonas aeruginosa* infection in offspring. *Alcoholism: Clinical and Experimental Research* 13:795-798, 1989.

Cicero, T.J.; Adams, M.L.; Giordano, A.; Miller, B.T.; O'Connor, L.; and Nock, B. Influence of morphine exposure during adolescence on the sexual maturation of male rats and the development of their offspring. *Journal of Pharmacology and Experimental Therapeutics* 256:1086-1093, 1991*a*.

Cicero, T.J.; Adams, M.L.; O'Connor, L.H.; Nock, B.; Meyer, E.R.; and Wozniak, D. Influence of chronic alcohol administration on representative indices of puberty and sexual maturation in male rats and the development of their progeny. *Journal of Pharmacology and Experimental Therapeutics* 255:707-715, 1991*b*.

Cloninger, C.R.; Sigvardsson, S.; Gilligan, S.B.; von Knorring A.L.; Reich, T.; and Bohman, M. Genetic heterogeneity and the classification of alcoholism. *Advances in Alcohol and Substance Abuse* 7(3/4):3-16. 1989.

Cohen, F.L. Paternal contributions to birth defects. *Nursing Clinics of North America* 21:49-64, 1986.

Durham, F.M., and Woods, H.M. *Alcohol and Inheritance: An Experimental Study*. Medical Research Council Special Reports Series. No. 168. London: H.M.S.O., 1932.

Ehlers, C.L.; Wall, T.L.; and Schuckit, M.A. EEG spectral characteristics following ethanol administration in young men. *Electroencephalography and Clinical Neurophysiology* 73:179-187, 1989.

Friedler, G. Effects of limited paternal exposure to xenobiotic agents on the development of progeny. *Neurobehavioral Toxicology and Teratology* 7:739-743, 1985.

Friedler, G., and Cicero, T.J. Paternal pregestational opiate exposure in male mice: Neuroendocrine deficits in their offspring. *Substance Abuse* 8:109-116, 1988.

Hegedus, A.M.; Alterman, A.I.; and Tarter, R.E. Learning achievement in sons of alcoholics. *Alcoholism: Clinical and Experimental Research* 8:330-333, 1984.

Henderson, G.I.; Patwardhan, R.V.; Joyumpa A.M.; and Schenker, S. Fetal alcohol syndrome: Overview of pathogenesis. *Neurobehavioral Toxicology and Teratology* 3:73-80, 1981.

Joffe, J.M., and Soyka, L.F. Paternal drug exposure: Effects on reproduction and progeny. *Seminars in Perinatology* 6:116-124, 1982.

Johnston, L.P.; O'Mally, P.M.; and Bachman, J.G. *National Trends in Drug Abuse and Related Factors Among American High School Students and Young Adults*, 1975-1986. National Institute on Drug Abuse. DHHS Pub. No. (ADM)87-1535. Washington, DC: Supt. of Docs., U.S. Govt. Print. Off., 1987.

MacDowell, E.C.; Lord, E.M.; and MacDowell, C.G. Heavy alcoholization and prenatal mortality in mice. *Proceedings of the Society for Experimental Biology and Medicine* 23:652-654, 1926.

Merikangas, K.R. The genetic epidemiology of alcoholism. *Psychological Medicine* 20:11-22, 1990.

Meyer, L.S., and Riley, E.P. Behavioral teratology of alcohol. In: Riley, E.P., and Vorhees, C.V., eds. *Handbook of Behavioral Teratology*. New York: Plenum Press, 1986. pp. 101-134.

Narod, S.A.; Douglas, G.E.; Nesmann, E.R.; and Blakey, D.H. Human mutagens: Evidence from paternal exposure. *Environmental and Molecular Mutagenesis* 11:401-415, 1988.

Obe, G.; Ristow, H.; and Herha, J. Effect of ethanol on chromosomal structure and function. In: Majchrowicz, E., and Noble, E.P., eds. *Biochemistry and Pharmacology of Ethanol*. Vol. 1. New York: Plenum Press, 1986. pp. 659-676.

Pickens, R.W.; Svikis, D.S.; McGue, M.; Lykken, D.T.; Heston, L.L.; and Clayton, P.J. Heterogeneity in the inheritance of alcoholism. *Archives of General Psychiatry* 48(1):19-28, 1991.

Randall, C.L., and Noble, E.P. Alcohol abuse and fetal growth in development. In: Mello, N.K., ed. *Advances in Substance Abuse*. Vol. 1. Greenwich, CT: JAI Press, 1980. pp. 327-367.

Scheiner, A.P.; Donovan, C.M.; and Bartoshesky, L.E. Fetal alcohol syndrome in child whose parents had stopped drinking. *Lancet* 1(8125):1077-1078, 1979.

Schuckit, M.A. Reactions to alcohol in sons of alcoholics and controls. *Alcoholism: Clinical and Experimental Research* 12:465-470, 1988.

Schuckit, M.A.; Butters, N.; Lyn, L.; and Irwin, M. Neuropsychologic deficits and the risk for alcoholism. *Neuropsychopharmacology* 1:45-53. 1987a.

Schuckit, M.A.; Gold, E.; and Risch, C. Plasma cortisol levels following ethanol in sons of alcoholics and controls. *Archives of General Psychiatry* 44:942-945, 1987b.

Schuckit, M.A.; Risch, S.C.; and Gold, E.O. Ethanol consumption, ACTH level, and family history of alcoholism. *American Journal of Psychiatry* 145:1391-1395, 1988.

Stockard, C.R., and Papanicolaou, G. A further analysis of the heredity transmission of degeneracy and deformities by the descendants of alcoholized mammals. I. *American Naturalist* 50:68-88, 1916.

Stockard, C.R., and Papanicolaou, G. A further analysis of the heredity transmission of degeneracy and deformities by the descendants of alcoholized mammals. II. *American Naturalist* 144- 177, 1918a.

Stockard, C.R., and Papanicolaou, G. Further studies on the modification of the germ-cells in mammals: The effect of alcohol on treated guinea-pigs and their descendants. *Journal of Experimental Zoology* 26:119-226. 1918b.

Tartar, R.E.; Jacob, T.; and Bremer, D.L. Specific cognitive impairment in sons of early onset alcoholics. *Alcoholism: Clinical and Experimental Research* 13:786-789, 1989.

Wozniak, D.F.; Cicero, T.J.; Kettinger, L.; and Meyer, E.R. Paternal alcohol consumption in the rat impairs spatial learning performance in male off-spring. *Psychopharmacology* 105:289-302, 1991.

Yazigi, R.A.; Odem, R.R.; and Polakoski, K.L. Demonstration of specific binding of cocaine to human spermatogenesis. *Journal of the American Medical Association* 266:1956-1959, 1991.

Chapter 23

Comparative Teratogenicity of Alcohol and Other Drugs

Prenatal exposure to alcohol or other drugs can impair physical, intellectual, and behavioral development. An understanding of how these drugs act and interact with one another and with lifestyle factors is necessary to plan effective prevention and intervention efforts.

The dangers of fetal alcohol exposure first came to light during the late 1960's. More recently, scientists have become aware of the relationship between other drugs and pregnancy outcome. This chapter compares the epidemiology of alcohol, marijuana, cocaine, and tobacco use among women of childbearing age and describes what is known about the effect of exposure to each drug during pregnancy.

Epidemiology of Alcohol Use

The National Institute on Drug Abuse (NIDA) conducted a national household survey of drug use in 1990, completing interviews with 9,259 people. Of all women surveyed, 78.7 percent reported they had drunk alcohol in their lifetime (NIDA 1991*a*). Sixty-one percent drank in the past year, and 44.1 percent drank in the past month. Women were generally light drinkers: 19 percent drank less often than once a month, and 20 percent drank monthly but less than once a week. In another national sample, of 5,221 respondents, a proportion of women drank more heavily: 25 percent drank at least once a week and 6 percent consumed five or more drinks weekly (Hilton 1988).

Excerpted from *Alcohol-Related Birth Defects*, National Institute on Alcohol Abuse and Alcoholism (NIAAA), NIH Pub. No. 94-3466, 1994.

Among women ages 18 to 25 and 26 to 34, 84.7 percent and 89.8 percent reported lifetime alcohol use, respectively (Table 23.1), and 53.3 percent and 55.2 percent reported alcohol use in the previous month, respectively.

In general among women, compared with nondrinkers, drinkers were young, Caucasian, and unmarried. Drinkers also had a higher education and income, worked full time outside the home, and were Jewish or Catholic. With the exception of religion, these same characteristics also described the heavy drinkers, defined as women who consumed two or more drinks a day or who had five or more drinks on an occasion (Day et al. 1993).

	Drug Use (%)		
Drug and Age Group	**Ever**	**Past Year**	**Past Month**
Alcohol			
18–25 years	84.7	74.6	53.3
26–34 years	89.8	74.7	55.2
Marijuana			
18–25 years	49.0	20.7	9.1
26–34 years	57.0	14.9	7.5
Tobacco			
18–25 years	65.0	35.6	27.1
26–34 years	78.7	41.2	35.2
Cocaine and Crack			
18–25 years	15.6	4.8	1.6
26–34 years	21.5	4.5	1.1
Crack			
18–25 years	1.7	1.1	—[1]
26–34 years	2.2	0.5	0.4

[1]Prevalence is too small for a precise statement.
SOURCE: National Institute on Drug Abuse 1991a.

Table 23.1. *Drug use among two age groups of young women according to the 1990 National Household Survey on Drug Abuse.*

Drinking during pregnancy has decreased dramatically in recent years. Serdula and colleagues (1991) reported a decline from 32 percent to 20 percent in the overall rate of alcohol use during pregnancy over a 3-year period from 1985 to 1988. Nevertheless, in this random, population-based study of 38,224 women, 1,712 of whom were pregnant,

25 percent of the pregnant women reported that they had drunk an alcoholic beverage in the previous month. Approximately 3 percent of the women fit the criteria for binge drinking (five or more drinks on one or more occasions during the past month), and 0.6 percent were classified as heavy drinkers (two or more drinks a day).

In a large multicenter study of the prevalence of psychiatric illness in the general population, 4.7 percent of the women interviewed met the criteria for alcohol abuse or dependence at some point in their lifetime (Helzer et al. 1991). The highest prevalence rates for both dependence and abuse were found among women in the childbearing years: 18 to 29 and 30 to 44 years of age (6.9 percent and 5.5 percent, respectively).

Effects of Alcohol Use

The effects of prenatal alcohol exposure occur along a continuum bounded by fetal alcohol syndrome (FAS) at the extreme end. FAS is defined in the infant by a pattern, or syndrome, of characteristics. Cardinal features of the syndrome include the following: (1) growth deficiency; (2) anomalies of brain structure and function, including intellectual deficits; and (3) abnormalities of the head and face (Sokol and Clarren 1989).

Abel and Sokol (1991) estimated the rate of FAS in the general population to be 0.33 cases per 1,000 births. However, FAS may be considerably underdiagnosed (Little et al. 1990) because of the difficulty in making the diagnosis and the unwillingness of clinicians to apply a stigmatizing label to affected children. Among alcoholic women, the risk of having a child with FAS is approximately 6 percent (Abel and Sokol 1987). (Throughout this article terms such as "alcohol abuse," "alcoholism," "moderate drinking," and "heavy drinking" are used. There is overlap among these terms in the alcoholism literature; therefore, the wording in each case is based on the terms used in the reference cited.)

Offspring of women who drink moderately during pregnancy may exhibit specific features of FAS without displaying the full syndrome. In the Maternal Health Practices and Child Development (MHPCD) Project, the exposed offspring were smaller in weight, height, and head circumference at 8, 18, and 36 months of age. (The Maternal Health Practices and Child Development Project is a program of research on the long-term effects of prenatal alcohol, marijuana, and cocaine exposure. Women were selected from a prenatal clinic population in the fourth month of pregnancy and followed up at the seventh prenatal month; delivery; 8 and 18 months; and 3, 6, and 10 years.) The effect of prenatal alcohol exposure on growth was still significant at 6 years of age, after considering the effects of the current environment, use of other drugs during pregnancy, nutrition, and sociodemographic factors (Day et al. in press *a*). The amount of alcohol consumed was directly proportional to the magnitude of the effect on growth. The specific physical characteristics that define FAS also are reported with a higher frequency among offspring exposed to alcohol prenatally in the absence of the complete syndrome (Day 1992).

The effects of prenatal exposure to low levels of alcohol on intellectual development also fall along a continuum. In general, alcohol exposure appears to be related to a small decrease in cognitive abilities. For example, one study found a decrement of seven IQ points in 7-year-old children who had been exposed to more than 1 ounce of alcohol per day before birth, compared with children who had been exposed to less than 1 ounce (Streissguth et al. 1990). School achievement scores in this and another study (Coles et al. 1991) also were related to prenatal alcohol exposure.

Children with FAS have been reported to have behavioral problems that persist through adulthood (Streissguth et al. 1991). Behavioral problems also have been reported, although not consistently, among offspring who were exposed to alcohol prenatally but who do not have FAS. These behavioral problems include attention deficits and impulsiveness (Brown et al. 1991).

Thus, offspring exposed to alcohol prenatally who do not have FAS may exhibit one or more of the defects associated with FAS or may exhibit all three major types of FAS defects but to a lesser degree.

Epidemiology of Marijuana Use

The rate of marijuana use in the United States peaked in the late 1970's and has since been decreasing. In the NIDA national survey, 10 percent of households reported marijuana use, making it the most commonly used illicit drug in the United States (NIDA 1991*b*).

Twenty-eight percent of all women have used marijuana in their lifetime, 8 percent reported marijuana use in the past year, and 4 percent reported use in the past month (NIDA 1991*a*). Women between the ages of 18 and 25 were the most likely to report current marijuana use; 9.1 percent of women ages 18 to 25 and 7.5 percent of women ages 26 to 34 had used marijuana in the last month (Table 23.1).

Overall, Caucasian women reported a higher lifetime prevalence of use, but African-American women were more likely to report current use than were Caucasian or Hispanic women.

Because no surveys of the general population have examined marijuana use during pregnancy, information can be obtained only from research studies of specific populations. However, the studied populations consist of relatively heavy drug users, whose use of marijuana does not represent that among the general population of pregnant women.

In the MHPCD project, Day and colleagues (1991) found that 30 percent of a random sample of 1,360 women reported marijuana use during pregnancy. These women were from an outpatient prenatal clinic that served a low-income, inner-city population. Another study, which interviewed women from prenatal clinics at two Denver hospitals, reported a prevalence rate of 34 percent (Tennes et al. 1985). In another low-income, inner-city sample, 23 percent of the women reported smoking marijuana and 16 percent of the women had positive urine screens for marijuana (Zuckerman et al. 1989).

Marijuana use may be lower in middle class samples. Fried and coworkers (1980) reported prevalence rates of 13 percent in the first trimester and 10 percent in the third trimester in a sample recruited from private obstetrical practices in Ottawa, Canada. However, toxicologic tests on women from 5 public health clinics and 12 private obstetrical offices in Pinellas County, FL, showed that among the women who attended the public clinics, 12.4 percent tested positive for marijuana-derived chemicals in urine, and 11.3 percent of the women in private care were positive for marijuana use (Chasnoff et al. 1990).

Women who use marijuana during pregnancy differ as follows from women who do not: they are more likely to be African-American, of lower socioeconomic status, less educated, younger, and unmarried. In addition, they more often use alcohol, tobacco, and other drugs (Day et al. 1993).

Effects of Marijuana Use

Although there have been reports of an association between prenatal marijuana exposure and smaller size at birth, these have been offset by reports that found no such effect. Growth deficits have not been found in studies with long-term followup (Fried and Watkinson 1988; Day et al. 1992). Similarly, recent data refute earlier reports of physical abnormalities resulting from prenatal marijuana exposure (Day et al. 1991; Astley et al. 1992).

Studies of the effects of prenatal marijuana exposure on the brain and on intellectual and behavioral development have been provocative. Researchers studying the electrical activity of the brain during sleep in a subset of newborns from the MHPCD project found significant differences between marijuana-exposed and nonexposed subjects (Scher et al. 1988). Disturbed sleep patterns were still significantly associated with prenatal marijuana exposure in 3-year-old children (Dahl et al. 1989).

Effects of marijuana exposure on the brain have been found in older children as well. In the MHPCD project, 3-year-old children showed significant effects of first- and second-trimester exposure to marijuana on the composite score of the Stanford-Binet Intelligence Scale (4th edition) as well as on those portions of the scale that measure short-term memory, verbal reasoning, and abstract/visual reasoning (Day et al. in press *b*). These children showed the same effects at age 6.

Fried and Watkinson (1990) reported on the behavioral development of children who were part of the Ottawa Prenatal Prospective Study. At 4 years of age, prenatal marijuana exposure was significantly associated with lower scores on both the verbal and the memory domains of the McCarthy Scales of Children's Abilities. Six-year-old children prenatally exposed to marijuana performed poorly on tasks requiring attention and were described by their mothers as impulsive and hyperactive (Fried et al. 1992). In the MHPCD project, behavior problems, including inattention and hyperactivity, also were significantly associated with prenatal exposure to marijuana among children ages 3 and 6.

Overall, the results suggest that prenatal exposure to marijuana has significant effects on sleep and, at older ages, on measures of intellectual development and behavior. There are few or no effects of prenatal exposure on growth or physical development.

Epidemiology of Cocaine Use

Cocaine use peaked in the United States between 1979 and 1985 and has decreased steadily since that time (NIDA 1991*a*). In the late 1970's, cocaine was predominantly used by Caucasians of middle class background who were well educated and employed (Gay 1981). With the advent of crack—a smokable form of cocaine that has a more intense effect—the proportion of Caucasian users has decreased, and

Comparative Teratogenicity of Alcohol and Other Drugs

the rate of cocaine use among minorities, people of lower socioeconomic status, and youth has increased.

In the 1990 NIDA survey, 9 percent of all women reported that they had ever used cocaine, 2 percent reported use in the past year, and 0.5 percent reported cocaine use during the past month (NIDA 1991*a*). Reported use in the past year was 4.8 percent and 4.5 percent for women ages 18 to 25 and 26 to 34, respectively (Table 23.1). Caucasian and Hispanic women reported similar lifetime rates of any cocaine use, and both were higher than the rates among African-Americans. Crack use in 1990 made up a small portion of the reported crack/cocaine use. Overall, 0.8 percent of all women reported any use of crack over their lifetime, 0.3 percent had used crack within the past year, and 0.1 percent within the past month.

However, current rates in the past year and the past month were higher among African-American and Hispanic women compared with Caucasian women. Crack use was highest among African-American women (NIDA 1991*a*). In the following sections, the term "cocaine use" includes both crack and cocaine use.

Studies in large urban hospitals have reported prevalence rates of cocaine use during pregnancy ranging from 8 to 17 percent. Neerhof and colleagues (1989) reported that 8 percent of all women admitted to the delivery unit of the Chicago Osteopathic Medical Center between 1986 and 1988 had positive urine screens for cocaine, whereas in Boston City Hospital, 17 percent of the women had either a positive urine screen or reported use on interview (Zuckerman et al. 1989). These high rates reflect the rise in the rates of crack and cocaine use among minority women and poor women in the inner city.

Women who used cocaine during pregnancy differed from nonusers as follows (Day et al. 1993): they were older, unmarried, and less educated. They had had more pregnancies and were more likely to have had previous induced abortions. They used more cigarettes, alcohol, marijuana, and other drugs during pregnancy; had a higher prevalence of sexually transmitted diseases; and were more likely to be HIV-positive.

Effects of Cocaine Use

There are few consistent effects of prenatal cocaine exposure. When the offspring of cocaine-using women are compared with the offspring of women not using drugs, the exposed offspring display a broad variety of abnormalities. However, when the offspring of drug-using women are compared with one another, few defects emerge that can be ascribed uniquely to cocaine.

Some reports associate cocaine use with pregnancy complications. Chasnoff (1988) found increased rates of preterm labor, precipitous labor, and abruptio placentae (premature detachment of the placenta) in a cocaine-using group compared with women who were not exposed to any drugs. In the MHPCD studies, however, there was no difference between cocaine users and nonusers in pregnancy, labor, or delivery complications (Richardson and Day 1991). Other studies have reported that women who used cocaine and who received adequate prenatal care did not differ in the rate of abruptio placentae from non-cocaine-using controls (MacGregor et al. 1989).

Prenatal cocaine exposure also has been associated with decreased length of gestation and increased rate of prematurity. However, researchers do not always control for the use of other drugs or for other factors associated with cocaine use and, therefore, the effects cannot conclusively be attributed to cocaine. Data from one prospective study showed no effect of cocaine use on gestational age when the correlates of cocaine use were controlled (Zuckerman et al. 1989). In addition, reports from the MHPCD project found no reduction in gestational age after accounting for such characteristics as race and the use of other drugs (Richardson and Day 1991).

Researchers have reported decreased weight, length, and head circumference in cocaine-exposed newborns (Chasnoff 1988), and Coles and coworkers (1992) found that the duration of cocaine exposure during pregnancy was associated with decreased birth weight. However, other studies found no effects of prenatal cocaine exposure on growth. Little and Snell (1991) reported that cocaine-exposed infants were smaller in weight, length, and head circumference than infants who were not exposed to either cocaine or alcohol. However, there were no significant differences in growth when the cocaine-exposed infants were compared with alcohol-exposed infants. Similar findings have been reported by Chasnoff and colleagues (1992).

In a recent report, Chasnoff and coworkers (1992) compared the offspring of three groups of women: cocaine, alcohol, and marijuana users; alcohol and marijuana users; and nonusers. The offspring were assessed at 3, 6, 12, 18, and 24 months. Infants in the two drug-exposed groups had smaller head circumferences than did the nonexposed infants at each followup point. However, the two drug-exposed groups did not differ from each other.

Most of the larger prospective studies have not found a relationship between prenatal cocaine exposure and physical defects. Richardson and Day (1991) reported no effects of prenatal cocaine exposure on either major or minor physical defects. Similarly, Zuckerman and coworkers (1989) found that cocaine exposure during pregnancy was not associated with physical development when associated factors were controlled for, and Chasnoff and colleagues (1988) found no significant differences in the number of physical anomalies between multiple-drug cocaine-exposed and multiple-drug non-cocaine-exposed infants.

Little is known about the effects of cocaine use on brain development because prospective studies have only begun recently. The Brazelton Neonatal Behavioral Assessment Scale (BNBAS) is used to measure the organization of the brain in the newborn and the infant's ability to interact socially. Cocaine-exposed newborns have been reported to perform differently than nonexposed newborns on the BNBAS (Chasnoff et al. 1987).

Richardson and colleagues (1993) found transient effects on the second day after birth that were gone by the third day. Other researchers found no differences on the BNBAS when controlling for factors associated with cocaine use. Neuspiel and colleagues (1991) administered the BNBAS at two time points, 1 to 3 days and 11 to 30 days of age, and found no significant differences. Coles and coworkers (1991) reported no effect of duration of prenatal cocaine use on the BNBAS 2 days after birth, although there were significant effects at 28 days. In the one longer term followup of exposed children (Chasnoff et al. 1992), no effects were found on development, as measured by the Bayley Scales of Infant Development, through 2 years of age, compared with children whose mothers used no drugs or drugs other than cocaine.

Cocaine users may experience unpleasant withdrawal symptoms upon terminating a period of heavy drug use. In adults, these symptoms may include decreased physical activity, lack of motivation, poor concentration, decreased libido, irritability, depression, and sleepiness (Herridge and Gold 1988). Withdrawal symptoms in newborns exposed prenatally may include jitteriness, poor muscle tone, and poor feeding. Van de Bor and colleagues (1990) reported that half of the cocaine-exposed offspring in their study exhibited signs of withdrawal, but another study found no differences in symptom levels when infants who had been exposed to heroin, methadone, and cocaine were compared with infants exposed to heroin and methadone (Ryan et al. 1987). Hadeed and Siegel (1989) found that cocaine-exposed and drug-free infants did not differ in the rates of jitteriness, poor muscle tone, or poor feeding, and Parker and coworkers (1990) reported no effect of cocaine use on jitteriness in full-term infants.

In summary, negative effects of prenatal cocaine exposure have not been substantiated. Although some investigators have demonstrated significant effects of cocaine use during pregnancy, almost all of these relationships disappear when factors such as prenatal care, lifestyle, and multiple drug use are assessed. This pattern can be noted for the effects of prenatal cocaine exposure on length of pregnancy, growth, and physical characteristics. Thus, previous reports may have misattributed poor pregnancy outcomes to prenatal cocaine exposure because of the failure to control for associated factors. It is reasonable to conclude, as have other researchers (Lutiger et al. 1991), that it is the lifestyle rather than the unique effect of cocaine exposure that leads to poorer outcomes in the offspring. However, there are few studies of the long-term effects of cocaine exposure, and judgment must be withheld until these data are available.

Epidemiology of Tobacco Use

Cigarette use approximates alcohol use in frequency. Using the 1990 National Household Survey on Drug Abuse data, 67.8 percent of all women reported ever smoking tobacco. Among women ages 18 to 25 and 26 to 34, 35.6 percent and 41.2 percent had smoked in the past year, respectively (Table 23.1). Of all the drugs discussed in this article, women are the least likely to decrease tobacco use during pregnancy (Day et al. 1993). In the MHPCD project, women who smoked cigarettes were more likely to be Caucasian, married, less educated, and users of alcohol and illicit drugs.

Effects of Tobacco Use

Maternal tobacco use during pregnancy has been associated with growth retardation in the offspring (Harrison et al. 1983; Kline et al. 1987). Birth weight decreases in direct proportion to the number of cigarettes smoked (Persson et al. 1978), and on average, smokers' babies are 150 to 250 grams lighter than the babies of nonsmokers (U.S. Department of Health, Education, and Welfare 1980). A few early studies found a long-term effect on growth, but the significance of these results is unclear because none controlled for alcohol or other drug use during pregnancy. More recent reports that have controlled for alcohol and other drug use have not found any long-term effect of prenatal tobacco exposure on growth or physical development (Day et al. 1992).

Comparative Teratogenicity of Alcohol and Other Drugs

Prenatal tobacco exposure may affect the brain. Data from the previously mentioned Ottawa Prenatal Prospective Study (Fried et al. 1992) show that tobacco exposure is related to impulsiveness and attention deficits in 6-year-olds. Another report, using a national sample, found that prenatal exposure to tobacco predicted an increased rate of behavior problems in children ages 4 through 11 (Weitzman et al. 1992). There also have been reports of small deficits in intellectual development (Fried and Watkinson 1990) and higher rates of hyperactivity (Naeye and Peters 1984).

Discussion

In summarizing the above findings, several comparisons can be made. Table 23.1 shows that for alcohol, marijuana, and cocaine, the highest rates of use are found among women of childbearing age. In this age population, the drug used most is alcohol, followed by tobacco, marijuana, cocaine, and crack. The rate of cocaine use is not as high among women of childbearing age as is generally believed; only 5 percent of women reported use within the past year. The prevalence of crack, by itself, is even smaller. By contrast, nearly 75 percent of the women reported alcohol use in the last year, so the ratio of cocaine use to alcohol use is approximately 1:15. Results of research studies also demonstrate a low ratio of cocaine use to alcohol use. In the MHPCD study, in a random sample of women attending a prenatal clinic, the ratio was 1:19 for the first trimester of pregnancy.

Assessing the relative effects of drug use is risky because of insufficient data. It is not possible to evaluate the relative dosages of each drug taken or the adequacy of measurement of exposure and outcomes. However, it is possible to compare the published data on known effects of exposure. Thus, prenatal alcohol exposure may have a broader range of effects—and more permanent effects—than prenatal exposure to other drugs. However, the long history of fetal alcohol research may make alcohol exposure appear more significant than other drug exposure, simply because more is known about it.

A more important point than the relative harmfulness of individual drugs is the effect of multiple drug use. As discussed above, women who use one drug are likely to use others as well, especially if they are heavy users. Data from the original representative sample of 1,360 women from the MHPCD project illustrate this overlap in drug use. Fifteen percent of the women reported drinking more than one drink per day during their first trimester of pregnancy. The mean average daily volume (ADV) for these women was 2.6 drinks compared with an ADV of 0.13 drinks for the women who drank less than one drink per day.

As shown in Table 23.2, 59 percent of the heavier drinkers used marijuana and 77 percent used tobacco, compared with rates of 17 percent and 33 percent, respectively, among the women who abstained from alcohol. Similarly, the rate of cocaine use was 8 percent among heavier drinkers, compared with 0.7 percent among abstainers, and the rate of other illicit drug use was 16 percent, compared with 2 percent among abstainers. Women who drank, but who drank less than a drink per day, were intermediate in their rates of other drug use. Thus, not only do drug-using women tend to use more than one drug, but the heavier users of any one drug are more likely to be users—and heavier users—of all other drugs.

Alcohol Use	Marijuana	Tobacco	Cocaine	Other Illicit Drugs
Daily	59	77	8	16
Less then daily	34	53	3	6
None	17	33	0.7	2

Table 23.2. Drug use by level of alcohol use among a sample of 1,360 Women. (These data are from the initial screening sample of 1,360 women in the Maternal Health Practices and Child Development Project. This cohort was a randomly selected sample of women attending an outpatient prenatal clinic.)

Researchers also have documented interactions among drugs. For example, Haste and coworkers (1991) found that the combination of tobacco and alcohol during pregnancy resulted in smaller offspring than the use of either drug separately. Similar findings were reported by Olson and colleagues (1991). Fried and O'Connell (1987) reported that marijuana use offset the negative effects of tobacco on birth weight. Similar, though statistically nonsignificant, findings have been reported from the MHPCD project (Day et al. 1992).

The study of the specific effects of each drug on the exposed offspring may provide valuable insight into the mechanisms of drug-related fetal damage. With this knowledge, women can be educated about the consequences of drug use during pregnancy. Such knowledge would also allow for more effective planning for the care of prenatally exposed children. In addition, it would allow the removal of pejorative terms such as "crack baby" and allow the placement of the relative effects of drug use into an appropriate perspective.

Women who use drugs during pregnancy have other characteristics that significantly affect the outcome of their pregnancy. Lifestyle, physical and mental health, nutrition, and socioeconomic status are all important predictors of pregnancy outcome. It is unclear whether drug effects occur independently or in interaction with these factors. An understanding of the total environment of the drug-using pregnant women is necessary to plan effective intervention and prevention efforts.

—by Nancy L. Day, PhD. and Gale A. Richardson, PhD.

Nancy L. Day, PhD., is associate professor of psychiatry, and Gale A. Richardson, PhD., is assistant professor of psychiatry, at the Western Psychiatric Institute and Clinic, Pittsburgh, Pennsylvania.

References

Abel, E., and Sokol, R. Incidence of fetal alcohol syndrome and economic impact of FAS-related anomalies. *Drug and Alcohol Dependence* 19:51-70, 1987.

Abel, E., and Sokol, R. A revised conservative estimate of the incidence of FAS and its economic impact. *Alcoholism: Clinical and Experimental Research* 15:514-524, 1991.

Astley, S.; Clarren, S.; Little, R.; Sampson, P.; and Daling, J. Analysis of facial shape in children gestationally exposed to marijuana, alcohol, and/or cocaine. *Pediatrics* 89:67-77, 1992.

Brown, R.; Coles, C.; Smith, I.; Platzman, K.; Silverstein, J.; Erickson, S.; and Falek, A. Effects of prenatal alcohol exposure at school age. II. Attention and behavior. *Neurotoxicology and Teratology* 13:369-376, 1991.

Chasnoff, I. Cocaine: Effects on pregnancy and the neonate. In: Chasnoff, I., ed. *Drugs, Alcohol, Pregnancy and Parenting*. Boston: Kluwer Academic Publishers, 1988. pp. 97-103.

Chasnoff, I.; Burns, K.; and Burns, W. Cocaine use in pregnancy: Perinatal morbidity and mortality. *Neurotoxicology and Teratology* 9:291-293, 1987.

Chasnoff, I.; Chisum, G.; and Kaplan, W. Maternal cocaine use and genitourinary tract malformations. *Teratology* 37:201-204, 1988.

Chasnoff, I.; Landress, H.; and Barrett, M. The prevalence of illicit drug or alcohol use during pregnancy and discrepancies in mandatory reporting in Pinellas County, Florida. *New England Journal of Medicine* 322:1202-1206, 1990.

Chasnoff, I.; Griffith, D.; Freier, C.; and Murray, J. Cocaine/polydrug use in pregnancy: Two-year follow-up. *Pediatrics* 89:284-289, 1992.

Coles, C.; Brown, R.; Smith, I.; Platzman, K.; Erickson, S.; and Falek, A. Effects of prenatal alcohol exposure at school age. I. Physical and cognitive development. *Neurotoxicology and Teratology* 13:357-367, 1991.

Coles, C.; Platzman, K.; Smith, I.; James, M.; and Falek, A. Effects of cocaine and alcohol use in pregnancy on neonatal growth and neurobehavioral status. *Neurotoxicology and Teratology* 14:23-33, 1992.

Dahl, R.; Scher, M.; Day, N.; Richardson, G.; Klepper, T.; and Robles, N. The effects of prenatal marijuana exposure: Evidence of EEG-sleep disturbances. *Journal of Developmental and Behavioral Pediatrics* 10:264, 1989.

Day, N. The effect of alcohol use during pregnancy. In: Zagon, I. and Sloikin, T., eds. *Maternal Substance Abuse and the Developing Nervous System*. Orlando, FL: Academic Press, 1992. pp. 27-44.

Day, N.; Sambamoorthi, U.; Taylor, P.; Richardson, G.; Robles, N.; Scher, M.; Stoffer, D.; Cornelius, M.; and Jasperse, D. Prenatal marijuana use and neonatal outcome. *Neurotoxicology and Teratology* 13:329-334, 1991.

Day, N.; Cornelius, M.; Goldschmidt, L.; Richardson, G.; Robles, N.; and Taylor, P. The effects of prenatal tobacco and marijuana use on offspring growth from birth through three years of age. *Neurotoxicology and Teratology* 14:407-414, 1992.

Day, N.; Cottreau, C.; and Richardson, G. The epidemiology of alcohol, marijuana, and cocaine use among women of childbearing age and pregnant women. *Clinical Obstetrics and Gynecology* 36:232-245, 1993.

Day, N.; Richardson, G.; Geva, D.; and Robles, N. Alcohol, marijuana and tobacco: The effects of prenatal exposure on offspring growth and morphology at age six. *Alcoholism: Clinical and Experimental Research*, in press a.

Day, N.; Richardson, G.; Goldschmidt, L.; Robles, N.; Taylor, P.; Stoffer, D.; Cornelius, M.; and Geva, D. The effect of prenatal marijuana exposure on the cognitive development of offspring at age three. *Neurotoxicology and Teratology*, in press b.

Fried, P., and O'Connell, M. A comparison of the effects of prenatal exposure to tobacco, alcohol, cannabis and caffeine on birth size and subsequent growth. *Neurotoxicology and Teratology* 19:79-85, 1987.

Fried, P., and Watkinson, B. 12- and 24-month neurobehavioral follow-up of children prenatally exposed to marijuana, cigarettes and alcohol. *Neurotoxicology and Teratology* 10:305-313, 1988.

Fried, P., and Watkinson, B. 36- and 48-month neurobehavioral follow-up of children prenatally exposed to marijuana, cigarettes and alcohol. *Neurotoxicology and Teratology* 11:49-58, 1990.

Fried, P.; Watkinson, B.; Grant, A.; and Knights, R. Changing patterns of soft drug use prior to and during pregnancy: A prospective study. *Drug and Alcohol Dependence* 6:323-343, 1980.

Fried, P.; Watkinson, B.; and Gray, R. A follow-up study of attentional behavior in 6-year-old children exposed prenatally to marijuana, cigarettes and alcohol. *Neurotoxicology and Teratology* 14:299-311, 1992.

Gay, G. You've come a long way, baby! Coke time for the new American lady of the eighties. *Journal of Psychoactive Drugs* 13:297-318, 1981.

Hadeed, A., and Siegel, S. Maternal cocaine use during pregnancy: Effect on the newborn infant. *Pediatrics* 84:205-210, 1989.

Harrison, G.; Branson, R.; and Vaucher, Y. Association of maternal smoking with body composition of the newborn. *American Journal of Clinical Nutrition* 38:757-762, 1983.

Haste, F.; Anderson, H.; Brooke, O.; Bland, J.; and Peacock, J. The effects of smoking and drinking on the anthropometric measurements of neonates. *Paediatric and Perinatal Epidemiology* 5:83-92, 1991.

Helzer, J.; Burman, A.; and McEvoy, L. Alcohol abuse and dependence. In: Robins, L., and Regier, D., eds. *Psychiatric Disorders in America: The Epidemiologic Catchment Area Study*. New York: The Free Press, 1991. pp. 81-115.

Herridge, P., and Gold, M.S. Pharmacological adjuncts in the treatment of opioid and cocaine addicts. *Journal of Psychoactive Drugs* 20(3):233-242, 1988.

Hilton, M. The demographic distribution of drinking patterns in 1984. *Drug and Alcohol Dependence* 22:37-47, 1988.

Kline, J.; Stein, Z.; and Hutzler, M. Cigarettes, alcohol and marijuana: Varying associations with birthweight. *International Journal of Epidemiology* 16:44-51, 1987.

Little, B., and Snell, L. Brain growth among fetuses exposed to cocaine in utero: Asymmetrical growth retardation. *Obstetrics and Gynecology* 77:361-364, 1991.

Little, B.; Snell, L.; Rosenfeld, C.; Gilstrap, L.; and Gant, N. Failure to recognize fetal alcohol syndrome in newborn infants. *American Journal of Diseases of Children* 144:1142-1146, 1990.

Lutiger, B.; Graham, K.; Einarson, T.; and Koren, G. Relationship between gestational cocaine use and pregnancy outcome: A meta-analysis. *Teratology* 44:405-414, 1991.

MacGregor, S.; Keith, L.; Bachicha, J.; and Chasnoff, I. Cocaine abuse during pregnancy: correlation between prenatal care and perinatal outcome. *Obstetrics and Gynecology* 74:882-885, 1989.

Naeye, R., and Peters, E. Mental development of children whose mothers smoked during pregnancy. *Obstetrics and Gynecology* 64:601-607, 1984.

National Institute on Drug Abuse. *National Household Survey on Drug Abuse: 1990 Population Estimates*. DHHS Pub. No. (ADM)91-1732. Washington, DC: Supt. of Docs., U.S. Govt. Print. Off., 1991*a*.

National Institute on Drug Abuse. *National Household Survey on Drug Abuse: Highlights 1990*. DHHS Pub. No. (ADM)91-1789. Washington, DC: Supt. of Docs., U.S. Govt. Print. Off., 1991*b*.

Neerhof, M.; MacGregor, S.; Retzky, S.; and Sullivan, T. Cocaine abuse during pregnancy: Peripartum prevalence and perinatal outcome. *American Journal of Obstetrics and Gynecology* 161:633-638, 1989.

Neuspiel, D.; Hamel, S.; Hochberg, E.; Greene, J.; and Campbell, D. Maternal cocaine use and infant behavior. *Neurotoxicology and Teratology* 13:229-233, 1991.

Olson, J.; Pereira, A.; and Olson, S. Does maternal tobacco smoking modify the effect of alcohol on fetal growth? *American Journal of Public Health* 81:69-73, 1991.

Parker, S.; Zuckerman, B.; Bauchner, H.; Frank, D.; Vinci, R.; and Cabral, H. Jitteriness in full-term neonates: Prevalence and correlates. *Pediatrics* 85:17-23, 1990.

Persson, P.; Grennert, L.; Gennser, G.; and Kullander, S. A study of smoking and pregnancy with special reference to fetal growth *Acta Obstetrica et Gynecologica Scandinavica* 78:33-39, 1987.

Richardson, G., and Day, N. Maternal and neonatal effects of moderate cocaine use during pregnancy. *Neurotoxicology and Teratology* 13:455-460, 1991.

Richardson, G.; Hamel, S.; Day, N.; and Goldschmidt, L. "Effects of Prenatal Cocaine Use on Neonatal Neurobehavioral Status." Paper presented at the Society for Behavioral Pediatrics, Providence, RI, Sept. 1993.

Ryan, L.; Ehrlich, S.; and Finnegan, L. Cocaine abuse in pregnancy: Effects on the fetus and newborn. *Neurotoxicology and Teratology* 9:295-299, 1987.

Scher, M.; Richardson, G.; Coble, P.; Day, N.; and Stoffer, D. The effects of prenatal alcohol and marijuana exposure: Disturbances in neonatal sleep cycling and arousal. *Pediatric Research* 24:101-105, 1988.

Serdula, M.; Williamson, D.; Kendrick, J.; Anda, R.; and Byers, T. Trends in alcohol consumption by pregnant women 1985-1988. *Journal of the American Medical Association* 265:876-879, 1991.

Sokol, R., and Clarren, S.K. Guidelines for use of terminology describing the impact of prenatal alcohol on the offspring. *Alcoholism: Clinical and Experimental Research* 13(4):597-598, 1989.

Streissguth, A.; Barr, H.; and Sampson, P. Moderate prenatal alcohol exposure: Effects on child IQ and learning problems at age 7 ½ years. *Alcoholism: Clinical and Experimental Research* 14:662-669, 1990.

Streissguth, A.; Aase, J.; Clarren, S.; Randels, S.; LaDue, R.; and Smith, D. Fetal alcohol syndrome in adolescents and adults. *Journal of the American Medical Association* 265:1961-1967, 1991.

Tennes, K.; Avitable, N.; Blackard, C.; Boyles, C.; Hassoun, B.; Holmes, L.; and Kreye, M. Marijuana: Prenatal and postnatal exposure in the human. In: Pinkert, T.M., ed. *Consequences of Maternal Drug Abuse*. National Institute on Drug Abuse Research Monograph No. 59. DHHS Pub. No. (ADM)85-1400. Washington, DC: Supt. of Docs., U.S. Govt. Print. Off., 1985. pp. 48-60.

U.S. Department of Health, Education, and Welfare. *Smoking and Health: A Report of the Surgeon General*. Public Health Service. DHEW Pub. No. (PHS)79-50066. Washington, DC: Supt. of Docs., U.S. Govt. Print. Off., 1980.

van de Bor, M.; Walther, J.; and Sims, M. Increased cerebral blood flow velocity in infants of mothers who abuse cocaine. *Pediatrics* 85:733-736, 1990.

Weitzman, M.; Gortmaker, S.; and Sobol, A. Maternal smoking and behavior problems of children. *Pediatrics* 90:342-349, 1992.

Zuckerman, B.; Frank, D.; Hingson, R.; Amaro, H.; Levenson, S.; Kayne, H.; Parker, S.; Vinci, R.; Aboagye, K.; Fried, L.; Cabral, H.; Timperi, R.; and Bauchner, H. Effects of maternal marijuana and cocaine use on fetal growth. *New England Journal of Medicine* 320(12): 762-768, 1989.

Chapter 24

A Long-Term Perspective of Fetal Alcohol Syndrome

Few people in their adolescent or adult years are diagnosed as having FAS. Studies have shown that most FAS patients outgrow the characteristic FAS facies after puberty. However, they may still suffer from mental handicaps and have poor age-appropriate life skills. Further research is needed to understand these patients' unique needs and to develop the most effective intervention strategies.

In the 20 years since fetal alcohol syndrome (FAS) was identified as a birth defect, relatively few studies have described adolescents and adults with this disability, although FAS is thought to be the leading known cause of mental retardation. Many practical problems exist in accruing a population of adolescent and adult patients with FAS and in following them systematically past childhood. Yet by examining the natural history of FAS, it should be possible to evaluate the long-term needs of these patients and to develop an appropriate set of lifetime interventions suitable to their disabilities.

Taking a historical perspective, this chapter reviews the pertinent literature, describing the findings of several long-term follow-up studies of children with FAS. It raises questions about the needs of adolescents and adults with FAS that should be addressed through future research and public policy.

Excerpted from *Alcohol-Related Birth Defects*, National Institute on Alcohol Abuse and Alcoholism (NIAAA), NIH Pub. No. 94-3466, 1994.

FAS: The Initial Research

FAS is growing up. It is now 20 years since Jones and Smith (1973) coined the term "fetal alcohol syndrome" to describe children who had a specific and visually recognizable pattern of characteristics, and in July 1993, the first baby in the world to receive a diagnosis of FAS at birth celebrated his 20th birthday. Children with similar characteristics had been independently identified in France (Lemoine et al. 1968) and in Seattle (Jones et al. 1973) as a specific subgroup of children born to alcoholic mothers.

The characteristics of FAS were identified as growth deficiency; specific physical anomalies, including a characteristic facies; and central nervous system (CNS) dysfunction. The CNS manifestations include delayed development, hyperactivity, motor incoordination, learning or attentional problems, seizures, mental retardation, and/or microcephaly (small head). These early insights on FAS suggested a biological cause for some of the problems seen in children of alcoholic mothers—and indicated that these problems could be prevented if women did not drink alcohol during pregnancy. (The term "alcoholic" has been defined in many ways. Here the term includes "alcohol abuse" and/or binge consumption but does not necessarily imply dependence.)

Two decades of laboratory research have validated these early findings on the causes of FAS. For example, experimental research has shown that alcohol is teratogenic across a wide variety of species and conditions of exposure, and it is the most commonly used known human teratogen in the world. (A teratogen is a substance that can affect a developing fetus, resulting in physical and neurological damage.) Alcohol also causes FAS, with an estimated prevalence of 1-3/1,000 live births (National Institute on Alcohol Abuse and Alcoholism 1990).

Early Research and Prevention Efforts

The early clinical reports of FAS by Lemoine and colleagues (1968) in western France and Jones and colleagues (1973) in Seattle were soon replicated by reports by Majewski and colleagues (1976) in western Germany, by Dehaene and colleagues (1977a) in northern France, and by Olegård and colleagues (1979) in Sweden. Like the initial reports, all of these studies in the 1970's described patients with FAS who were infants and young children. Because these children with FAS were mostly functioning within the borderline and retarded range of intellectual development, FAS soon became recognized as one of the

A Long-Term Perspective of Fetal Alcohol Syndrome

three most prevalent causes of mental retardation with a known etiology—and the only one that was entirely preventable.

This knowledge stimulated the development of important programs in the late 1970's, designed to demonstrate methods to prevent FAS and to intervene in maternal alcohol abuse during pregnancy (Rosett et al. 1980; Rosett and Weiner 1981; Little and Streissguth 1981; Little et al. 1984, 1985). The United States Government initiated two important policies: an official government warning by the Surgeon General against drinking alcoholic beverages during pregnancy or when planning a pregnancy (Public Health Service 1981), and the labeling of alcoholic beverage containers with a warning about the risk of birth defects associated with drinking alcohol during pregnancy (Public Law 100 690, 1988). It is impossible to know how many children were helped as a result of these official policies, but it is probably a large number. Research projects such as those by Little and colleagues (1984), Rosett and colleagues (1980), and Larsson and colleagues (1985) have clearly demonstrated that curtailing alcohol use during pregnancy does improve pregnancy outcome.

Initially, researchers thought that the CNS effects of FAS were primarily manifested as mental retardation or microcephaly. There was an implicit assumption that the treatment and service needs of patients with FAS would be like those of patients with Down syndrome. (As a result of decades of research, a network of support services and special cradle-to-grave programs exists nationwide to accommodate the special needs of Down syndrome patients.) However, FAS did not turn out to be like Down syndrome. Children with FAS manifest a wide range of intellectual abilities, and no early biological marker has yet appeared to help identify those at risk. Clinicians who continued to work with patients with FAS as they grew up realized that they often behaved very differently than patients with Down syndrome, often getting into trouble in their communities, in their schools, and with their families. This awareness led us to the next set of research studies.

Adolescent Manifestations of FAS

As early as the mid-1970's, Smith made the diagnosis of FAS in two young men who were examined for the first time as adults; both were mentally retarded. Their facial photographs and IQ profiles were published in 1978 (Clarren and Smith 1978; Streissguth et al. 1978). In 1981, Iosub and colleagues described longitudinal data on three siblings with FAS who had been diagnosed in childhood. The two who had reached maturity had small heads, short palpebral fissures (eye openings), borderline to mild mental retardation, but variable growth deficiency; one was growth deficient only for height, the other only for weight.

During the first decade of FAS research, most clinicians seemed reluctant to make the initial diagnosis in adolescents and adults. This was understandable, as all the early patients identified were young children; the classic FAS face was the face of a young child. Only patients with the most classic manifestations of FAS were identified initially as adolescents and adults. It was only when we were able to present systematic longitudinal data on the first children with a diagnosis of FAS that we were able to see how the physical features (the primary markers for the syndrome) changed with age, which makes initial identification more difficult in older patients. This first long-term FAS followup study (Streissguth et al. 1985) was a 10-year followup of the 11 children identified in Seattle in 1973. It revealed that the facial morphology of many persons with FAS changed as they matured. Longer noses and bigger chins often gave their faces a coarser look after puberty, a finding that has been confirmed by several other studies (Spohr et al. 1987, 1993; Lemoine and Lemoine 1992; Majewski 1993). Girls in particular tended to put on weight at this time, and their weight-to-height age ratio changed from low to high.

Does this mean that FAS attenuates in adolescents? Absolutely not. The decreasing specificity of the face and the growth deficiency after puberty only explains why initial identification of people with FAS after puberty can be more difficult. In FAS, the physical features are only the markers for the CNS deficits. As many studies of alcohol teratogenesis have demonstrated, the brain is the most vulnerable organ in the body to the effects of prenatal alcohol exposure (West 1986; Goodlett and West 1992; Streissguth et al. 1993). Although the physical features associated with FAS may change in adolescence, the CNS problems continue, often with more severe repercussions than those experienced in early childhood.

In this 10-year followup study (Streissguth et al. 1985), we also examined the intellectual and behavioral outcomes of these first children with FAS. Of the original 11, 2 had died, and 8 were available for followup. Four were functioning in the borderline-to-dull normal range of intelligence (IQ scores of 76 to 86), and four were clearly mentally retarded, with IQ scores of 20 to 57. (Most IQ tests have a mean of 100 [100 is considered normal] and a standard deviation of 15 points. An IQ of less than 70 is usually considered to reflect mental retardation, and IQ scores of 70 to 85 are considered to be in the borderline range.) The four who were mentally retarded were appropriately managed by schools and society, were in stable foster or adoptive situations, and were in appropriate programs for the mentally retarded, according to accepted guidelines (none were institutionalized).

The four who were *not* officially "mentally retarded" were the ones who seemed headed for trouble in the community, and subsequent observations confirmed this. One boy dropped out of school for the entire fifth grade year and only resumed school after moving to a different State. One girl dropped out of middle school and had a baby soon afterwards. The girl with the highest IQ and whose rearing background had seemed to be the most stable and supportive, ran away from home, lived a transient lifestyle, and became an unmarried teenage mother. The fourth has now been lost to followup. It is apparent that having a higher IQ did not assure these children a higher level of well-being; in a sense, it was not an "advantage." This paradox motivated our next FAS followup study.

Long-Term Consequences of FAS

Studies of adolescents and adults with FAS now have been conducted in several countries. The results show that FAS has lifelong consequences, with outcomes often more complex than those anticipated based on the fact that many patients with FAS are mentally retarded.

We published the first major data-based study of the long-term consequences of FAS in adolescents and adults in 1991 (Streissguth et al. (1991*a*). This study, which involved 61 patients who ranged in age from 12 to 40 (mean age 17 years), confirmed that the physical features of FAS are less distinctive after puberty. Four characteristics of the facial phenotype were noted: (1) continued growth of the nose in two dimensions (height of the nasal bridge and nasal length from root to tip); (2) continued growth of the midfacial region corrected the earlier midfacial hypoplasia; (3) improved soft-tissue modeling of the philtrum and upper lip; and (4) continued growth of the chin. In terms of growth deficiency, 25 percent of the adolescent and adult patients with FAS were not growth deficient for weight, and only 16 percent were not growth deficient for height; 28 percent were not microcephalic. Although the average IQ score of the adolescents and adults was 66, the range of intellectual development was broad; 42

percent had IQ scores not technically in the retarded range. This last finding has serious implications for the availability of appropriate services in schools and the community.

An additional study demonstrated general stability of IQ scores across a 5-year interval ending in adolescence or adulthood (Streissguth and Randels 1991*b*). Although these patients' average academic functioning was at the second to fourth grade level, some did read and spell at a fifth grade level or beyond. A particular deficit in arithmetic skills was noted, which seemed related to difficulty with abstractions such as time and space, cause and effect, and generalizing from one situation to another. The severity of their arithmetic disability, often masked by superficial verbal skills, appeared to be central to their difficulty with independent living and poor judgment and their generally dysfunctional lives (Streissguth et al. 1991*a*).

In an attempt to document and quantify the type of adaptive living deficits noted clinically in our 1985 study, we used the Vineland Adaptive Behavior Scales (VABS) for the larger study of adolescents and adults. Although these patients had an average chronological age of 17 years, their overall level of adaptive functioning was at the 7-year-old level. Of the three domains measured by the VABS, the patients performed best on daily living skills (at an average 9-year-old level) and most poorly on socialization skills (at an average 6-year-old level). On average, these patients also showed significant difficulty with communication, as measured by the VABS. Only a few patients had age-appropriate daily living skills; none were age appropriate in terms of socialization or communication skills. Even patients with FAS or fetal alcohol effects (FAE) who were not technically retarded were frequently characterized on the VABS by such items as failing to consider consequences of their actions, lacking appropriate initiative, being unresponsive to subtle social cues, and lacking reciprocal friendships (Streissguth et al. (1991*a*).

In 1992, LaDue and colleagues published an additional report on this cohort, subsequently expanded to 92 patients, with a mean age of 18.4 years (age range 12 to 42). On a symptom checklist developed for this study, 80 percent of the patients were identified by their caretakers as having attentional problems, 73 percent had memory problems, and 72 percent were or had been hyperactive. On the VABS, 58 percent of the patients were identified as having maladaptive behavior scores in the "significant" range. This is a much higher proportion of patients with severe behavior problems compared with, for example, patients with Down syndrome (e.g., Harris 1988).

A Long-Term Perspective of Fetal Alcohol Syndrome

Long-Term FAS Followup Studies From Europe

Reports from three sites in Germany and one in France have in general confirmed the findings of the Seattle studies. The long-term mental and behavioral consequences of FAS are serious, yet the patients are more difficult to recognize from their physical characteristics as they mature.

In 1992, Lemoine and Lemoine published an important study involving a 30-year followup of Lemoine's original patients from Nantes, France. Many were found in state institutions as adults. Lemoine found that the facial dysmorphology changed radically in many patients, with the small nose and small chin of childhood giving way to a very elongated face with a large nose, a large chin, and coarse features. Lemoine had originally classified his patients in terms of severity of effects; those with the most severe growth deficiency and the most severe physical findings were called severe (75 percent of these patients had clear physical malformations). Others who had characteristic facial features and less severe growth deficiency were called mild (only 10 percent of these patients had physical malformations).

Lemoine found that severity of diagnosis was related to cause of death in patients with FAS. Among the 50 patients with severe FAS, 5 were known to have died, and 4 of these had died as children from severe cardiac problems or from a condition in which there is not enough oxygen in the body's tissues (anoxia). Among the 28 patients with mild FAS in childhood, 2 had committed suicide as adults, and 5 others had attempted suicide.

Lemoine found that mental problems constituted the most severe manifestations of FAS in adulthood, including both intellectual retardation and behavioral problems. He described persistent behavior problems that prevented these patients from effectively using their intellectual potential and even their manual skills. He reported from his clinical observations that patients with FAS often could not focus on their work or their work environment because of their immaturity, considerable instability, and refusal to cooperate. Restlessness and hyperactivity concealed their lack of assurance and initiative and their need for assistance and protection. Although apparently euphoric and excited, they also were fearful, anxious, and depressed. Some were jokesters and comics; others were irritable and aggressive.

Lemoine also reported his observations on 16 additional former patients whom he had seen as children but had not classified as FAS. They had not had the characteristic physical features, although they had psychomotor retardation and alcoholic mothers. As adults, these patients also had significant behavior problems and were described as unable to stay focused on any activity. Six of these 16 patients were found in centers for the moderately disabled as adults. In the course of following up his former patients as adults, Lemoine also noted that 10 of the alcoholic mothers of the children he had diagnosed with FAS had undergone treatment for alcoholism and subsequently given birth to normal children who grew into normal adults.

Based on evaluations of his adult patients and on additional patients identified through the records as children of alcoholic mothers, Lemoine estimated that in five centers serving moderately disabled patients, 20 percent of the population were born to alcoholic mothers (25 of these 33 patients had severe FAS, 8 were without dysmorphic characteristics, and none were classified as mild FAS). In three institutions serving younger and less severely affected children and adolescents, he estimated that 14 percent of the population were born to alcoholic mothers (of these 42 patients, 6 were dysmorphic and 36 were not).

Lemoine concluded that there are severe long-term psychological problems associated with FAS that indicate the need for long-term professional services for these patients, even when they lack the characteristic dysmorphic features. These are the first known data that have attempted to address the prevalence of alcohol-related birth defects in institutions treating disabled persons.

Several studies from Germany also have described the lessening of the growth deficiency and the dysmorphic features associated with FAS as the patients mature physically (Spohr et al. 1987, 1993; Majewski 1993). Stability of IQ over time and the lack of general improvement in school status among adolescents also have been noted by Spohr in a study of 60 children with FAS who ranged in age from 8 to 15 years (1993).

In an important set of studies from Berlin, Steinhausen, a psychiatrist, and Spohr, a pediatrician, have been following a group of children with FAS as they grow older. In addition to confirming the diminished specificity of the facial features and growth deficiency with increasing age, these researchers also have documented the wide range of IQ scores, the general stability of IQ scores over time, and the general absence of change in IQ scores in an improved milieu (Spohr et al. 1987, 1993; Steinhausen et al. 1993, 1994).

What makes these Berlin studies unique is their attempt to quantify the behavioral disabilities often alluded to in the clinical descriptions of persons with FAS, particularly as they approach puberty and maturity. In two recent papers on the psychopathology of FAS, Steinhausen and colleagues (1993, 1994) used structured psychiatric interviews and the Achenbach Child Behavior Checklist, and accompanying Teacher Form, to examine profiles of psychiatric symptomatology. Changes in profiles of psychiatric symptomatology were examined across three ages: preschool, early school age (6 to 12 years), and late school age (13 years and older). Hyperkinetic disorders were the most frequent type of psychopathology at both the pre-school and the early school age period in a group of 27 children examined at both times. By the early school years, earlier problems such as enuresis (urinary incontinence) and eating disorders declined greatly, whereas speech disorders, emotional disorders, and unusual habits and stereotypic behaviors doubled in magnitude, characterizing approximately 45 to 50 percent of the sample.

Although unusual habits and stereotypic behaviors decreased by the late school years, emotional disorders, followed by hyperkinetic disorders, remained present in more than 50 percent of the 33 patients examined at both early and late school years. Conduct disorders remained constant in this group, at around 20 percent. Data from the Achenbach scales revealed attention-deficit problems as the most frequent problem, followed by social relationship problems, with the same pattern manifest at both examinations during the school age period. Both parent and teacher Achenbach scales revealed attentional and social problems to be the most prominent peaks in the symptom profiles. Although boys tended to have higher psychopathology scores than girls, there was little difference in the type of symptoms manifested in children with FAS within these age ranges.

Future Directions for FAS Research

In the past few years, long-term followup studies of patients with FAS have been leading the field in a new direction. No longer can FAS be viewed as just a childhood disability—the changing needs of this population must be considered as they enter the adolescent years, which will (often for the first time) most clearly differentiate them from their peers. It is in early adolescence that many persons with FAS (even prior to a diagnosis) begin to express the feeling that they do not "think quite like everybody else." It is at this age that parents may begin to realize that "just trying harder" is not the whole solution.

No longer can FAS be viewed as just another type of mental retardation. Not only are there many patients with FAS whose intellectual abilities fall well within the normal range, but they also are displaying an increasing and unsettling degree of recognizable psychopathology. Questions remain about the specific etiology of the psychopathology and behavioral disorders. Although it is always tempting to attribute psychopathology to adverse environments—and children with FAS have a greater likelihood of some adversity in their backgrounds—most followup studies of patients with FAS find a weaker than expected relationship.

Clinicians continue to see some patients with FAS who have severe cognitive deficits lasting into adulthood but who have not had adverse rearing environments. Clinicians also continue to see extremely variable outcomes in terms of secondary psychopathology and secondary disabilities that are not easily accounted for by either the level of the patients' overall intellectual ability or the status of their rearing environment. These unsettling discrepancies demonstrate the need for more research: research on the affected patients themselves, research on their genetic predispositions, and research on effective ways to modify and improve behavioral outcome in individual patients.

A recent report of differential outcomes in dizygotic twins (fraternal twins) of alcoholic mothers should stimulate further investigation of the interaction of genetic and teratogenic influences on development (see Streissguth and Dehaene 1993). The almost complete absence of any literature on scientifically based interventions (either pharmacological or behavioral) should prompt researchers to study effective interventions for patients with FAS. It is hoped that the curious oversight by which FAS is not systematically addressed in the literature on children of alcoholics will be resolved so that more studies will focus (as Werner [1986] has done) on individual differences in children of alcoholic mothers and children of alcoholic fathers.

Documentation of prenatal alcohol exposure history should be a necessity in all studies of children of alcoholics, because both short-term (Day 1992) and long-term (Streissguth et al. 1994) consequences of prenatal alcohol exposure per se, even in the absence of maternal alcoholism or alcohol problems, has been reported from several cohort studies. Understanding the specific types of neuropsychological deficits that underlie FAS psychopathology will be an important challenge for the future, as will the complex interactions between individual levels of cognitive deficit and adverse and therapeutic environments.

The clinical work of the past 20 years also has suggested that what were thought to be suitable environmental interventions and educational opportunities for populations of retarded children (such as those with Down syndrome), are often not effective for patients with FAS. In particular, existing treatment and rehabilitative strategies seem less effective for people with FAS who are not classifiable as mentally retarded and for those whose mild cognitive deficits are compounded by attentional deficits or emotional instability.

Understanding the specific characteristics and needs of patients with FAS/FAE will permit development of the most appropriate interventions. Ideally such studies will not focus just on the preschool years and on academic attainment but will take a lifespan approach, with the goal of developing productive citizens who are capable of contributing to society at their own level of endowment. Recognizing the individual and specific needs of groups of patients with different types and etiologies of disabilities is an important current focus in developmental disabilities research (see Burack et al. 1988; Hodapp and Dykens 1991, 1992). This approach is needed for patients with FAS, who often have multidisciplinary problems that involve the home, the schools, the health care system, vocational training, the criminal justice system, and the community.

More and more, the behavioral characteristics of FAS appear broad and diverse rather than tightly constrained around a narrow cognitive dimension. Although some overlap between FAS and existing psychiatric nomenclature has been observed (see Shaywitz et al. 1980; Nanson 1992 and Nanson and Hiscock 1990 on attention deficits and childhood autism), FAS seems to have been largely ignored both in the psychiatric literature and in the psychiatric clinics in the United States. Steinhausen is the only psychiatrist who has published continuing followup studies (e.g., Steinhausen et al. 1993, 1994) that assess specific psychopathologic outcomes in patients with FAS. The recent study by Lemoine and Lemoine (1992) demonstrates the need for understanding prenatal alcohol exposure and FAS as a potential cause of psychiatric disability.

Diagnostic issues in the field are far from resolved. Not only does the diagnosis of FAS include recognizing a wide range of individual capabilities and differences, but there also are many fetal alcohol-affected children whose condition is not diagnosable because of the absence of specific facial characteristics. Without a diagnosis, such individuals often cannot receive the services they require.

As experimental animal studies accrue, an increasing body of research demonstrates both the early and the lifelong behavioral effects of alcohol in offspring who are neither growth deficient nor malformed (see Goodlett and West 1992; Riley 1990; Means et al. 1989). Even prospective longitudinal human cohort studies are showing a variety of behavioral problems at lower doses of alcohol than are necessary to produce physical effects (Day 1992; Streissguth et al. 1993). Further studies that emphasize the behavioral characteristics of alcohol teratogenesis are needed. By and large, it is the behavior and not the growth deficiency or anomalies that present the primary problems to the patients themselves, their families, and society.

The body of research reviewed here, all generated during the past 20 years about a developmental disability that previously had been unknown, is extensive. The research did not lead in the direction initially anticipated when FAS was first identified. Patients with FAS are not all mentally retarded, and their behavioral problems are often more debilitating than their cognitive deficits would suggest.

Acknowledgments

The author would like to thank her dysmorphology colleagues (the late Dr. David W. Smith, and Drs. Kenneth Lyons Jones, James W Hanson, Sterling K. Clarren, Jon Aase, and David F. Smith) for their diagnostic acumen and collaboration. She also thanks Drs. Robin A. LaDue, Heather Carmichael Olson, Karen Kopra-Frye, and Ruth E. Little and Ms. Sandra P. Randels for their collaboration in these studies at the Fetal Alcohol and Drug Unit. Cara C. Ernst, Sue Lippek, and Barbara O'Hara are gratefully acknowledged for technical assistance. Finally, she thanks the patients and their families, who have been such a source of inspiration over the past 20 years.

—by Ann P. Streissguth, PhD.

Ann P. Streissguth, PhD., is professor and director of the Fetal Alcohol and Drug Unit, Department of Psychiatry and Behavioral Sciences, University of Washington. Seattle, Washington.

The writing of this article was supported in part by National Institute on Alcohol Abuse and Alcoholism grant AA01455-01-19, Indian Health Service grant 282-92-0009, Centers for Disease Control and Prevention grant R04/CCR008515-01-03, and gifts through the Seattle Foundation.

References

Burack, J.A.; Hodapp, R.M.; and Zigler, E. Issues in the classification of mental retardation: Differentiating among organic etiologies. *Journal of Child Psychology and Psychiatry* 29(6):765-779, 1988.

Clarren, S.K., and Smith, D.W. The fetal alcohol syndrome. *New England Journal of Medicine* 298(19):1063-1067, 1978.

Day, N.L. Effects of prenatal alcohol exposure. In: Zagon, I.S., and Slotkin, T.A. eds. *Maternal Substance Abuse and the Developing Nervous System*. San Diego: Academic Press, 1992. pp. 27-43.

Dehaene, P.; Samaille-Villette, C.; Samaille, P.–P.; Crépin, G.; Walbaum, R.; Deroubaix, P.; and Blanc-Garin, A.–P. Le syndrome d'alcoolisme fœtal dans le nord de la France. [Fetal alcohol syndrome in the north of France.] *Revue l'Alcoölisme* 23(3):145-158, 1977a.

Goodlett, C.R., and West, J.R. Fetal alcohol effects: Rat model of alcohol exposure during the brain growth spurt. In: Zagon, I.S., and Slotkin, T.A., eds. *Maternal Substance Abuse and the Developing Nervous System*. San Diego: Academic Press, 1992 pp. 45-75.

Harris, J.C. Psychological adaptation and psychiatric disorders in adolescents and young adults with Down syndrome. In: Pueschel, S.M., ed. *The Young Person With Down Syndrome: Transition From Adolescence to Adulthood*. Baltimore: Paul Brookes, 1988. pp. 35-51.

Hodapp, R.M., and Dykens, E.M. Toward an etiology-specific strategy of early intervention with handicapped children. In: Marfo, K., ed. *Early Intervention in Transition: Current Perspectives on Programs for Handicapped Children*. New York: Praeger Publishers, 1991. pp. 41-60.

Hodapp, R.M., and Dykens, E.M. The role of etiology in the education of children with mental retardation. *McGill Journal of Education* 27:165-173, 1992.

Iosub, S.; Fuchs, M.; Bingol, N.; Stone, R.K.; and Gromisch, D.S. Long-term follow-up of three siblings with fetal alcohol syndrome. *Alcoholism: Clinical and Experimental Research* 5(4):523-527, 1981.

Jones, K.L., and Smith, D.W. Recognition of the fetal alcohol syndrome in early infancy. *Lancet* 2(7836):999-1001, 1973.

Jones, K.L.; Smith, D.W.; Ullelend, C.N.; and Streissguth, A.P. Pattern of malformation in offspring of chronic alcoholic mothers. *Lancet* 1(7815):1267-1271, 1973.

LaDue, R.A.; Streissguth, A.P.; and Randels, S.P. Clinical considerations pertaining to adolescents and adults with fetal alcohol syndrome. In: Sonderegger, T.B., ed. *Perinatal Substance Abuse: Research Findings and Clinical Implications*. Baltimore: The Johns Hopkins University Press, 1992. pp. 104-131.

Larsson, G.; Bohlin, A.–B.; and Tunell, R. Prospective study of children exposed to variable amounts of alcohol in utero. *Archives of Disease in Childhood* 60:316-321, 1985.

Lemoine, P., and Lemoine, PH. Avenir des enfants de mères alcooliques (´tude de 105 cas retrouvés à l'âge adulte) et quelques constatations d'intérêt prophylactique. *Annales de Pediatrie* 39:226-235, 1992.

Lemoine, P.; Harousseau, H.; Borteyru, J.P.; and Menuet, J.C. Les enfants de parents alcooliques: Anomalies observees. A propos de 127 cas. [Children of alcoholic parents: Anomalies observed in 127 cases.] *Ouest Medical* 21:476-482, 1968.

Little, R.E., and Streissguth, A.P. Effects of alcohol on the fetus: Impact and prevention. *Canadian Medical Association Journal* 125(2): 159-164, 1981.

Little, R.E.; Young, A.; Streissguth, A.P.; and Uhl, C.N. Preventing fetal alcohol effects: Effectiveness of a demonstration project. In: *Mechanisms of Alcohol Damage in Utero*. Ciba Foundation Symposium 105. London: Pitman, 1984. pp. 254-274.

Little, R.E.; Streissguth, A.P.; Guzinski, G.M.; Uhl, C.N.; Paulozzi, L.; Mann, S.L.; Young, A.; Clarren, S.K.; and Grathwohl, H.L. An evaluation of the pregnancy and health program. *Alcohol Health & Research World* 10(1):44-53, 71, 75, 1985.

Majewski, F. Alcohol embryopathy: Experience in 200 patients. *Developmental Brain Dysfunction* 6:248-265, 1993.

Majewski, F.; Bierich, J.R.; Löser, H.; Michaelis, R.; Leiber, B.; and Bettecken, F. Zur Klinik und Pathogenese der Alkohol-Embryopathie: Bericht über 68 Fälle. [Diagnosis and pathogenesis of alcohol embryopathy: Report of 68 cases] *Münchener Medizinische Wochenschrift* 118(50):1635-1642, 1976.

Means, L.W.; McDaniel, K.; and Pennington, S.N. Embryonic ethanol exposure impairs detour learning in chicks. *Alcohol* 6(4):327-330, 1989.

Nanson, J.L. Autism in fetal alcohol syndrome: A report of six cases. *Alcoholism: Clinical and Experimental Research* 16(3):558-565, 1992.

Nanson, J.L., and Hiscock, M. Attention deficits in children exposed to alcohol prenatally. *Alcoholism: Clinical and Experimental Research* 14(5):656-661, 1990.

National Institute on Alcohol Abuse and Alcoholism. *Seventh Special Report to the U.S. Congress on Alcohol and Health*. DHHS Pub. No. (ADM) 90-1656. Washington, DC: Supt. of Docs., U.S. Govt. Print. Off. 1990.

Olegård, R.; Sabel, K.G.; Aronsson, M.; Sandin, B.; Johansson, P.R.; Carlsson, C.; Kyllerman, M.; Iversen, K.; and Hrbek, A. Effects on the child of alcohol abuse during pregnancy. *Acta Paediatrica Scandinavica Supplement* 275:112-121, 1979.

Public Health Service. Surgeon General's advisory on alcohol and pregnancy. *FDA Drug Bulletin* 11(2):9-10, 1981.

Public Law 100-690, 100th Cong. 2d. sess. Nov. 18, 1988. Alcoholic Beverage Labeling Act of 1988.

Riley, E.P. The long-term behavioral effects of prenatal alcohol exposure in rats. *Alcoholism: Clinical and Experimental Research* 14(5):670-673, 1990.

Rosett, H.L., and Weiner, L. Identifying and treating pregnant patients at risk from alcohol. *Canadian Medical Association Journal* 125(2):149-154, 1981.

Rosett, H.L.; Weiner, L.; Zuckerman, B.; McKinlay, S.; and Edelin, K.C. Reduction of alcohol consumption during pregnancy with benefits to the newborn. *Alcoholism: Clinical and Experimental Research* 4(2):178-184, 1980.

Shaywitz, S.E.; Cohen, D.J.; and Shaywitz, B.A. Behavior and learning difficulties in children of normal intelligence born to alcoholic mothers. *Journal of Pediatrics* 96(6):978-982, 1980.

Spohr, H.L., and Steinhausen, H.C. Follow-up studies of children with fetal alcohol syndrome. *Neuropediatrics* 18(1):13-17, 1987.

Spohr, H.L.; Willms, J.; and Steinhausen, H.C. Prenatal alcohol exposure and long-term developmental consequences. *Lancet* 341(8850): 907-910, 1993.

Steinhausen, H.C.; Willms, J.; and Spohr, H.L. Long-term psychopathological and cognitive outcome of children with fetal alcohol syndrome. *Journal of the American Academy of Child and Adolescent Psychiatry* 32(5):990-994, 1993.

Steinhausen, H.C.; Willms, J.; and Spohr, H.L. Correlates of psychopathology and intelligence in children with fetal alcohol syndrome. *Journal of the American Academy of Child and Adolescent Psychiatry* 35:323-331, 1994.

Streissguth, A.P., and Dehaene, P. Fetal alcohol syndrome in twins of alcoholic mothers: Concordance of diagnosis and IQ. *American Journal of Medical Genetics* 47:857-861, 1993.

Streissguth, A.P., and Little, R.E. *Alcohol: Pregnancy and the Fetal Alcohol Syndrome*. Krock Foundation Slide Curriculum on Alcoholism, Unit 9: Alcohol and Pregnancy. Timonium, MD: Milner-Fenwick, Inc., 1994.

Streissguth, A.P.; Herman, C.S.; and Smith, D.W. Stability of intelligence in the fetal alcohol syndrome: A preliminary report. *Alcoholism: Clinical and Experimental Research* 2(2):165-170, 1978.

Streissguth, A.P.; Clarren, S.K.; and Jones, K.L. Natural history of the Fetal Alcohol Syndrome: A ten-year follow-up of eleven patients. *Lancet* 2:85-91, 1985.

Streissguth, A.P.; Aase, J.M.; Clarren, S.K.; Randels, S.P.; LaDue, R.A.; and Smith, D.F. Fetal alcohol syndrome in adolescents and adults. *Journal of the American Medical Association* 265(15):1961-1967, 1991*a*.

Streissguth, A.P.; Randels, S.P.; and Smith, D.F. A test-retest study of intelligence in patients with fetal alcohol syndrome: Implications for care. *Journal of the American Academy of Child and Adolescent Psychiatry* 30(4):584-587, 1991*b*.

Streissguth, A.P.; Bookstein, F.L.; Sampson, P.D.; and Barr, H.M. *The Enduring Effects of Prenatal Alcohol Exposure on Child Development: Birth Through 7 Years, a Partial Least Squares Solution*. Ann Arbor, MI: University of Michigan Press, 1993.

Streissguth, A.P.; Sampson, P.D.; Carmichael Olson, H.; Bookstein, F.L.; Barr, H.M.; Scott, M.; Feldman, J.; and Mirsky, A.F. Maternal drinking during pregnancy: Attention and short-term memory in 14-year-old offspring: A longitudinal prospective study. *Alcoholism: Clinical and Experimental Research* 14(1):202-218, 1994.

Werner, E.E. Resilient offspring of alcoholics: A longitudinal study from birth to age 18. *Journal of Studies on Alcohol* 47(1):34-40, 1986.

West, J.R., ed. *Alcohol and Brain Development*. New York: Oxford University Press, 1986.

Chapter 25

Tracking the Prevalence of Fetal Alcohol Syndrome

Surveillance programs allow the tracking of the prevalence of a condition over time. Tracking the prevalence of FAS poses particular problems, however, as there is no "gold standard" of diagnosis. To evaluate the effectiveness of prevention efforts, surveillance techniques must be refined.

Fetal alcohol syndrome (FAS) is a birth defect that causes significant lifetime disabilities (Abel 1990). But unlike many other birth defects, FAS, which is caused by maternal alcohol abuse during pregnancy, is preventable (Abel 1990). In fact, prevention of FAS is a national health priority included in the *Healthy People 2000* objectives for health promotion and disease prevention (U.S. Department of Health and Human Services 1990 [USDHHS]). The specific health objective is to reduce the rate of FAS to no more than 1.2 cases per 10,000 live births by the year 2000.

Baseline data for this objective were derived from a national hospital-based epidemiologic surveillance program of birth defects — the Birth Defects Monitoring Program (BDMP) of the Centers for Disease Control and Prevention (CDC). Although the rate of 5.2 cases per 10,000 live births in 1992 seems to be an increase over the baseline rate of 2.2 cases per 10,000 (USDHHS 1990), it more likely represents improvements over recent years in recognition and reporting of FAS at birth.

Excerpted from *Alcohol-Related Birth Defects*, National Institute on Alcohol Abuse and Alcoholism (NIAAA), NIH Pub. No. 94-3466, 1994

In this chapter, we review the challenges of developing simple and efficient State-based and national epidemiologic surveillance that can track what progress is being made toward meeting the *Healthy People 2000* objective for FAS.

Epidemiologic Surveillance

CDC defines epidemiologic surveillance as the ongoing systematic collection, analysis, and interpretation of health data that are essential to the planning, implementation, and evaluation of public health practice (Thacker et al. 1989). Such surveillance is closely integrated with timely dissemination of these data to anyone who requires this information. To monitor progress in meeting the FAS prevention objective, epidemiologic surveillance is needed to evaluate changes in the rate of FAS over time.

Methodological Problems

Diagnosing FAS. Developing surveillance of FAS presents unique challenges Because there is no simple, objective laboratory test for diagnosing FAS, diagnosis is based primarily on clinical definitions developed for the purpose of clinical practice and research (Sokol and Clarren 1989). To meet the clinical FAS case definition, the patient must exhibit symptoms in each of the following three categories: (1) prenatal or postnatal growth retardation; (2) central nervous system abnormalities; and (3) characteristic abnormal facial features (dysmorphology), including short palpebral fissures (eye openings), an elongated midface, a long and flattened philtrum (area between the nose and mouth), and a thin upper lip. It is also helpful to determine if the patient was exposed prenatally to alcohol, but diagnosis can still be made if such information is unavailable (Sokol and Clarren 1989).

Applying these diagnostic criteria requires expertise in recognizing dysmorphic features. Moreover, the clinical features of a child with FAS may change with age (Streissguth et al. 1991; see Chapter 24). There is encouraging evidence that the clinical recognition and reporting of FAS is improving (CDC 1993a). However, such improvements may prove troublesome by clouding the true changes in the rate of FAS over time.

Collecting data. CDC includes FAS in its two birth-defects surveillance programs. The first program is the BDMP, which relies on reported hospital discharge diagnoses of newborns that use the *International Classification of Diseases, Ninth Revision, Clinical Modification* (ICD-9-CM) (World Health Organization 1989). This program started monitoring FAS after 1979 when the ICD-9 introduced a code (760.71) that could be applied to the syndrome.

The second program is the Metropolitan Atlanta Congenital Defects Program (MACDP) (Lynberg et al. 1990), which started in 1968 and is the oldest active case-ascertainment birth-defects surveillance program in the United States. It monitors all births occurring in the five-county metropolitan Atlanta area—currently about 38,000 per year. The MACDP, unlike the BDMP, uses multiple sources to identify diagnoses of FAS in newborns and infants, including obstetrical, nursery, and pediatric logs. In addition, the MACDP identifies cases of FAS diagnosed through the first year of life, not solely at birth.

Because the BDMP, the MACDP, and other birth-defects surveillance programs examine only the medical records rather than the children directly, they rely on clinicians recognizing the condition and recording the diagnosis in the patient's medical record. Further, the BDMP relies on the diagnosis of FAS during the newborn's hospital admission and the recording of that diagnosis in the baby's discharge record. The MACDP, on the other hand, detects diagnoses mentioned anywhere in a medical record, throughout the first year of a child's life.

Designing a Surveillance Program

Three important attributes of a successful surveillance program are sensitivity, predicted value positive, and representativeness (Klaucke 1992). These are defined and discussed below.

Sensitivity of Surveillance

Sensitivity is a measure of how well the surveillance program detects cases of a condition. The greater the percentage of cases identified, the greater the chance to identify true changes in the rate of the condition over time.

Underdiagnosis. A case definition that only captures some of the FAS cases will decrease the surveillance program's sensitivity. Sensitivity also will be decreased when surveillance is based only on clinical recognition of FAS, because the condition may sometimes be hard to discern. For example, the facial features that are characteristic of

FAS can be missed by clinicians who may not be familiar with dysmorphology (Morse et al. 1992).

During a 6-year period, a separate longitudinal study examined prenatal exposure to alcohol in a large metropolitan hospital in Atlanta (Cordero et al. 1990). The study examined babies born at the hospital between 1980 and 1986, using a systematic checklist specific to the features of FAS. The concurrence of the study and the MACDP surveillance program allowed a comparison of their rates of diagnosis. Only 38 percent of the FAS cases diagnosed by the longitudinal study also were diagnosed by the MACDP (Cordero et al. 1990). This may indicate a lack of clinical recognition, a failure to record findings in the medical record, the use of variable criteria for the case definition, or a combination of all of these by the MACDP program.

Underreporting of diagnosis. Another potential bias is that FAS may be recognized and recorded in medical records at different rates in different populations. About 75 percent of all recorded cases of FAS in the MACDP came from a large inner-city hospital that serves the poor and uninsured. Between 1975 and 1989, the inner-city hospital reported 88 FAS cases out of 98,000 births, whereas a comparable large suburban hospital reported 3 cases out of 72,000 births over the same period. Although it is possible that the rate of FAS in the two hospitals truly is different, lack of recognition of FAS, not recording the diagnosis, and bias in suspecting diagnosis should be evaluated as potential reasons for the difference.

In another study, which looked at the rate of diagnosis of FAS by pediatricians, a survey in Massachusetts found that among pediatricians who reported ever making a diagnosis of FAS, 9 percent also reported not recording the diagnosis in the medical record (Morse et al. 1992). The reasons for not recording the diagnosis were not explored. Regardless of whether the diagnosis is missed or not recorded, both events decrease the sensitivity of FAS surveillance and therefore will cause the underestimation of the rate of FAS.

Using a limited population. The child's age when the diagnosis of FAS is made also may affect the sensitivity of the surveillance program. Surveillance of FAS based on newborn diagnosis will likely have a low sensitivity, because some affected newborns may have subtle facial abnormalities, inapparent central nervous system deficits, and normal birth weight (Abel and Sokol 1991). In addition, clinical, behavioral, and facial features may vary with the age of the child beyond the newborn period (Streissguth et al. 1985). In the MACDP, about 78 percent of the FAS cases were diagnosed during the newborn period (unpublished data). Surveillance programs that focus on the diagnosis of FAS at a specific age may tend to have lower sensitivity than others that cover all age groups.

In summary, several factors will affect the sensitivity of FAS surveillance. They include underdiagnosis, lack of recording of the diagnosis in the medical record, the possibility of stereotyping populations, inclusion of a limited population subset, and a restrictive case definition.

Predictive Value Positive

A good surveillance program for FAS must identify the rate of true cases of FAS. Each case recorded using the surveillance case definition should have a high probability of being a true case of FAS. Predictive value positive (PVP) is the measure of how accurately cases are diagnosed given the nature of the case definition. FAS presents a particularly challenging situation for estimating PVP because there is no known "gold standard" for diagnosis. Even knowledgeable dysmorphologists often disagree about clinical diagnoses of FAS.

Low PVP. A case definition that allows inclusion of noncases will decrease the PVP of the surveillance. For example, if an FAS surveillance program uses a case definition of intrauterine growth retardation and a history of maternal alcohol abuse only but not the dysmorphic facial features, it is likely that many cases included under that definition may not meet the clinical criteria of FAS.

Clinical features in each of the three categories of the current case definition are not unique to FAS; they may result from many different causes. For example, the general definition of intrauterine growth retardation is weight and length below the 10th percentile for gestational age. Using this definition, about 10 percent of all newborns would meet this criterion, most of whom will not have FAS.

High PVP. Selecting a case definition that has a high PVP may decrease the sensitivity of the surveillance program. One can develop a definition for a condition that has such a high PVP that there is little doubt that each recorded case is a true case of the condition. Such a specific definition, however, also may miss many true cases, thereby greatly lowering the program's sensitivity.

An example of this dilemma is a report of the sensitivity and PVP of isotretinoin embryopathy, or birth defects caused by maternal use of retinoic acid. The case definition with the highest PVP had a sensitivity of only about 16 percent (i.e., 84 percent of all true cases were missed) (Lynberg et al. 1990). However, the case definition avoided counting false cases. If the intent of the surveillance is to follow the trends of a condition, without trying to ascertain its incidence, such an approach may be adequate. In the situation of FAS, however, determining the incidence is quite important, given the current *Healthy People 2000* objective and the potential use of the surveillance as a registry that may track access of services to affected children.

Representativeness

Representativeness is the ability of the surveillance program to reflect accurately the occurrence of the condition over time in the population of interest.

A major purpose of FAS surveillance on a national level is to gauge the trends in the U.S. population. Representativeness ensures that the picture painted by the surveillance program reflects the picture of the Nation. For example, using data from the BDMP, Chávez and colleagues (1988) found that the reported rate of FAS varies by race and ethnic group. If the surveillance is not population based, as with the case of the BDMP, and the racial and ethnic distribution does not reflect that of the general population, the findings may not be generalized except with appropriate adjustments.

The rate of FAS in a population is dependent on the rate of maternal alcohol abuse during pregnancy. If a specific sub-population included in the surveillance program has a rate of alcohol abuse during pregnancy different from that of the general population, the representativeness of the surveillance also will be affected. Stereotyping that affects the program's definition or diagnosis of FAS also can affect representativeness.

Estimating the Extent of the Problem

The Estimates

The estimated birth prevalence of FAS among newborns identified through the BDMP increased from about 1 case per 10,000 live births in 1979 to 5.2 cases per 10,000 live births in 1992 (Figure 25.1) (CDC

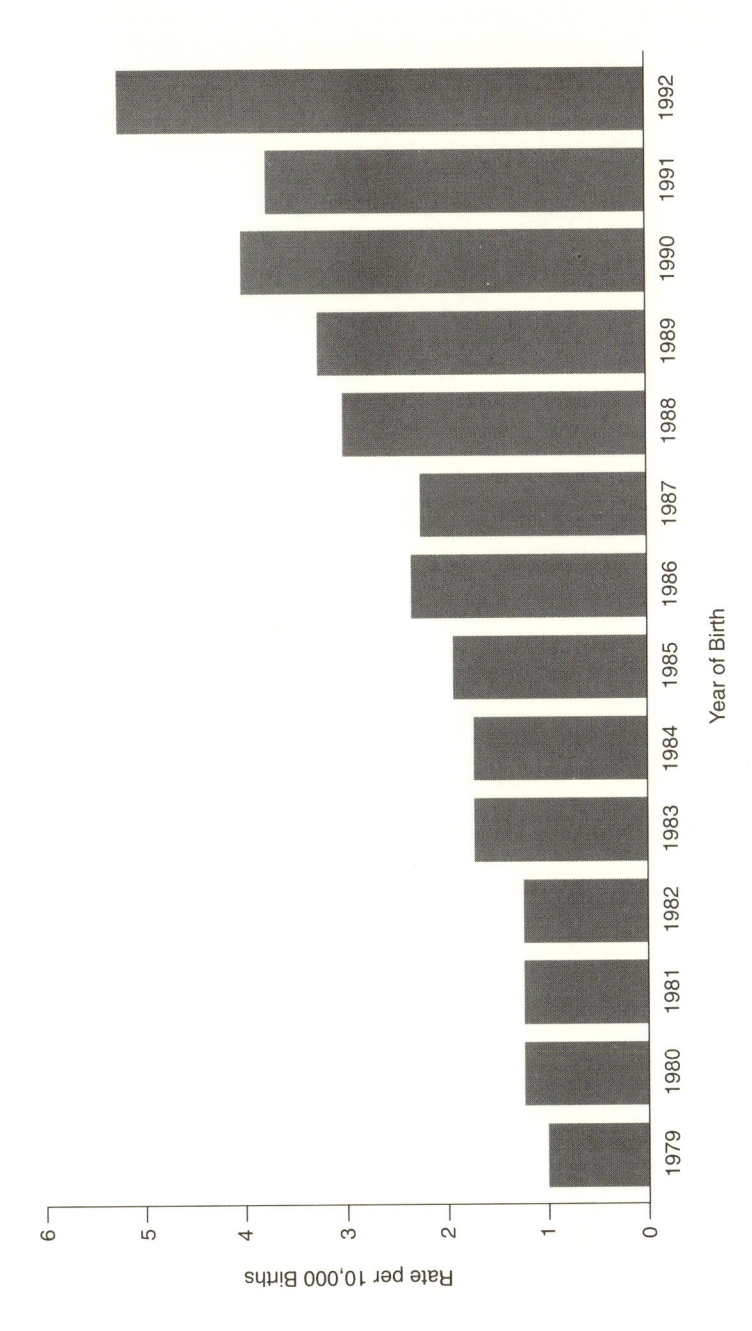

Tracking the Prevalence of Fetal Alcohol Syndrome

Figure 25.1. Reported incidence rate of fetal alcohol syndrome, by year of birth, from the Birth Defects Monitoring Program of the Centers for Disease Control and Prevention, 1979-1992.

1993a). As mentioned above, the BDMP is based on doctors recording the ICD-9-CM FAS diagnosis code at discharge from the hospital of birth, and the program has not been evaluated in terms of its sensitivity and PVP. In 1992, the MACDP reported a rate of 3.3 cases per 10,000 live births. Both programs crudely estimate the average incidence of FAS for the reporting period 1979-1992 as 2 cases per 10,000 live births (Lynberg and Edmonds 1992). It is difficult to tell whether the reported increase during the last decade represents a true increase or the increased awareness and improved reporting among health care professionals. Interestingly, Serdula and colleagues (1991) reported that between 1985 and 1988, the percentage of women who drank during pregnancy actually *declined*. However, this decline was not evident for less educated women and women under age 25 years.

Abel and Sokol (1991) estimated the rate of FAS to be 3.3 cases per 10,000 live births. This estimate is based on the results of 15 prospective studies and 4 surveillance studies from Australia, New Zealand, Sweden, the United Kingdom, and the United States (Abel and Sokol 1991). None of these studies was population based. (An earlier study of Abel and Sokol [1987] that surveyed 19 published epidemiologic studies worldwide reported an overall rate from all studies of 1.9 cases of FAS per 1,000 live births [i.e., 19 cases per 10,000 live births].)

Limitations of the Estimates

Potential limitations of the CDC data sources include decreased sensitivity arising from decreased recognition of FAS in newborns (CDC 1993a), possible failure to incorporate the FAS diagnosis into the medical records (CDC 1993b), and the possible inappropriate use of the ICD-9-CM FAS code for reporting prenatal exposure to alcohol. The MACDP and the BDMP were designed primarily to monitor major birth defects in infants—to identify structural birth defects that are evident at birth or have significant clinical manifestations during the first year of life. They were not designed to track syndromes such as FAS that have few major birth defects.

In their estimate, Abel and Sokol (1991) did not use data that were population based, and they did not include minorities, Native Americans in particular. This omission may underestimate the rate of FAS. A recent survey of FAS among Native Alaskans reported an FAS rate of 21 cases per 10,000 live births (CDC 1993b).

Improving FAS Surveillance

Given the limitations of current national FAS surveillance, researchers must improve it by systematically determining the strengths and shortcomings of existing surveillance, for example, through evaluation of the sensitivity, PVP, and representativeness of these existing programs. In addition to improving the national surveillance program, researchers should focus attention on State-based FAS surveillance. The proportion of hospitals participating in the BDMP is declining, and participation in some States is insufficient to estimate rates of FAS for these States.

The first task in improving surveillance is to develop a uniform case definition of FAS that optimally balances sensitivity with precision and can be used for surveillance. This should be followed by uniformity in application of the case definition. Also, the development of sensitive and specific screening instruments, including biologic markers, could contribute greatly to better epidemiologic data in this field. The second task is to ensure uniformity in methods of reporting data and in surveillance programs to receive the data. The combined effort of all concerned with the prevention of FAS will help make improved surveillance of FAS a reality.

Acknowledgments

The authors would like to thank Joseph Hollowell and J. David Erickson for their review and comments.

—by José F. Cordero, M.D., M.P.H.;
R. Louise Floyd, D.S.N., R.N.;
M. Louise Martin, D.V.M., M.S.;
Margarett Davis, M.D., M.P.H.;
and Karen Hymbaugh, M.P.A.

José E. Cordero, M.D., M.P.H., is assistant director for science; R. Louise Floyd, D.S.N., R.N., is chief of the Fetal Alcohol Prevention Section; M. Louise Martin, D.V.M., M.S., is chief of the Surveillance Unit; Margarett Davis, M.D., M.P.H., is medical epidemiologist; and Karen Hymbaugh, M.P.A., is behavioral scientist in the Division of Birth Defects and Developmental Disabilities, National Center for Environmental Health, Centers for Disease Control and Prevention, Atlanta, Georgia.

References

Abel, E.L. *Fetal Alcohol Syndrome*. Oradell, NJ: Medical Economics Company Inc., 1990.

Abel, E.L., and Sokol, R.J. Incidence of fetal alcohol syndrome and economic impact of FAS related anomalies. *Drug and Alcohol Dependence* 19(1):51-70, 1987.

Abel, E.L., and Sokol, R.J. A revised conservative estimate of the incidence of FAS and its economic impact. *Alcoholism: Clinical and Experimental Research* 15(3):514-524, 1991.

Centers for Disease Control and Prevention. Fetal alcohol syndrome—United States, 1979-1992. *Morbidity and Mortality Weekly Report* 42:339-341, 1993*a*.

Centers for Disease Control and Prevention. Linking multiple data sources in fetal alcohol syndrome surveillance—Alaska. *Morbidity and Mortality Weekly Report* 42:312-314, 1993*b*.

Chávez, G.F.; Cordero, J.F.; and Becerra, J.E. Leading major congenital malformations among minority groups in the United States, 1981-1986. *Morbidity and Mortality Weekly Report: CDC Surveillance Summaries* 37:17-24, 1988.

Cordero, J.F.; Tosca, M.; Falek, A.; Coles, C.; Smith, I.; and Fernhoff, P. The sensitivity of surveillance systems in detecting fetal alcohol syndrome (FAS) and alcohol related defects (ARD) (Abstract). *Proceedings of Greenwood Genetics Center* 9:88, 1990.

Klaucke, D.N. Evaluating public health surveillance systems. In: Halperin, W.; Baker, E.L.; and Monson, R.R., eds. *Public Health Surveillance*. New York: Van Norstand Reinhold, 1992. pp. 26-41.

Lynberg, M.C., and Edmonds, L.D. Surveillance of birth defects. In: Halperin, W.; Baker, E.L.; and Monson, R.R., eds. *Public Health Surveillance*. New York: Van Nostrand Reinhold, 1992.

Lynberg, M.C.; Khoury, M.J.; Lammer, E.J.; Waller, K.O.; Cordero, J.F.; and Erickson, J.D. Sensitivity, specificity, and positive predictive value of multiple malformations in isotretinoin embryopathy surveillance. *Teratology* 42:513-520, 1990.

Morse, B.A.; Idelson, R.K.; Sachs, W.H.; Weiner, L.; and Kaplan, L.C. Pediatricians' perspectives on fetal alcohol syndrome. *Journal of Substance Abuse* 4(2):187-195, 1992.

Serdula, M.; Williamson, D.F.; Kendrick, J.S.; Anda, R.F.; and Byers, T. Trends in alcohol consumption by pregnant women: 1985 through 1988. *Journal of the American Medical Association* 265(7):876-879, 1991.

Sokol, R.J., and Clarren, S.K. Guidelines for use of terminology describing the impact of prenatal alcohol on the offspring. *Alcoholism: Clinical and Experimental Research* 13(4):597-598, 1989.

Streissguth, A.P.; Clarren, S.K.; and Jones, K.L. Natural history of the fetal alcohol syndrome: A 10-year follow-up of eleven patients *Lancet* 2(8446):85-91, 1985.

Streissguth, A.P.; Aase, J.M.; Clarren, S.K.; Randels, S.P.; LaDue, R.A.; and Smith, D.F. Fetal alcohol syndrome in adolescents and adults. *Journal of the American Medical Association* 265:1961-1967, 1991.

Thacker, S.B.; Berkelman, R.L.; and Stroup, D.F. The science of public health surveillance. *Journal of Public Health Policy* 10:187-203, 1989.

U.S. Department of Health and Human Services. *Healthy People 2000: National Health Promotion and Disease Prevention Objectives*. DHHS Pub. No. (PHS)91-50212. Washington, DC: Supt. of Docs., U.S. Govt. Print. Off., 1990.

World Health Organization. *International Classification of Diseases, 9th Revision, Clinical Modification*. Vol. 1. Ann Arbor, MI: Commission on Professional and Hospital Activities, 1989.

Part Five

Other Congenital Disorders

Chapter 26

Congenital Heart Defects

How the Heart Works

The heart (Figure 26.1) is a muscular four-chambered organ that lies under the sternum, or breastbone. It is usually easy to feel the apex or tip of the heart in the left side of the chest, just below the nipple. In young children, because the chest wall is thin, you can often see the heart beating. If you feel your own pulse or heartbeat while you are sitting relaxed, you will find that the rate is somewhere between fifty and eighty beats per minute. The beats follow one another regularly, although if you take a deep breath the rate speeds up a little as you breathe in and slows as you breathe out. The rate of the heart varies with age and with the demands of the body. A baby's heart rate is likely to be faster than an adult's, probably around 100 beats per minute. A young baby's heart rate will al also vary more than an adult's, and changes in rate will occur more quickly.

How the Heart Develops in the Embryo and Fetus

All defects in the heart and all types of heart disease are caused by some disturbance in the development or functioning of one of the

---

Neill, Catherine A., MD; Clark, Edward B., MD; and Clark, Carleen, RN. *The Heart of a Child*. pp 36-37, 41-45, 76-76, 80-82, 94-95, 97-106, 109-11, 113-18, 331, and 313-23; Figures 2.2 and 5.1. ©1992. The Johns Hopkins University Press. Reprinted with permission.

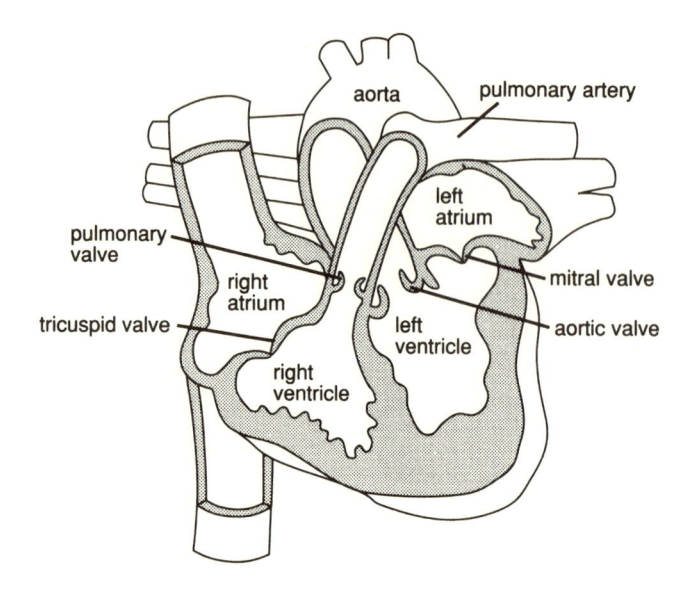

Figure 26.1. *The Normal Heart. The normal heart is separated into right and left sides by walls (septa); each heart chamber has a wall around it consisting of a delicate membrane, the pericardium (not labeled); a layer of muscle, the myocardium (shown shaded); and a smooth inner lining, the endocardium (not labeled). The normal heart has four valves, the tricuspid and pulmonary valves on the right, the mitral and aortic valves on the left.*

parts of the normal heart. The heart begins as a simple, almost primitive structure, quite different from the complex four-chambered organ that is the center of a child's circulation. It begins with two tubes that appear side by side in the midline of the embryo; these tubes join or fuse together and produce the early heart tube. This cardiac tube, made of muscle cells only about three to five cell layers thick, becomes the cardiac muscle or myocardium. The myocardial (heart muscle) cells surround a collection of complex proteins called cardiac jelly, which later plays a big role in forming the heart valves. The cardiac tube is lined with a delicate single layer of cells that will later become the inner lining of the heart, or endocardium.

By the seventeenth day, the mitochondria have been supplied with enzymes that power the movement or contraction of the primitive myocardial cells, and the heart of the embryo has begun to beat. (The genetic and chemical processes controlling these amazingly rapid changes are now being studied in chick embryos and other models.)

Congenital Heart Defects

Looping of the Heart: Looping Defects

By the twenty-third day after conception the human embryo is 2.2 millimeters long. The heart tube now has four layers: the endocardium, the myocardium, the cardiac jelly, and an outer layer of cells called the pericardium. The heart now twists or loops toward the right. This looping of the heart is under very strong genetic control; only very occasionally does the loop go in the opposite direction. When this happens we say that a looping defect is present. This is the first thing that can go wrong in the fetus's developing heart.

By the time the embryo is five millimeters long (approximately twenty-seven days) blood is already circulating from the heart to the rest of the embryo, although the oxygen and nutrition needed for fetal growth continue to come from the placenta, which will supply these needs until the time of birth. The heart tube is now folding on itself. The receiving chamber, or atrium, now lies nearer to the embryo's head than does the pumping chamber, the primitive ventricle. The ventricle leads into a large single vessel called the truncus arteriosus, or truncus, which later divides into two vessels, the aorta and the pulmonary artery.

Cardiac Jelly to Endocardial Cushions: Endocardial Cushion Defects

The cardiac jelly becomes more elaborate and helps to form the endocardial cushions. These cushions gradually thin out and play an important part in forming the delicate yet tough heart valves and part of both septa. In one serious form of heart defect, this jelly does not separate properly: it seems somehow to have been wrongly programmed. As a result, a complete atrioventricular canal remains in the center of the heart. This canal is normal in embryos of about nine millimeters or thirty days, but if still present at birth, it can cause much difficulty. Such atrioventricular canal defects are frequent in Down syndrome.

The Developing Aorta and Pulmonary Artery: Conotruncal Defects

Some important cells have moved into the upper pole of the heart tube from the primitive nervous system and the arches that form the head and neck. These migrating ("neural crest") cells later take part in forming the connection between the heart and the lungs. At the same time as the ventricles are beginning to separate, changes are taking place in the truncus and in the area of the heart leading from the ventricle to the truncus. The changes in this conotruncal area are complicated and are still the subject of some argument. However, two important events are known to occur. First, a spiral wall or septum grows vertically in the conotruncus, separating it into two arteries, the aorta and the pulmonary artery. These two arteries form by equal division and are approximately equal in size. Second, the artery to the lungs, or pulmonary artery, comes to lie in front of the aorta and to join the right ventricle. When this spiraling goes awry, a conotruncal defect is the result.

Septation of the Walls of the Heart and Development of the Heart Valves: Septal Defects and Heart Flow Defects

Between the twenty-seventh and thirty-seventh days of development the two atria become separated by a wall, the atrial septum. However, this wall continues to have a small opening in it—called the foramen ovale because of its oval shape—and blood can pass between the atria until the time of birth. A wall grows between the ventricles, made up partly of muscle and partly of tissues coming from the cardiac jelly. The growth of the walls separating the right and left sides of the heart is called septation. Septal defects—failure of completion of the atrial or ventricular septum—are among the most common childhood heart problems.

The aortic and pulmonary valves develop from endocardial cushion tissue as the truncus is dividing. At first the valves are little bumps or ridges in the truncus wall; then they thin out to become thin delicate valves, each with three cusps that meet perfectly as they close. These valves develop during the time that the embryo is growing from fourteen to forty millimeters in length, so they are still forming while most of the heart has already developed into the four chambers needed for life outside the womb.

The size of the two ventricles is critically important to life after birth. If the right ventricle is too small, not enough blood reaches the lungs. Even worse, if the left ventricle is too small, too little blood will reach the body. Our present understanding is that the two ventricles divide equally early in embryonic life, probably by seven weeks, when the embryo is fourteen to fifteen millimeters long. If something disturbs the normal flow of blood through the early heart, the growth of that particular chamber may be affected.

During life in the womb, the right ventricle is the dominant one. Most of the blood returning to the fetal heart bypasses the lungs, reaching the left ventricle through the hole in the atrial septum (the foramen ovale), or it passes from the pulmonary artery to the aorta through the ductus arteriosus. The foramen ovale and the ductus arteriosus are important during life in the womb, but they normally close soon after birth.

Atrial Septal Defects (ASD)

An ASD is an opening or defect in the middle part of the wall between the right and left atrium. It usually occurs in otherwise healthy children, more often in girls than in boys.

In the womb there is always a small opening in the fetus's atrial septum. Because of its oval shape, this opening is called the foramen ovale (*foramen* = opening). Before birth, blood flows from the right atrium to the left through the foramen. At birth the pressure in the left atrium rises, and blood flow through the foramen ends; eventually the foramen seals off completely. If blood flow into the right ventricle is lower than normal before birth, however, more blood is forced through the atrial septum and a larger than normal opening persists after birth. This is an ASD. Because the pressure is higher in the left atrium than the right after birth, blood flows from the left to the right atrium. As a result of excessive blood flow into the right side of the heart, the right atrium and ventricle and the pulmonary artery all dilate, becoming larger than normal to accommodate the extra blood.

Ventricular Septal Defects

A ventricular septal defect (VSD) is an opening or defect in the wall or septum between the right and left ventricle. Most VSDs are in the upper part of the septum, where the septum is thin like a parchment or membrane; they are often called membranous or perimembranous VSDs. It is not surprising they are so frequent, because closure in this area requires at least four different structures to join perfectly together, so there are many possibilities for mistiming. The lower part of the septum is thicker and contains more muscle fibers than the upper membranous part; a defect low in the septum is called a muscular VSD.

Patent Ductus Arteriosus

Patent ductus arteriosus is a persistence after birth of the fetal channel or ductus that has joined the aorta and the pulmonary artery. In the fetus, blood flows from the pulmonary artery to the aorta down the ductus, but at birth the muscle in the wall of the ductus normally tightens up or constricts because it is sensitive to the new, higher level of oxygen in the blood. Blood thus stops passing through the ductus a few hours after birth. However, the ductus may remain open after birth, either in a small premature infant whose ductus muscle is not mature enough to react to changes in oxygen (the most usual case) or, much less frequently, in a full-term infant whose ductus muscle is defective.

Immediately after birth, blood flow through the ductus is usually from the aorta to the pulmonary artery because the pressure in the aorta is now higher. Only if there is a severe lung problem does blood flow from the right side of the heart to the left side, as it did before birth.

Occasionally, all three types of defect occur together, and the child has an open (patent) ductus and both an ASD and a VSD. Fortunately, all three of these defects can usually be repaired in surgery at the same time.

Valves of the Heart

In infants in whom septation (the division of the heart into two sides) is normal, the valves or the chambers on one side or the other may fail to develop properly, probably because blood flow through the heart has been disturbed in some way before birth. Usually such obstruction is caused by thickening of one or more of the heart valves: if the valve leading into or out of a ventricle is badly malformed, the ventricle itself may fail to grow and at birth may be too small to take over its role as an effective pumping chamber. When the tricuspid or pulmonary valve, the pulmonary artery, or the right ventricle is abnormal, we say that a right-heart flow defect is present. Such defects range from a mild bicuspid pulmonary valve to the severe problem of a hypoplastic (small) right ventricle, which requires treatment immediately after birth. When the obstruction involves the left side of the heart, the mitral or aortic valve, or the aorta or the left ventricle, a left-heart flow defect is present. These defects also vary a great deal in severity, from a mild bicuspid aortic valve to the life-threatening hypoplastic left ventricle.

Conotruncal Defects

In the normal heart, blood returning from the body passes to the right ventricle, the pulmonary artery, and then to the lungs to receive a new supply of oxygen. The conotruncal area of the heart provides this vital connection between heart and lungs. When this area has not developed normally before birth, blood does not reach the lungs as it should and oxygen levels in the blood are too low. This low oxygen level in the arteries and tissues of the body results in a blue color known as cyanosis, from the Greek word cyan (blue).

The skin of newborn babies often shows a bluish color immediately after birth, but after a few vigorous cries the lungs fill with oxygen and the blueness disappears. A baby who remains persistently blue, even after the administration of oxygen, is said to be cyanotic. Cyanosis is sometimes caused by a problem in the lungs requiring treatment with a ventilator. In other infants cyanosis is due to a conotruncal heart defect, usually either tetralogy of Fallot or transposition of the great arteries. All conotruncal defects are serious and require surgery, which can now usually be performed in the first weeks or months of life.

Tetralogy of Fallot

Tetralogy of Fallot (named for the nineteenth-century French cardiologist Arthur Fallot) is the most usual cause of cardiac cyanosis, occurring in about three of every ten thousand children born. Successful treatment first became available more than forty years ago; a number of adults who are now leading healthy lives were born with this defect and had successful surgery.

The word *tetralogy* (from the Greek tetra, four) implies correctly that there are four defects. Two of these are of major importance. The first, pulmonary stenosis, is an obstruction of blood flow to the lungs resulting from a narrowing of the outflow area connecting the right ventricle to the pulmonary artery. It usually affects the pulmonary valve and the infundibular area below the valve. The more severe the pulmonary stenosis, the less blood reaches the child's lungs with each heartbeat, and the worse the cyanosis or blueness. The second important defect is a large ventricular septal defect, causing blood to mix freely between the two ventricles (Figure 26.2).

In addition to the two major defects, tetralogy includes two minor, or secondary, defects. The first is an overriding aorta. The term overriding

Congenital Disorders Sourcebook

means that the ventricular septal defect lies immediately beneath the aorta, so the aorta "overrides" both the right and the left ventricle. The aorta receives blue venous blood from the right ventricle mixed with normal, fully oxygenated blood from the left ventricle, a mix that results in cyanosis. The other minor defect is thickening of the right ventricular wall, or right ventricular hypertrophy, which develops when the ventricular septal defect is large and causes equal pressure in the right and left ventricles; the wall of the right ventricle then becomes thickened or hypertrophied as a result of this high pressure.

Variants of tetralogy of Fallot are important, because they may affect the timing of surgical repair and how much can be accomplished in one operation.

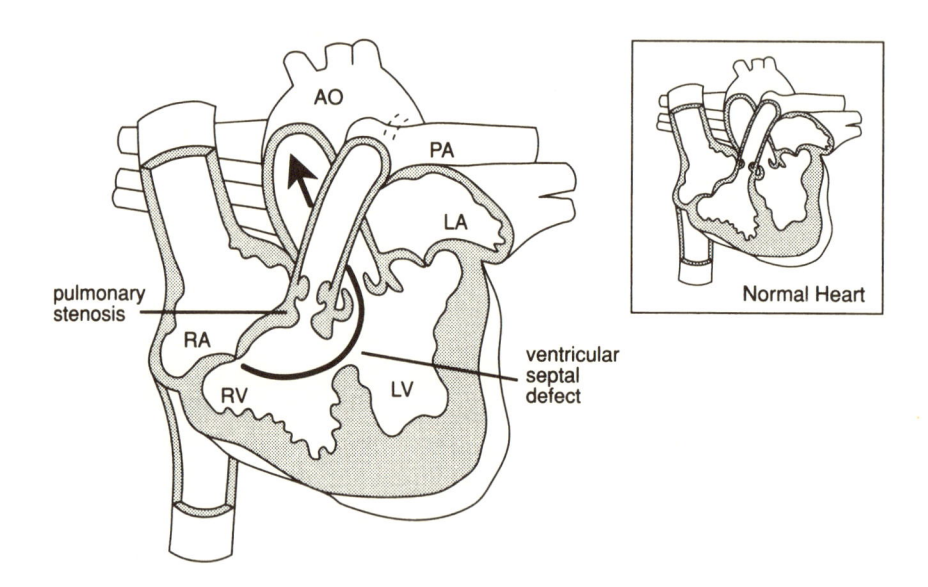

Figure 26.2. Tetralogy of Fallot. Pulmonary stenosis is present below the pulmonary valve, so blood flow from the right ventricle (RV) to the pulmonary artery (PA) is obstructed. Blue venous blood is shown with the arrow to pass from the right ventricle through the large ventricular septal defect into the aorta (AO). Because the aorta is connected to both ventricles, it is said to be overriding. The wall of the right ventricle is thickened (right ventricular hypertrophy).

Transposition

Transposition is also referred to as transposition of the great arteries and sometimes, as d-transposition (*d* is short for the Latin *dextro*, right), a medical shorthand term meaning that the aorta is transposed from its normal position and lies to the right of the pulmonary artery. (In *levo-* or *l*-transposition, the aorta is connected to the right ventricle but lies to the left of the pulmonary artery; this is a rare condition not discussed in this chapter.)

In transposition the great arteries are wrongly connected with the heart. The aorta connects to the right ventricle (receiving blue venous blood from it) instead of to the left. The pulmonary artery is connected to the left ventricle, which receives red blood full of oxygen. Venous blood returning to the heart passes normally into the right ventricle but then is routed back to the aorta. In transposition, blood coming back from the body does not reach the lungs for a fresh supply of oxygen.

Transposition is a serious defect of the heart, but it has seen a more dramatic change in outlook than any other single heart problem. Until the mid-1960s infants with transposition died from complications of low blood oxygen (hypoxia) before their first birthday. It is now possible for some such infants to receive successful correction of transposition in the first few days of life. They go home a healthy pink color and with their great arteries no longer transposed.

Other Conotruncal Defects

Rarer defects in the conotruncal area of the heart include double outlet right ventricle, truncus arteriosus, and aortopulmonary window.

Double Outlet Right Ventricle. In double outlet right ventricle both the aorta and the pulmonary artery arise from the right ventricle; a large ventricular septal defect is usually also present. Some of these babies have severe pulmonary stenosis and are intensely blue. Many of them can eventually have successful surgery, but usually more than one operation is needed. Additional defects outside the heart are common in such cases, so this remains a challenging and difficult type of heart defect. When there is no pulmonary stenosis the baby often does not appear blue but is in heart failure. It is sometimes possible to correct the defect in a one-stage operation, but often in such cases two procedures are needed.

Truncus Arteriosus. Truncus arteriosus is a rare condition in which the aorta and pulmonary artery have failed to separate and remain joined as one big artery leaving the heart, overriding a large ventricular septal defect. Successful surgery to separate the two vessels is now possible in early infancy. The surgery is difficult and often requires the use of an artificial valve. These children need careful follow-up even after successful surgery. Infants born with truncus arteriosus often have a poorly developed thymus gland and other features of Di George syndrome (a condition with a cluster of defects), which may complicate their course before and after surgery.

Aortopulmonary Window. Aortopulmonary window, a rare condition, is rather like a truncus, but less severe. In this condition there are separate aortic and pulmonary valves. The defect is between the aorta and the pulmonary artery a little after they leave the heart. Defects outside the heart are unusual in children with aortopulmonary window, and surgery (requiring a heart-lung machine) is usually quite successful.

Further advances in fetal echocardiography will help us identify the early stages of conotruncal defects during the mother's pregnancy, and eventually, perhaps, we will be able to treat them before birth. Most important of all, as we learn more about the interactions between the developing heart and the nervous system, we will learn why some children are born with multiple handicaps, and how these tragedies can be avoided.

Endocardial Cushion Defects

Early in the development of the fetal heart, specialized tissue in the center of the heart helps form the tricuspid and mitral valves; it also plays a part in closing the lower part of the atrial septum and the top of the ventricular septum. When this tissue does not develop as it should, an endocardial cushion defect results. Sometimes the term atrioventricular septal defect is used to describe an endocardial cushion defect. Atrioventricular canal defect is also an appropriate term, because there is a wide opening, a freely flowing canal, between the left and right sides of the heart. The defect may be mild or moderate in its effects or extremely serious. In the severe form, a complete atrioventricular canal defect, heart failure may start in early infancy, and surgery is usually recommended before the first birthday to avoid complications from high pressure in the lungs. Milder or partial forms of the defect, involving mainly the atrial septum, cause much less trouble, and surgery is usually performed during early childhood, before the child begins school.

Congenital Heart Defects

Ostium Primum Atrial Septal Defect

In the mildest form of an atrioventricular canal defect the ventricular septum is almost normal; only the lower part of the atrial septum is missing, and there is usually also an abnormality of the mitral valve. The mitral valve appears to have a cleft in it; it fails to close completely with each heartbeat, allowing some blood to leak back from the left ventricle to the left atrium. Because the principal problem here is in the lower atrial septum, this is sometimes called an ostium primum type of atrial septal defect. Between the most severe and the mildest forms of this anomaly are a number of intermediate atrioventricular canal defects; they vary in the size of the hole in the center of the heart and in the degree of severity of leaking or insufficiency of the mitral and tricuspid valves.

Complete Atrioventricular Canal Defect

In some children the development of the heart has been arrested at a very early stage. The specialized endocardial cushions in the center of the primitive heart have failed to grow and separate in a normal way. The heart has a major defect: there is a large open space in the center of the heart, and therefore blood can pass back and forth between the left and right atria and the left and right ventricles, as it is not intended to do. The lower atrial septum is missing and so is the upper part of the ventricular septum. As if this were not problem enough, the tricuspid valve, on the right, and the mitral valve, on the left, are incomplete and thus allow blood to leak back from the ventricles into the atria.

Babies who have endocardial cushion defects may show a number of different symptoms:

- A heart murmur is usually, *but not always*, audible from birth.
- Feeding is slower than normal; the slowness increases between the ages of 1 and 6 months.
- Signs of heart failure—rapid breathing, slow growth, and sweating—may appear.
- Chest infections are frequent, sometimes leading to pneumonia.

Diagnosis can be surprisingly difficult because the heart murmur may not be loud. Occasionally the defect is found before birth by means of fetal echocardiography; after birth the defect is often found during evaluation of a newborn baby who has been recognized as having Down syndrome.

The heart murmur in such conditions is variable, but many other signs indicate that a serious heart problem exists. The baby's breathing is rapid, the heart is overactive, and the right ventricle can be felt to be enlarged and pumping too hard. An electrocardiogram shows an abnormal pattern seen in almost no other defect. An echo-Doppler shows the defect in the center of the heart and shows that the mitral and tricuspid valves are badly formed and leaky. Cardiac catheterization is sometimes recommended to permit the doctor to see the valves even more clearly and to measure the pressure in the lungs.

The delay in the onset of symptoms is related to changes in the small arteries of the lungs. Immediately after birth the pressure in the infant's lung arteries remains very high, so circulation, although abnormal, is balanced. Somewhere between one and six months after birth the pressure in the lung arteries falls somewhat, allowing blood to move from the left side of the heart into the right ventricle and the lungs. The heart rapidly enlarges, the lungs become more congested every day, and the baby becomes exhausted during feeding. The heart murmur usually becomes louder at the same time. In this precarious state, the baby is ultrasensitive to any viral illness that is going around. A particular virus known as the *respiratory syncytial virus* may invade the infant's congested lungs and lead to severe pneumonia, while the rest of the family experiences what seems like a cold or a mild attack of flu.

It is impossible to discuss complete atrioventricular canal defects without mentioning their very strong association with Down syndrome. More than 60 percent of all complete atrioventricular canal defects occur in infants with Down syndrome, and more than 30 percent of infants with Down syndrome have this defect. Because a heart murmur may be quite faint, any breathing difficulty the baby has can be mistakenly blamed on the characteristics of Down syndrome itself.

Atrioventricular Canal Defect with a Hypoplastic Ventricle

When one of the ventricles (usually the left) fails to grow properly before birth, the baby is born with both a small (hypoplastic) left ventricle and a complete atrioventricular canal defect. This atrioventricular canal defect with a hypoplastic ventricle is sometimes referred to as an "unbalanced atrioventricular canal," meaning there is no normal balance or ratio between the two ventricles. By any name, this is

Congenital Heart Defects

an extremely serious defect. Occasionally a Norwood type of operation [a complex procedure in which the aorta is joined to the pulmonary artery] will help, but successful treatment in such cases remains the exception.

Other Congenital Heart Defects

Looping Defects

A looping defect of the heart occurs very early in development. In the normal looping process, the heart lies in the left side of the chest. Powerful genetic forces control this looping process and are responsible for the fact that nearly everyone's heart is located in the left side of the chest.

Some parts of the body are symmetrical and others are one-sided, or asymmetrical. There is a striking contrast between the asymmetry of the inside of the body (the left-sided heart, the right-sided liver) and the symmetry of the outside of the body (the limbs, the facial features, and the ears). Externally, our right and left sides are essentially mirror images. But inside, the heart is on the left, the liver on the right. There is only one appendix, and almost everyone knows that the appendix is in the right side of the lower abdomen. The asymmetry is programmed into the genetic function of development. Work with a special strain of mice in which the normal asymmetry has been disturbed has shown that there is a gene controlling place or position (*situs*). In the great majority of humans and mammals, the heart is in the left side of the chest, the liver in the right side of the abdomen. But in some, the position of the liver, stomach, and other abdominal organs is the opposite of normal (*situs inversus*, or turned around). Sometimes position is really mixed up, almost scrambled, with the liver in the center of the abdomen, the stomach misplaced, and even the appendix's place unpredictable. This condition is known as **heterotaxy**—that is, different or other than normal.

If the gene controlling the place of the abdominal organs is faulty or missing, chance takes over: half the hearts loop to the right, half to the left. In humans, looping defects are usually familial, although sometimes the family pattern is very difficult to track down. Many family studies suggest that the gene for abnormal position in humans is inherited (autosomal recessive). If parents have one child with abnormal position of one or more organs, there is approximately one chance in four that a later child will be similarly affected.

Anomalies of the Pulmonary Venous Return

In the normal heart all four pulmonary veins enter the left atrium separately, two from the right lung and two from the left lung. In abnormal or anomalous pulmonary venous return, some or all of the pulmonary veins connect to the right atrium instead of the left; sometimes they connect directly with the right atrium but more often they connect to a vein outside the heart, which then leads to the right atrium. How do the strange connections come about?

When the pulmonary veins are forming in the primitive lung bud of the embryo the atrium has not separated into two sides, and the small veins from the lung are very close to two large veins that drain into the right atrium. The veins grow toward the left atrium, an embryological process described as "targeted growth." If something happens to disturb this targeted growth—perhaps the embryo has a faulty gene, or a toxin causes a transient disturbance in embryo chemistry—the veins may miss the left side of the primitive atrium and end up joined to one of the body veins or connected directly to the right atrium.

Coronary Artery Abnormalities

Normally, the right and left coronary arteries arise from the aorta and supply oxygen and nutrients to the heart. There has been a great surge in the number of detailed X-ray pictures of the coronary artery tree since coronary artery bypass surgery became widely used. A surprising number of people who have been healthy into their fifties, or even their eighties, are found to have missing or misplaced coronary artery branches. This is not our topic, although it does point to a need for continuing work on coronary artery embryology and development. Here we will describe briefly some rare coronary defects that can lead to difficulty in infancy or childhood.

Anomalous Origin of the Left Coronary Artery from the Pulmonary Artery. An infant with anomalous origin of the left coronary artery from the pulmonary artery seems quite healthy at birth and usually has no heart murmur or anything to direct attention to the heart. During the early months of life, however, trouble begins. As the pressure in the lung arteries falls, blood begins to flow backward: it begins flowing from the aorta down the right coronary artery, in the normal way, but then flows back up the left coronary artery to

Congenital Heart Defects

the pulmonary artery. This condition is often described as a "coronary steal," meaning that good oxygen-containing blood is being stolen from the heart muscle by the abnormal flow into the pulmonary artery.

The child's first symptom is usually difficulty in feeding. At somewhere between 3 and 6 months of age the infant stops feeding eagerly, and often cries and seems colicky after feeding only a few minutes. Sometimes during feeding the child sweats, struggles, and draws the knees up, suggesting that the infant is in severe pain. We believe that these babies feel the kind of agonizing pain felt by an older patient with angina pectoris. Other times the pain will be less obvious, but the baby's sweating, difficulty in feeding, and slow growth cause the parents to seek medical attention.

This condition can be a very difficult problem to recognize; many normal babies have episodes of being colicky and only very, very, occasionally is their discomfort caused by heart problems. The parents' account of the infant's sweating and pain may be the clues that alert the nurse or physician to the defect. Sometimes the enlargement of the heart can be detected when the physician examines the baby. Heart murmurs are very faint, so early detection by this means is not easy.

Once a heart problem is suspected, chest X-ray, EKG, and echo-Doppler studies will be helpful. The chest X-ray confirms that the heart, particularly the left ventricle, is larger than normal. The EKG may show a quite specific set of changes, exactly like those seen in a middle-aged person who is having a severe heart attack. This infarct pattern on the EKG occurs because the heart muscle of the left ventricle is getting insufficient oxygen and nutrients; the blood that should supply the muscle is going into the pulmonary artery is being "stolen." Even though the baby is only 2 or 3 months old, some of the muscle of the vital left ventricle is dead or dying. The echo-Doppler shows three important things: first, the enlargement of the right coronary artery, which has dilated in an effort to increase the flow of blood to the damaged heart; second, the extend of damage to the heart muscle (often seen); and third, the abnormal course of the blood flow back up into the pulmonary artery. Cardiac catheterization is sometimes needed if the echo-Doppler findings are not conclusive or if an additional defect is suspected.

Abnormal Course of the Left Coronary Artery. The left coronary artery usually comes off the left side of the aortic root. In perhaps one in a million people, it comes instead from the *right* side of the aorta and has to twist its way between the aorta and the pulmonary artery.

Although this unusual course does not cause any heart murmur or anything that leads to a suspicion of heart disease, during strenuous exercise the artery may become twisted on itself, resulting in sudden severe chest pain. For some reason, possibly because teenagers exercise more strenuously, this happens most often in adolescence and seldom in early childhood. A combination of exercise electrocardiography and echo-Doppler testing can identify the problem. If a cardiac catheter test confirms the artery's abnormal course, surgery to reroute the coronary artery is usually recommended, because the defect occasionally leads to the sudden death of an otherwise healthy teenager engaged in strenuous exercise. Surgical treatment may relieve the problem completely, provided that the heart muscle has not already been too badly damaged.

Fistulas

A fistula is an abnormal channel, or communication, between two structures that are not ordinarily joined.

Coronary Artery Fistula. A coronary artery fistula is an abnormal communication between one of the coronary arteries and the inside of a ventricle or atrium. Usually a loud and unusual heart murmur is heard; thus the condition generally is noticed by the pediatrician and so comes quickly to the attention of a cardiologist. If the fistula is quite large, the heart may become enlarged or signs of heart failure may appear.

In most babies this defect can be recognized on an echo-Doppler test, but generally a cardiac catheter test is performed so the surgeon can be certain of the best approach to take. If the fistula is very small surgical repair is not considered necessary, but the usual treatment is surgical and is very successful. In surgery the fistula is closed where it enters the heart chamber, usually with a small patch, so little if any damage is done to the coronary artery itself. Children who have this operation can become as active as normal children.

Arteriovenous Fistula of the Vein of Galen. An abnormal communication between an artery and a vein, known as an arteriovenous fistula can be present before birth and may be discovered by a fetal echocardiogram; it can also occur almost anywhere in the body, but is found most often in the brain and sometimes in the liver. If the fistula is large, the baby can develop heart failure even before birth.

Congenital Heart Defects

The most usual fistula, a cerebral arteriovenous fistula of the vein of Galen, lies between the arteries and veins inside the brain. A baby born with this problem has a large heart and becomes ill with heart failure very rapidly, as blood rushes through the abnormal communication in the center of the brain. It is an extremely serious problem. Once the defect is recognized, from the heart murmur and from echo-Doppler tests, treatment is attempted by specialists in neurology; some infants have been helped by the insertion of tiny coils into the artery that feeds the fistula, in an effort to close off the abnormal channel. Successful treatment is, so far, infrequent. Fistulas elsewhere in the body can more often be treated effectively, either by surgery or by insertion of balloons or coils in the catheterization laboratory.

Tumors of the Heart (Rhabdomyomas)

Most heart tumors in infants are caused by clusters of overgrown muscle cells, known as rhabdomyomas. These benign tumors are nearly always a sign that the baby has a neurological disorder called tuberous sclerosis. Because fetal echocardiography is now widely used, many of these tumors are discovered before birth. A few lead to obstruction of one of the heart valves and need surgery after birth, but most require no treatment and become smaller as the baby grows. The baby with tuberous sclerosis needs careful follow-up.

Oncocytic Cardiomyopathy

Oncocytic cardiomyopathy, a disorder called by many different names, is somewhere in a gray zone between heart muscle disease and an unusual heart tumor. In this condition there are tiny collections of cells in the wall of the ventricle that can set off abnormal heart rhythms. A baby with this problem may have repeated attacks of rapid heart rate (tachycardia) and may respond poorly to the usual medications. Specialized catheter tests can pinpoint the exact location of the abnormal cells in the ventricle: treatment, which in some cases has been remarkably successful, consists of surgical removal or freezing. In most cases, the child will then grow normally.

Ectopia Cordis

In ectopia cordis the heart grows partly or even completely on the outside of the chest wall. It is usually also badly formed in some other way, usually with a defect resembling tetralogy of Fallot. This is perhaps the only heart defect that can be diagnosed with no special skill or knowledge: there is no mistaking it. It is rarely successfully treated by surgery; fortunately, the defect is rare.

Summary

Most rare congenital heart problems can be treated surgically when necessary. As new knowledge is gained about normal heart development, many rare defects are beginning to be understood, and even greater successes in treatment should follow in the next decade. The gene for heterotaxy has been discovered in the mouse model, and this discovery has given researchers a great incentive to look closely at the genes that control the looping of the human heart. Some babies with total anomalous pulmonary venous return have an abnormality of chromosome 22; this discovery is stimulating research into the genes that control the targeted growth of the normal pulmonary veins toward the left atrium. As for the coronary arteries, much still needs to be learned about their normal development and why some arteries are more prone than others to atherosclerosis in middle age. Rare defects can sometimes provide significant clues to common and severe problems.

Groups That Can Help

Family support groups can be a source of comfort, information, and friendship. One family support group in Maryland, Big Hearts for Little Hearts, can be reached through the Division of Pediatric Cardiology at the Johns Hopkins Hospital, 600 N. Wolfe Street, Baltimore, Maryland 21205. In the Rochester, New York, area, contact Helping Hearts, Division of Pediatric Cardiology, Box 631, University of Rochester Medical Center, Rochester, New York 14642.

A list of local family support groups can be obtained from the local affiliate of the American Heart Association (check the business pages of the telephone book) or by writing to the Council of Cardiovascular Disease in the Young, American Heart Association, National Center, 7320 Greenville Avenue, Dallas, Texas 75231. The American Heart Association will also provide booklets about specific topics on request.

Glossary

Acidosis: The accumulation of acid products in the blood after either a severe episode of oxygen lack or failure of the circulation.

Acquired heart disease: A heart problem that is not due to a congenital defect, but that appears or is acquired after birth, such as rheumatic heart disease or myocarditis.

Aneurysm: A ballooning out of the wall of an artery or vein or of the heart wall due to weakening of the wall by injury or disease or to some abnormality dating from birth.

Angina pectoris: Chest pain due to heart disease. A condition in which the heart muscle doesn't receive enough blood, usually due to coronary insufficiency.

Angiocardiography: An X-ray examination of the blood vessels or chambers of the heart. A special fluid (called "contrast material" or "dye"), visible to X-ray, is injected into the bloodstream. Also called angiography; the X-ray pictures made are called angiograms. Cineangiography is the recording of angiograms on cinefilm.

Angioplasty: A procedure sometimes used to dilate (widen) narrowed arteries. A catheter with a deflated balloon on its tip is passed into the narrowed artery segment, the balloon inflated, and the narrowed segment widened.

Aorta: The large artery that receives blood from the heart's left ventricle and distributes it to the body.

Aortic valve: The heart valve between the left ventricle and the aorta. It normally has three flaps, or cusps; when only two cusps are present the valve is said to be "bicuspid."

Aphasia: The inability to speak, write, or understand spoken or written language because of brain injury or disease.

Arrhythmia (or dysrhythmia): An abnormal rhythm of the heart.

Arteriography: A testing procedure, similar to angiography, in which an X-ray-opaque dye is injected into the bloodstream and pictures of arteries (usually the coronary arteries) are taken and studied to see if the arteries are damaged.

Arterioles: Small, muscular branches of arteries. When they contract, they increase resistance to blood flow, and blood pressure in the arteries increases.

Arteriosclerosis: Commonly called "hardening of the arteries," the term refers to a variety of conditions that cause artery walls to thicken and lose elasticity.

Artery: Any one of a series of blood vessels that carry blood from the heart to the various parts of the body. Arteries have thick, elastic walls that can expand as blood flows through them.

Atherosclerosis: A form of arteriosclerosis in which the inner layers of artery walls become thick and irregular due to deposits of fat, cholesterol, and other substances. These deposits, sometimes called "plaques," cause the arteries to narrow and the flow of blood through them is reduced.

Atresia: A complete failure of development of a structure normally present and open at birth, as in pulmonary valve atresia (affecting the heart), or intestinal atresia (affecting part of the intestine).

Atria (singular, atrium): The two upper holding chambers of the heart. The right atrium receives blood from the body; the left atrium receives blood returning from the lungs via the pulmonary veins.

Atrial septal defect: A congenital defect in the atrial septum. Most defects are in the middle part of the septum (ostium secundum defect); some are in the upper part of the septum, often with abnormal drainage of the right pulmonary veins (sinus venosus defect). A defect low in the atrial septum with an abnormal mitral valve, a form of endocardial cushion defect, is sometimes referred to as an ostium primum.

Atrial septum: The wall or septum dividing the right from the left atrium.

Atrioventricular (AV) node: A small mass of specialized conducting tissue at the bottom of the right atrium through which the electrical

Congenital Heart Defects

impulse stimulating the heart to contract must pass to reach the ventricles.

Atrioventricular canal defect (also endocardial cushion defect or atrioventricular septal defect): A congenital defect in which the mitral and tricuspid valves are abnormal and defects are present between the atria and ventricles. Large defects are called "complete atrioventricular canal defects." "Incomplete" or partial defects, including ostium primum, affect mostly the atrial septum and are less severe.

Atrium: See atria.

Bacterial endocarditis: A bacterial infection of the heart lining or valves. It occurs more often in people with abnormal heart valves or congenital heart defects than in those with normal hearts. Bacterial endocarditis prophylaxis (BE prophylaxis) means precautions taken to prevent endocarditis.

Balloon catheter: A specialized catheter used to dilate a narrowed structure in the circulation: See angioplasty and valvuloplasty.

Blood pressure: The force or pressure exerted by the heart in pumping blood; the pressure of blood in the arteries.

Blue babies: Babies who have a blue tinge to their skin (cyanosis) resulting from insufficient oxygen in the arterial blood; this blue color often indicates a heart defect.

Bradycardia: Slow heart rate.

Bronchial arteries: See collateral circulation.

Capillaries: Microscopically small blood vessels between arteries and veins that distribute oxygenated blood to the body's tissues.

Cardiac: Pertaining to the heart.

Cardiac arrest: Cessation of the heartbeat.

Cardiac catheterization: The process of examining the heart by introducing a thin tube (catheter) into a vein or artery and passing it into the heart.

Cardiac jelly: A substance found early in heart development that helps to form the framework on which the heart valves are formed.

Cardiology: The study of the heart and its functions in health and disease.

Cardiomyopathy: A disorder of the muscle of the heart.

Cardiopulmonary resuscitation (CPR): A technique combining chest compression and mouth-to-mouth breathing, used during cardiac arrest to keep oxygenated blood circulating in the body.

Cardiovascular: Concerning the heart and blood vessels.

Cerebral embolism: A blood clot formed in one part of the body and then carried by the bloodstream to the brain, where it lodges in an artery.

Cerebral thrombosis: Formation of a blood clot in an artery that supplies part of the brain.

Cholesterol: A fat-like substance manufactured in the body and found in foods from animal sources, such as whole-milk dairy products, meat, fish, poultry, animal fats, and egg yolks.

Cineangiogram: See cineangiography.

Cineangiography (also called cineangiocardiography): The technique of taking moving pictures, known as cineangiograms, to show the passage of an X-ray opaque dye through blood vessels.

Circulatory system: System comprising the heart and blood vessels, responsible for the circulation of the blood.

Closed-heart surgery: Surgery that does not require the heart-lung machine and is performed on blood vessels in the chest but outside the heart itself.

Clot (also blood clot): A jelly-like mass of blood tissue formed by clotting factors in the blood. Clots stop the flow of blood from an injury. Clots also can form inside an artery whose walls are damaged by atherosclerotic buildup and can cause a heart attack or stroke.

Congenital Heart Defects

Coarctation: Narrowing of the aorta where the pulmonary artery and aorta are joined by the ductus arteriosus.

Collateral circulation: A system of smaller arteries, closed under normal circumstances, that may open up and start to carry blood to part of the heart when a coronary artery is blocked. These arteries can serve as alternate routes of blood supply. Collateral vessels in the lungs (bronchial arteries) may be found in severely blue (cyanotic) children.

Complex heart defects: Abnormalities of the heart in which there are several defects, so that one of the ventricles or pumping chambers has failed to develop; or in which a major artery or heart valve is completely blocked (atretic). Children with such defects usually need several operations.

Computerized axial tomography (CAT) scan: A specialized X-ray technique producing a three-dimensional image using a rotating X-ray beam.

Congenital: Refers to conditions existing at birth.

Congenital heart defect: Malformation of the heart or its major blood vessels present at birth.

Congestive heart failure: See heart failure.

Conotruncal area: The part of the heart joining the right ventricle to the pulmonary artery. If the conotruncal area does not develop normally, blood flow between heart and lungs is disturbed and blueness or cyanosis occurs.

Coronary arteries: Two arteries arising from the aorta that arch down over the top of the heart, branch, and provide blood to the heart muscle.

Coronary artery disease: Conditions that cause narrowing of the coronary arteries so blood flow to the heart muscle is reduced.

Coronary bypass surgery: Surgery to improve blood supply to the heart muscle.

Coronary thrombosis: Formation of a clot in one of the arteries that conduct blood to the heart muscle. Also called coronary occlusion.

Cyanosis: Blueness of the skin and body tissues caused by insufficient oxygen in the blood.

Defibrillator: An electronic device that helps reestablish normal contraction rhythms in a malfunctioning heart.

Diabetes (also diabetes mellitus): A disease in which the body doesn't produce or properly use insulin. Insulin is a hormone that the body needs to convert sugar and starch into the energy needed in daily life.

Diastole: The time when the ventricles, the pumping chambers of the heart, relax and receive blood from the atria, the receiving chambers.

Diastolic blood pressure: The lowest blood pressure measured in the arteries, measured when the heart muscle is relaxed between beats.

Digitalis (also digoxin, digitoxin): A drug that strengthens the contraction of the heart muscle, slows the rate of contraction of the heart, and promotes the elimination of fluid from body tissues. Digitalis is often used to treat heart failure and also to treat certain arrhythmias.

Diuretic: A drug that increases the rate at which urine forms by promoting the excretion of water and salts.

Doppler-echocardiography: See echocardiography.

Doppler shift: A sound, such as the sound of a siren or train whistle, increases in pitch as it approaches and decreases as it moves away. This change in pitch or frequency, the Doppler shift, is used to calculate the speed or velocity of the source of sound and sound waves.

Ductus arteriosus: An artery present before birth that connects the aorta and pulmonary artery. The ductus normally closes shortly after birth; if it remains open (patent ductus arteriosus), medical or surgical treatment may be necessary.

Echocardiography: A diagnostic method in which pulses of sound are transmitted into the body and the echoes returning from the surfaces of the heart and other structures are electronically plotted and recorded. In Doppler-echocardiography the speed with which the waves travel can be measured, allowing for measurements of pressure changes across the heart valves. Doppler color flow mapping superimposes color on the image received back from the heart; this color is useful in showing the direction of blood flow across valves or through small defects in the heart, which might otherwise be difficult to detect.

Echo-Doppler: See echocardiography.

Edema: Swelling due to an abnormally large amount of fluid in body tissues.

Elective referral: A nonemergency consultation about a heart murmur or other medical problem.

Electrocardiogram (EKG): A graphic record of electrical impulses produced by the heart.

Electroencephalogram (EEG): A graphic record of the electrical impulses produced by the brain.

Electrophysiologic study (EPS): A detailed, highly specialized study of the conducting system of the heart performed in the cardiac catheterization laboratory.

Embolus: A blood clot that forms in a blood vessel in one part of the body and then is carried to another part of the body.

Endocardial cushions: Formed in part from the cardiac jelly, the cushions form the infrastructure for the developing valves of the heart.

Endocardium: The smooth inner lining of the heart wall, lying between the heart muscle (myocardium) and the blood inside the heart chambers.

Endothelium: The smooth inner lining of many body structures, including the heart and blood vessels.

Enzyme: A complex organic substance capable of speeding up specific biochemical processes in the body.

Exercise testing: A study of how much exercise an individual can do compared to others of the same age and size with normal hearts; the test is done using either a treadmill or a stationary bicycle, while the EKG, blood pressure, and breathing are monitored.

Extrasystole: An extra heartbeat, a form of arrhythmia, usually not needing treatment.

Fetal Doppler-echocardiography: A detailed examination of the baby's heart while the baby is still in the mother's womb. This test may be done in a specialized center (in addition to the usual ultrasound tests for the baby's growth), if there is any reason to suspect an abnormality of the rhythm or structure of the developing heart.

Fibrillation (also atrial or ventricular fibrillation): Rapid, uncoordinated contractions of individual heart muscle fibers. The heart chamber involved can't contract all at once and pumps blood ineffectively, if at all.

Fibrin: A protein in the blood that enmeshes blood cells and other substances during blood clotting.

Foramen ovale: A small opening in the atrial septum present before birth.

Gradient: A change in pressure across a heart valve or between different heart chambers.

Health team: The group of professionals helping the child and the family achieve heart health.

Heart attack: Death of or damage to an area of the heart muscle due to a reduced supply of blood to that area. Also myocardial infarction, coronary occlusion.

Heart block: When the heartbeat does not pass normally from the atrium to the ventricles, heart block is present. This is a form of abnormal heart rhythm (arrhythmia).

Congenital Heart Defects

Heart failure: The inability of the heart to pump out all the blood that returns to it. This failure results in a backup of blood in the veins that lead to the heart and sometimes an accumulation of fluid in the lungs and various parts of the body.

Heart-lung machine: An apparatus that oxygenates and pumps blood while a person's heart is opened for open-heart surgery.

Heredity: The genetic transmission of a particular quality or trait from parent to offspring.

Heterotaxy: Abnormal arrangement of the heart and the abdominal organs, often with multiple defects in the heart and absent or multiple spleens.

High blood pressure: A chronic increase in blood pressure above its normal range.

High-density lipoprotein (HDL): A carrier of cholesterol believed to transport cholesterol away from the tissues to the liver, where it can be excreted.

Holter monitoring (ambulatory electrocardiography): The EKG is recorded on tape over twenty-four to seventy-two hours, then analyzed for arrhythmias or other abnormalities.

Hypertension: High blood pressure.

Hypoplastic: Too small or poorly developed. In the most severe heart flow defects, either the right or the left ventricle may be hypoplastic and incapable of functioning normally.

Hypoxia: Too low a level of oxygen in the blood and tissues of the body.

Incidence: The number of new cases of a disease that develop in a population during a specified period of time, such as a year.

Interrupted aortic arch: An extreme form of coarctation of the aorta.

Invasive: Entering the body. Cardiac catheterization and angiography are sometimes called "invasive" procedures, because a catheter is introduced into the body through a vein or artery. By contrast, echocardiography or magnetic resonance imaging are described as "noninvasive," because nothing is introduced into the body.

Ischemia: Decreased blood flow to an organ, usually due to constriction or obstruction of an artery.

Ischemic heart disease: Also called coronary artery disease and coronary heart disease. This term is applied to heart ailments that are caused by narrowing of the coronary arteries and that therefore are characterized by a decreased blood supply to the heart.

Kawasaki disease (syndrome): An acute illness of children characterized by fever, rash, swelling, and inflammation of various parts of the body. The coronary arteries or other parts of the heart are affected in 20 percent of children with this disease.

Left-heart flow defect: A congenital abnormality affecting the ventricle or the valves and arteries on the left side of the heart, due to abnormal flow patterns during embryonic life.

Lipid: A fatty substance insoluble in blood.

Lipoprotein: A lipid surrounded by a protein; the protein makes it soluble in the blood.

Looping: Looping of the heart, so that the heart apex points to the left, occurs early in development; when the process is abnormal a cardiac looping defect occurs.

Low-density lipoprotein (LDL): The main carrier of harmful cholesterol in the blood.

Lumen: The opening of a tube, such as a blood vessel.

Magnetic resonance imaging (MRI) (also called nuclear magnetic resonance): An imaging method using radio frequency pulses in a magnetic field to define body structures.

Mitral valve: The heart valve between the left atrium and left ventricle. It has two flaps, or cusps.

Congenital Heart Defects

Mucocutaneous lymph node syndrome: See Kawasaki disease.

Murmur (heart murmur): An extra sound between the two normal heart sounds "lub" and "dup." Most murmurs in children are innocent, but some indicate a heart problem needing treatment.

Myocardial infarction: See heart attack.

Myocardium: The muscular wall of the heart that contracts to pump blood out of the heart and relaxes when the heart refills with returning blood.

Obesity: The condition of being significantly overweight.

Open-heart surgery: Surgery performed on the opened heart while the bloodstream is diverted through a heart-lung machine. Also called cardiopulmonary bypass surgery.

Ostium primum defect: See atrial septal defect.

Oximetry (pulse oximetry): A technique for measuring the oxygen saturation in the blood.

Pacemaker or sinus (sinoatrial) node: A small mass of specialized cells in the right atrium of the heart that produces the electrical impulses that cause contractions of the heart. The term "artificial pacemaker" is applied to an electrical device that can substitute for a defective natural pacemaker and control the beating of the heart by transmitting a series of rhythmical electrical discharges.

Pericarditis: Inflammation of the pericardium.

Pericardium: The membrane forming the outer lining of the heart, separating the myocardium, or heart muscle, from the lungs and other structures in the chest.

Platelets: One of three kinds of formed elements found in the blood. Platelets aid in the clotting of the blood.

Pulmonary: Pertaining to the lungs.

Pulmonary artery: The artery carrying blood from the heart to the lungs.

Pulmonary atresia: Failure of development of the pulmonary valve or the pulmonary artery.

Pulmonary blood flow: The flow of blood into the lungs with each heartbeat. The amount of flow depends on the size of the child, increasing with age. It is normally equal to the flow of blood to the body (systemic blood flow).

Pulmonary valve: The valve between the right ventricle and the pulmonary artery. The pulmonary valve, like the aortic valve, opens and closes with each heartbeat. The valve usually has three leaflets or cusps; when two leaflets are present the pulmonary valve is said to be "bicuspid."

Rheumatic heart disease: Damage done to the heart, particularly to the heart valves, by one or more attacks of rheumatic fever.

Right-heart flow defect: A congenital abnormality of the ventricle, or the valves and arteries on the right side of the heart, due to abnormal flow patterns during embryonic life.

Rubella: A viral illness, commonly known as German measles, that causes fever and a rash. When a woman develops rubella during her first three months of pregnancy, the exposed baby may be born with heart defects and other problems.

Septation: The process of development of the septa of the heart, resulting in the four separate chambers of the normal newborn heart.

Septum (plural septa): The wall dividing the heart chambers into right and left sides. The atrial septum separates the right from the left atrium; the ventricular septum separates the two ventricles.

Stenosis: Narrowing or obstruction of a valve or opening, which may be present from birth (as in pulmonary valve stenosis) or follow rheumatic heart disease (as in mitral stenosis).

Streptococcal infection: A bacterial infection, usually in the throat, resulting from the presence of an unusual form of streptococcus.

Congenital Heart Defects

Syndrome: A combination of problems or defects often seen together.

Systemic blood flow: The flow of blood to the body with each heartbeat. The amount of flow increases as the child grows.

Systole: The time when the ventricles contract and pump blood out to the body and the lungs.

Systolic blood pressure: The highest blood pressure measured in the arteries, measured when the ventricle is contracting and pumping blood to the body during systole.

Tachycardia: Fast heart rate.

Tetralogy of Fallot: A conotruncal heart defect with a large ventricular septal defect and pulmonary stenosis, leading to cyanosis.

Thrombosis: The formation or presence of a blood clot (thrombus) inside a blood vessel or cavity of the heart.

Tricuspid atresia: Failure of development of the tricuspid valve, associated with a hypoplastic right ventricle.

Truncus arteriosus: A conotruncal defect in which a single artery or trunk leaves the heart, due to a failure of the normal embryonic division of the truncus into the aorta and pulmonary artery.

Valvuloplasty: Dilation of a narrowed valve using a balloon catheter.

Vascular: Pertaining to the blood vessels.

Vein: Any one of the vessels of the vascular system that carry blood from various parts of the body back to the heart.

Ventricle: One of the two lower (pumping) chambers of the heart. The left ventricle pumps blood to the body, the right ventricle to the lungs.

Ventricular hypertrophy: Thickening (hyper, too much; troph, growth) of the muscle forming the wall of the ventricle. Ventricular hypertrophy is usually a response to some obstruction in the heart or blood vessels, but is sometimes part of a heart muscle disease (cardiomyopathy).

Ventricular septal defect: See ventricular septum.

Ventricular septum: The wall separating the right from the left ventricle. If the wall is incomplete, a ventricular septal defect is present; the defect may lie in the upper part of the wall (membranous or perimembranous defect) or lower down the wall, in the muscular ventricular septum.

Viral myocarditis: Inflammation of the myocardium with a virus; this inflammation sometimes leads to a chronic disease of the heart muscle, cardiomyopathy.

Chapter 27

Twin-Twin Transfusion Syndrome

Twin-Twin Transfusion Syndrome (TTTS) is a complication which develops in about 15 percent of identical twin pregnancies. Approximately 6,000 babies born each year in the United States are affected. TTTS occurs only when twins (or higher-order pregnancies) share a single placenta with blood vessel connections which allow free passage of blood from one twin into the other. If the blood pressures differ in the two individual twins connected by these placental vessels, then one twin will tend to "steal" blood from the other. (Blood will flow out of the high-pressure side into the side with a lower blood pressure.)

This "stealing" can lead to relative under-nourishment for one twin, causing him to grow more slowly than his co-twin. Birthweights may differ by several pounds, and the twins will definitely have different blood counts at birth.

In severe cases, the "donor" twin becomes very anemic, and the "recipient" twin becomes overloaded with fluid and develops heart failure. The recipient twin will also produce excessive amounts of urine, overdistending the bag of water with too much amniotic fluid (polyhydramnios).

Polyhydramnios increases the risk of early labor and the number of maternal complications. Without treatment, the most likely outcome is death of both twins either in the womb or because of extremely early delivery. If severely affected twins survive, birth defects or cerebral palsy can result from the disordered blood flow experienced in the womb.

"Promising News about TTTS," *Twins Magazine*, March/April 1996. Source: http://www.twinsmagazine.com/mar96pre.html; reprinted with permission.

Because identical (monozygotic) twins begin as a single conception, TTTS can occur. A few days after conception, the developing embryo is a microscopic ball of cells which can split apart to form two groups of cells. When the split occurs early enough, before the third day of development, the resulting groups are able to grow into perfectly-formed and genetically identical twins. If the split occurs later, the ball of cells may split incompletely.

A dramatic example of this is "Siamese" or conjoined twins, in which the incomplete splitting occurs around day 12 to 14, and the twins are born attached to one another, often sharing several vital organs. Conjoined twins are rare, but a portion of the placenta is shared in about two-thirds of identical twin pregnancies. Often placental sharing has no adverse consequence for the twins, but if one or more "high-pressure" arteries from one twin happens to be connected to a "low-pressure" vein in the other twin's placenta, then TTTS can result.

Symptoms

Excessive weight gain, very rapid growth of the uterus, or the sudden onset of severe swelling (edema) are symptoms which might suggest that TTTS is occurring. More often it occurs without symptoms, and it is only diagnosed when an ultrasound examination shows excessive fluid around one twin and no fluid around the other. Other conditions can mimic TTTS—for instance, twin fetuses would have very different amounts of fluid if only one fetus had an infection, a genetic problem, or a sick placenta.

When severe TTTS occurs early in pregnancy, termination of the pregnancy is frequently recommended, since the prognosis for the twins is so poor, and because the mother's health is at increased risk when carrying twins with severe polyhydramnios. In recent years, techniques have been developed to abort only one of the fetuses, with the hope that this would give the other a chance at life. As you can imagine, neither of these decisions is easy for a doctor to recommend, nor for a parent to make.

Fortunately, several treatments have been developed which increase the odds that one or even both fetuses will survive. Various drugs have been given to the mother in order to improve the function of the twins' hearts and avoid heart failure. Another drug, indomethacin, has been prescribed to reduce the urine production by the fluid-overloaded, recipient twin, thereby decreasing the polyhydramnios and reducing the risks inherent in extremely premature delivery.

Alternatively, obstetricians have aggressively drained the excessive amniotic fluid by inserting a needle through the mother's abdomen into the bag of water (amniocentesis). Quarts or even gallons of fluid are removed, and the procedure may need to be repeated every few days. Repeated amniocentesis seems to reduce the risks of prematurity and, in some cases, miraculously end the stealing of blood across the placenta.

No Longer a 'Hopeless' Complication

Perhaps the most promising treatment, and the only one which addresses the root cause of TTTS, involves laser surgery to divide the connecting blood vessels in the placenta. Julian Delia, M.D., presently on the faculty of the Medical College of Wisconsin in Milwaukee, developed this experimental procedure. The mother is given anesthesia, and a thin, telescope-like device called a fetoscope is inserted through the mother's abdomen and into the bag of water containing the excessive fluid. The placental vessels which are connecting one twin to the other can be seen through the fetoscope. Dr. Delia then fires a surgical laser at these vessels through the fetoscope to seal or cauterize the connections.

Dr. Delia has treated over 40 pregnancies to date, and almost two-thirds of the twins have survived. Almost all of the survivors are completely healthy. I have personally participated in about a half dozen of these cases; the reversal of TTTS after laser surgery can be quite dramatic! Another group of physicians at King's College in London, England, used laser surgery in 45 pregnancies complicated by TTTS. Fifty-three percent of the twins survived, with at least one baby surviving in 71 percent of the twin pregnancies.

It is thrilling that TTTS is not longer a "hopeless" complication. None of the treatments works perfectly, and each approach presents some risk to the mother or her babies. The success rates are likely to increase, however, as we gain experience and learn more about the syndrome.

—by Kenneth Ward, M.D.

Kenneth Ward, M.D., of Salt Lake City, Utah, specializes in high-risk obstetrics and genetics, and directs the DNA Diagnostic Laboratory at the University of Utah School of Medicine. He is the father of two.

Chapter 28

Hirschsprung's Disease

There are a number of diseases that are well-known to the medical community but relatively unknown to the public. Congenital megacolon is one such disease. Congenital megacolon is more commonly known as Hirschsprung's disease, named for Dr. Harold Hirschsprung who made the first clinical diagnosis.

What is Hirschsprung's?

Hirschsprung first described it fully in 1888. He established it as a clinical entity with autopsy findings from two patients. Hirschsprung had no real clue as to the cause of the disease, but began the inquiry into what is still a very intriguing disease, even to the pediatric surgical community today.

The first signs of this disease include abdominal distention, or swelling. Also, meconium, or the first stools of a newborn consisting of cellular debris, mucous and bile pigments, may not be passed in the first 24 to 48 hours of life. In some cases, the infant may pass meconium, but distention and vomiting still will occur. Distention may be followed by vomit containing bile, and the infant may become pale and very lethargic.

Infants with failure to pass meconium may be diagnosed as having a small bowel obstruction due to another cause. Some infants will

"What Is Hirschsprung's Disease?" *Ostomy Quarterly*, (29)2, 1992:39-41; © United Ostomy Association, reprinted with permission. For more information contact: United Ostomy Association, 36 Executive Park, Suite 120, Irvine, CA 92614; (800) 826-0826.

evacuate their colon on rectal examination, and the unwary physician may dismiss the situation as a meconium plug and not investigate further.

In a normal colon, there are nerves and ganglia, or structures containing collections of nerve cells. These regulate the involuntary wavelike movements, called peristalsis, that push contents of the digestive tract along. With Hirschsprung's disease, the ganglia are absent in a variable portion of the colon and rectum. This absence interrupts the relaxation phase that is a normal part of peristalsis, and the bowel remains in spasm, acting as an obstruction.

Statistics

The incidence of this disease is about one in every 5,000, and there is no link to race. Although Hirschsprung's is usually diagnosed in newborns and infants, diagnosis may occasionally be delayed until adulthood. It is estimated Hirschsprung's disease accounts for 20 percent to 25 percent of newborns with intestinal obstructions. Hirschsprung's is four times more common in boys than in girls. However, in cases where aganglionosis, or the lack of ganglia, extends beyond the sigmoid colon, the ratio drops below three to one.

The extent of aganglionosis varies with each patient. Aganglionosis always involves the rectum and extends upward to the lower end of the colon. Some researchers believe that the nerves do not reach the rectum in this disease. It may involve only the area close to the sphincter, or it may affect the entire colon and/or small intestine. Seventy-five percent of children with Hirschsprung's disease have only the rectum and a small portion of the colon involved. The other 25 percent have more colon involved. Of that 25 percent, only 8 percent have the entire colon or part of the small intestine affected.

The likelihood of other unrelated malformations with Hirschsprung's disease is higher than in the normal population. Nearly every known congenital malformation can be observed in patients affected by this disease. Some more common birth defects are Down's syndrome, urological malformations, cardiovascular defects, cystic fibrosis, facial hypoplasia and cleft palate.

Diagnosis

Although distention, vomiting, paleness and recurring bouts of enterocolitis (inflammation of the colon and small intestine) may suggest

Hirschsprung's Disease

the diagnosis, there is a more accurate way of making a positive diagnosis. When there is a concern that Hirschsprung's disease could be present, a combination of techniques are used for diagnosis. The first of these is manometry. Electromanometry is a relatively new investigative method by which pressure changes within hollow muscular organs of the gastrointestinal tract and the bladder can be registered. These pressure changes can be transformed into electrical impulses and, after appropriate amplification, are registered by a recorder. Recording pressure changes allows for evaluation of the function of the anorectal muscle.

Another diagnostic tool is the barium enema. The chemical barium is used as an opaque medium for X-ray examination of the gastrointestinal tract. The barium enema will show the involved rectum and colon to be very narrow with colonic dilatation above the narrowed area, like that which Hirschsprung found in his autopsy reports.

This X-ray can frequently provide a clear-cut zone of transition between the aganglionic segment and the normal segment. Occasionally, the results of the enema are inconclusive.

The third, and most conclusive, test used is the rectal section biopsy. The simple nature and low risk of this test procedure make it the test of choice. In this test, a small portion of rectal tissue is removed for examination. Microscopically, a determination can be made whether or not ganglia are present in the lower rectal region of the colon.

Treatment

Once a test confirms the presence of Hirschsprung's disease, decisions for treatment can be made. Although colostomy was originally unpopular, it has proven to be the most effective initial treatment in pediatric surgical practice today.

Surgical management of patients with Hirschsprung's disease varies depending on the patient's age and physical condition. Prompt treatment of newborns is critical. Following diagnosis, a colostomy is made in the normal segment of the colon adjacent to the transition zone. The proper place for the colostomy can only be found by biopsy of the colon wall.

The colostomy gives the infant an opportunity to recuperate from his obstruction and grow. The decision to resect the infant's colon and reconstruction of the rectum depends on a variety of circumstances. This operation is scheduled around the first year of life or 20 lbs., depending on the child and the extent of the disease.

Complications

Problems after surgical treatment of Hirschsprung's disease include constipation, chronic diarrhea and enterocolitis. Enterocolitis, which can break down the intestinal lining, remains the No. 1 cause of death among patients with Hirschsprung's disease. A survey of the American Academy of Pediatrics showed a 30 percent mortality rate among patients with enterocolitis, a statistic that has not changed in 20 years.

Enterocolitis is more common among patients who have a large portion of their intestine involved, but it does occur even in cases where the disease is limited to the rectum. Repeated bouts of enterocolitis separated by intervals of relative good health is a pattern seen from time to time after surgery.

The exact cause of the incorrect development of ganglia in the colon and rectum is speculative. Some researchers have theorized that the disease is related to environmental factors, such as maternal, nutritional deficiencies, irradiation, measles, thalidomide or other compounds. As yet, these have not been confirmed. In some patients, the disease is clearly related to genetics. In cases where parent and child have been affected, the mother is more often affected than the father.

Emotional Support

Chronic or recurring illness due to such a disease can be an emotionally traumatic experience for both the child and his parents. When hospitalization is necessary, careful handling of the situation is imperative. Hospitalization is advised only when care cannot be provided at home, and every attempt should be made to make the ill child feel secure.

With such a traumatic experience, support is necessary for the parents as well. Sharing experiences with others in similar situations can help prepare the parents for potential complications. Parents must quickly learn the subtle signs of oncoming illness for their own child. They must learn how to apply an ostomy pouch and how to care for the stoma and the skin around it.

Infants with additional problems may come home with a heart or respiration monitor and may require a variety of medications. Parents are frequently required to learn infant cardiopulmonary resuscitation (CPR). The responsibility of caring for any child is great, but

Hirschsprung's Disease

with a chronically ill child, this responsibility may be much more demanding and require the commitment of the entire family.

Following successful surgical treatment of Hirschsprung's disease, children have the opportunity to grow and develop normally. Of course, there is the risk of postoperative surgical complications, but these must be analyzed by the surgeon and gastroenterologist, and systematically treated.

—by Lori L. Batchelor

Lori L. Batchelor is executive vice president of the Fort Worth, TX, Area Chapter of the United Ostomy Association and a member of the national UOA Board of Directors. She has served as liaison for UOA with the American Hirschsprung's Disease Association for two years. Lori is the mother of a son, Brandon, who has Hirschsprung's. Medical advisement for this article was provided by pediatric surgeon Timothy Black MD, of Cook-Fort Worth Children's Medical Center.

Chapter 29

Clubfoot and Other Pediatric Foot Deformities

In the challenging field of pediatric orthopedics, the physician must learn to distinguish the abnormal from the wide variations of normal and avoid the mistake of improperly labeling a condition that neither merits nor requires correction. The extremely wide variations of normal body shape and function change spontaneously with age, and seemingly abnormal conditions at birth can resolve or improve over time, while other conditions are considered abnormal if they persist into adulthood. Normal variations can often be a source of great concern to parents, grandparents, friends and neighbors of perfectly healthy children.[1]

Once the specific area of concern is examined and the correct diagnosis made, the primary care physician must also perform a general musculoskeletal screening examination. For example, a child with metatarsus adductus must be examined carefully to rule out an accompanying congenital dislocation of the hip. After the general screening examination, the primary care physician must determine whether referral to a pediatric orthopedic surgeon is appropriate.

According to Staheli,[2] treatment is appropriate if the following three criteria are met: the therapy must be necessary, it must be effective, and the benefits must outweigh the accompanying risks and potential adverse psychosocial effects. Some normal orthopedic variants do not resolve as the child grows but are not serious enough to cause disability and thus do not necessitate corrective surgery. Ineffective

---

"Diagnosis and Treatment of Pediatric Foot Deformities," *American Family Physician*, March 1993 v47 n4 p883(7). Reprinted with permission.

treatment of conditions with a history of spontaneous resolution should be avoided. For example, corrective shoes, exercises and braces are not effective in the majority of cases.

Nearly all interventions can have negative aspects that must be weighed against the proposed benefits. Factors to consider include radiation exposure, financial cost, poor self-image, limited play function and the loss of opportunities to develop interpersonal and motor skills, the intrinsic risks of surgery (such as infection and exposure to anesthesia) and the prospect of worsening the disability. Observation is more appropriate than placebo treatments for parents who demand therapy for a "condition" that is a normal variant. Most parents respond positively to reassurance and the offer of close follow-up after a thorough examination and careful diagnosis.[2]

Etiology

Deformities (or deformations) occur when abnormal mechanical forces distort tissues. Deformation can be defined as an abnormality in the shape, position or form of a body or body part, caused partly by intrinsic or extrinsic mechanical molding.[3] Hypomobility of the fetus secondary to a defect in the nervous system is an example of intrinsic molding (increased susceptibility to deformation), while uterine constraint is an extrinsic force.

Deformation can occur either prenatally or postnatally; other forms of dysmorphogenesis (i.e., malformations, disruptions, dysplasias) originate before birth. Deformation is rarely familial and, unlike other types of birth defects, may resolve spontaneously or after simple therapy. The musculoskeletal system is particularly susceptible to deformation. A list of factors causing fetal constraint and resultant deformation can be found in Table 29.1.[3,4]

Deformities (or deformations) such as metatarsus adductus, calcaneovalgus foot and some forms of clubfoot, are extremely common. Once a foot deformity is identified, a search should be made to detect other deformations, such as torticollis or congenital dislocation of the hip. Intrinsic anomalies of the central nervous system, bone or muscle should be considered if the gestational history fails to confirm the presence of extrinsic compression, includes a history of teratogenic exposure or contains the rare family history of deformation. Deformation not associated with intrinsic anomaly usually has an excellent prognosis because the infant is no longer exposed to the deforming force.[3] Table 29.2 lists conditions known to cause foot deformities.[5]

Table 29.1. Risk Factors for Foot Deformation

Intrauterine compression
  Multiple gestation
  Uterine leiomyoma
  Uterine malformation

Uterine compression
  Increased muscle tone
  Oligohydramnios
  Macrosomia
  Nonvertex presentation

Extrauterine compression
  Small maternal pelvis
  Prominent maternal lumbar spine
  Tight abdominal musculature

Maternal hypertension (mechanism unknown)[4]

General fetal hypotonia
  Diseases of the central and peripheral nervous systems
  Congenital muscle diseases

Congenital muscle imbalance (myelomeningocele)

Family history (clubfoot, dislocated hip)

(Derived from Dunne and Clarren,[3] and Dunne.[4])

Diagnosis

The calcaneovalgus foot (a cause of out-toeing), metatarsus varus or metatarsus adductus (a cause of in-toeing) and talipes equinovarus (clubfoot) are the three most common neonatal foot deformities.[5]

Feet in neonates often look very much alike, but disorders can easily be distinguished by seeking and documenting three variables. First, the foot should be examined from the side to see if it is in an abnormal, fixed equinus position (tiptoe/ tight-heel-cord/plantar-flexed).

Table 29.2. Conditions Associated with Foot Deformities

Arthrogryposis
Brain tumor
Cerebral palsy
Charcot-Marie-Tooth disease
Duchenne's muscular dystrophy
Friedreich's ataxia
Sacral agenesis
Spina bifida
Sacral lipoma
Spinal cord tumor

(Derived from Wenger and Leach.[5])

A normal neonatal foot can easily be dorsiflexed above the neutral position (90 degrees). Second, the sole of the foot should be viewed from below to see if it is shaped like a kidney bean (deviated medially) or like a banana (deviated laterally). Third, the heel should be held in the neutral position and viewed from behind to check for heel varus (medial deviation) or heel valgus lateral deviation).

Calcaneovalgus Foot

The calcaneovalgus foot is the most common neonatal foot deformity. It is the result of positional confinement *in utero*. The foot has a banana-shaped sole (lateral deviation), dorsiflexes quite easily because of a stretched, abnormally long heel cord and has a heel that deviates laterally. Prognosis is excellent; most cases improve spontaneously and rapidly. Parents who are uncomfortable with the prescription of observation alone may be encouraged to exercise the child's foot at each diaper change by stretching the ligaments and dorsal tendons.

In the rare instance that the foot remains severely deformed, corrective casts are applied. If the calcaneovalgus foot can only be partially corrected, a flexible flatfoot results. The severe, resistant calcaneovalgus foot must be differentiated from a congenital vertical talus (congenital convex pes valgus), which is associated with neurologic disorders such as spina bifida or arthrogryposis in about 50 percent of cases. The vertical talus foot has a "rocker-bottom" appearance, with a tight heel cord.[5]

Metatarsus Adductus

The terms "metatarsus adductus" and "metatarsus varus" are used synonymously in practice, although they describe slightly different variations of the forefoot. In both cases, the heel deviates laterally, the sole is kidney-shaped (medial deviation) and the foot is easily dorsiflexed[5]. The incidence of metatarsus adductus is two cases in 1,000 live births.[1] Metatarsus adductus may be bilateral or unilateral and is probably secondary to *in utero* confinement. Often an infant presents with "windblown feet" (both feet pointing in the same direction), in which one foot has calcaneovalgus while the other has metatarsus adductus.[5]

Metatarsus adductus usually improves during the first two months of life, and 85 percent of cases fully resolve spontaneously.[6] The newborn examination should document the severity of the metatarsus adductus, which is classified as (1) mild/flexible, (2) moderate/fixed or (3) severe/rigid.[5] Associated deformities such as congenital dislocation of the hip should also be ruled out.

Parents should be taught how to stretch the child's foot by firmly holding and stabilizing the heel to prevent more heel valgus and stretching the forefoot laterally, holding for a count of five (the baby may wince but should not cry). The exercise should be performed five times at each diaper change.[5]

Mild, flexible metatarsus adductus should rapidly improve by two months of age. Moderate, fixed metatarsus adductus generally is not corrected with stretching alone, and the feet are still deformed at two months of age. To determine the extent of deformity, the child is held in a standing position, because weight-bearing makes the deformity even more obvious.

A pediatric orthopedic surgeon should be consulted when children with moderate fixed metatarsus adductus are approaching two months of age, so that the need for serial corrective casts can be determined. A child should be referred for possible casting by no later than four months of age, if possible, so that the foot is still pliable. By six months of age, foot stiffness and vigorous kicking make correction by serial casting difficult. The most common reasons cited for treating metatarsus adductus are prevention of bunions and calluses of the base of the fifth metatarsal as an adult, although treatment is controversial.[5] Rapid correction of metatarsus adductus can be obtained by applying three or four plaster casts every one to two weeks.[7]

Severe, rigid metatarsus adductus includes a fixed-joint deformity of the midfoot that does not respond to conservative therapy. Infants with this rare condition should be referred for serial corrective casting in the first few weeks of life to take advantage of neonatal ligamentous laxity resulting from exposure to maternal hormones. Corrective surgery is sometimes required, usually at two to four years of age.[5]

A moderate case of metatarsus adductus is occasionally accompanied by a persistent extreme adduction (medial deviation) of the great toe, or metatarsus primus varus. Application of shoes and socks is difficult, and surgical release of the abductor hallucis tendon may be necessary at six to 18 months of age.[5]

Clubfoot

Clubfoot is characterized by the inability to dorsiflex, the presence of heel varus (medial deviation) and a sole that is kidney-shaped when viewed from the bottom. Mild cases can be attributed to deformation caused by intrauterine compression, while more severe, fixed cases are usually secondary to underlying anatomic abnormalities, such as an abnormal talus.

Accompanying deformities such as congenital dislocation of the hip must be ruled out, and the child must be examined carefully for an underlying neurologic or muscular disorder such as spina bifida, myotonic dystrophy or arthrogryposis. Newborns with clubfoot should be referred as soon as possible for corrective serial casts starting in the first week of life to take advantage of residual neonatal ligamentous laxity. Significant correction can be obtained with four to eight casts applied one week apart.

Some physicians try to maintain correction with shoes connected to a device such as a Denis Browne splint. The splint and shoes are worn continuously for several months and then during naps and nighttime sleeping until the child is one year old or surgical correction is attempted. Severe clubfoot requires surgery (posteromedial release) late in the first year of life if full correction is to be achieved. The proportion of children requiring major surgery varies from 75 percent, if full anatomic, radiographic and clinical correction is attempted, to less than 50 percent, if mild radiographic and clinical deformity is accepted.[5]

Flexible Flatfoot

The flexible flatfoot is extremely common, with an incidence ranging [upwards] from 7 percent.[8] The condition is often hidden by normal

Clubfoot and Other Pediatric Foot Deformities

adipose tissue in the infant foot and usually becomes noticeable after a child begins to stand. The most common etiology of the flexible flatfoot is ligamentous laxity, which allows the foot to sag with weight bearing. Children often have accompanying hyperextension of fingers, elbows and knees, as well as a family history of flatfoot and ligamentous laxity.

The child with flexible flatfoot secondary to ligamentous laxity can form a good arch when asked to stand on tiptoe. The heel rolls into a varus position (medial deviation) on tiptoe, and good strength of the ankle and foot muscles is assured.[5]

Flexible flatfoot may be secondary to a tight heel cord and muscular dystrophy, mild cerebral palsy (deep tendon reflexes are increased) or congenital tightness of the heel cords (normal deep tendon reflexes). A stiff and painful flatfoot is unusual and may be attributed to trauma, occult infection, a foreign body, tarsal coalition, bone tumors, Kohler's disease (osteochondrosis of the tarsal navicular bone) or other disorders. Radiographs are not routinely obtained for the diagnosis of flexible flatfoot but are useful in the examination of a stiff, painful flatfoot, which requires orthopedic referral.[1,5,8]

Treatment of the flexible flatfoot is controversial.[1,5] In the past, corrective shoes were modified in an attempt to improve the arch. Custom orthotics worn in normal shoes were tried, without documented success. In 1979, a survey by Staheli and Giffin[9] revealed that most pediatricians and pediatric orthopedic surgeons did not prescribe orthotic inserts or corrective shoes for children with flatfoot. A randomized, prospective study of 129 children with flexible flatfoot, comparing aggressive treatment using corrective shoes or orthotic inserts with no treatment, found no benefit from treatment.[10] Some physicians recommend that children with flexible flatfoot wear well-fitted tennis shoes and recommend special shoes only for children who complain of persistent pain or have such a severe deformity that regular shoes are worn out after a few weeks.[5]

Corrective Shoes

The 1979 survey by Staheli and Giffin[9] demonstrated for the first time that corrective shoes are not recommended by the majority of pediatricians and orthopedic surgeons for pediatric lower extremity deformities.

Most high-top leather infant shoes are made to fit children with metatarsus adductus and do not fit the straight inner border of a normal foot. These shoes are expensive and quickly outgrown. Staheli and Giffin[9] suggest that a properly fitted infant or child shoe should be straight and not exert any inward medial or lateral pressure on the toes. The shoe should be broad enough so the toes assume a natural, noncompressed position when the child is standing. Inexpensive shoes meet these requirements. High-topped shoes are only recommended when the child first begins to walk and is in danger of stepping out of a low-cut shoe.

—by Catherine A. Churgay

Catherine A. Churgay, M.D. is a clinical instructor in the Department of Family Practice at the University of Michigan Medical School, Ann Arbor, where she received her medical degree and served as co-chief resident

References

1. Salter RB. *Textbook of disorders and injuries of the musculoskeletal system*. 2d ed. Baltimore: Williams & Wilkins, 1983: 101-44.

2. Staheli LT. Philosophy of care. *Pediatr Clin North Am* 1986; 33:1269-75.

3. Dunne KB, Clarren SK. The origin of prenatal and postnatal deformities. *Pediatr Clin North Am* 1986; 33:1277-97.

4. Dunne PM. The influence of the intrauterine environment in the causation of congenital postural deformities with special reference to congenital dislocation of the hip [Thesis]. Cambridge, Eng.: Cambridge University, 1969.

5. Wenger DR, Leach J. Foot deformities in infants and children. *Pediatr Clin North Am* 1986; 33:1411-27.

6. Staheli LT. Torsional deformity. *Pediatr Clin North Am* 1986; 33:1373-83.

7. Ponseti IV, Becker JR. Congenital metatarsus adductus: the results of treatment. *J Bone Joint Surg* [Am] 1966; 48:702-11.

8. Barry RJ, Scranton PE Jr. Flat feet in children. *Clin Orthop Rel Res* 1983; 181:68-75.

9. Staheli LT, Giffin L. Corrective shoes for children: a survey of current practice. *Pediatrics* 1980; 65:13-7.

10. Wenger DR, Mauldin D, Speck G, Morgan D, Lieber RL. Corrective shoes and inserts as treatment for flexible flatfoot in infants and children. *J Bone Joint Surg [Am]* 1989; 71:800-10.

Chapter 30

Cleft Lip and Cleft Palate

Background Information

Nature of Cleft Lip and Cleft Palate

If you are like most parents, you may be hearing about clefts for the first time and so some explanation may be helpful. In simple terms a *cleft* is a separation of parts or segments of the lip or roof of the mouth which are usually joined together during the early weeks in the development of an unborn child. A *cleft lip* is a separation of the two sides of the lip and often includes the bones of the maxilla (upper jaw) and/or the upper gum. It looks as though there is a split in the lip and upper gum.

Figure 30.1 illustrates a normal lip and labels parts of the lip and base of the nose. A cleft lip can range from a slight notch in the vermilion (red portion of the lips) to a complete separation of the lip extending into the nose and affecting the side of the nose (nasal alae). When there is a cleft lip, we frequently find that the alveolar ridge (upper gum) is also separated. Clefts of the lip may occur on one or both sides, again with varying degrees of severity. If the cleft occurs

---

This chapter includes two documents produced by the Cleft Palate foundation: "Selected Bibliography," © 1996 and *Cleft Lip and Cleft Palate: The First Four Years*, © 1989. This publication is being revised and will be available in the fall of 1997. Please contact the Cleft Palate Foundation at 1-800-24-CLEFT to receive an updated version. Both documents reprinted with permission.

on one side, it is called a *unilateral cleft lip* (Figure 30.2). If the cleft occurs on both sides of the lip, it is called a *bilateral cleft lip* (Figure 30.2).

Figure 30.3 illustrates a normal palate and labels parts of the palate that you may hear discussed. A *cleft palate* is an opening in the roof of the mouth and can vary in severity. A cleft palate does not mean that the palate is "missing" although it may sometimes look that way. It means the two sides of the palate did not fuse or join together as the unborn baby was developing. In some children, the cleft may involve only the uvula (the small, V-shaped portion at the back of the palate which hangs down into the throat) and the velum (muscular soft palate). This is called an *incomplete cleft palate* (Figure 30.3). In other children, the cleft may extend the entire length of the palate, from back to front, or from the uvula and the velum to just behind the alveolar ridge. This is called a *complete cleft palate* (Figure 30.4). A complete cleft palate may involve one (unilateral) or both sides of the palate (bilateral).

Since the lip and palate develop separately, it is possible for a child to have a cleft lip, a cleft palate, or both cleft lip and palate.

Cause of Cleft Lip and Palate and Its Frequency

It is natural for parents to wonder why the cleft occurred and what may have caused this condition. While many possible causes are being investigated through research, no single cause of cleft lip, cleft palate, or both has been identified. We do know that the majority of clefts appear to be due to a combination of inherited factors (genes) probably interacting with certain "environmental" factors. Clefting occurs very early in a pregnancy and represents a problem over which a pregnant woman has no control. Most families want to know the chances of having another child with a cleft. Because each family is different, this question is best answered by your own doctor or by specialists known as genetic counsellors. These specialists may be physicians who concentrate on the study of genetics and birth defects (dysmorphology) or by persons with a masters or doctoral degree in genetics. The Cleft Palate Foundation has a booklet providing more information on the *Genetics of Cleft Lip and Palate*.

Clefts of the lip and palate are among the most common of all birth defects and occur in all racial and ethnic groups. Approximately one out of every 700 to 750 children born alive has a cleft lip and/or cleft palate.

Cleft Lip and Cleft Palate

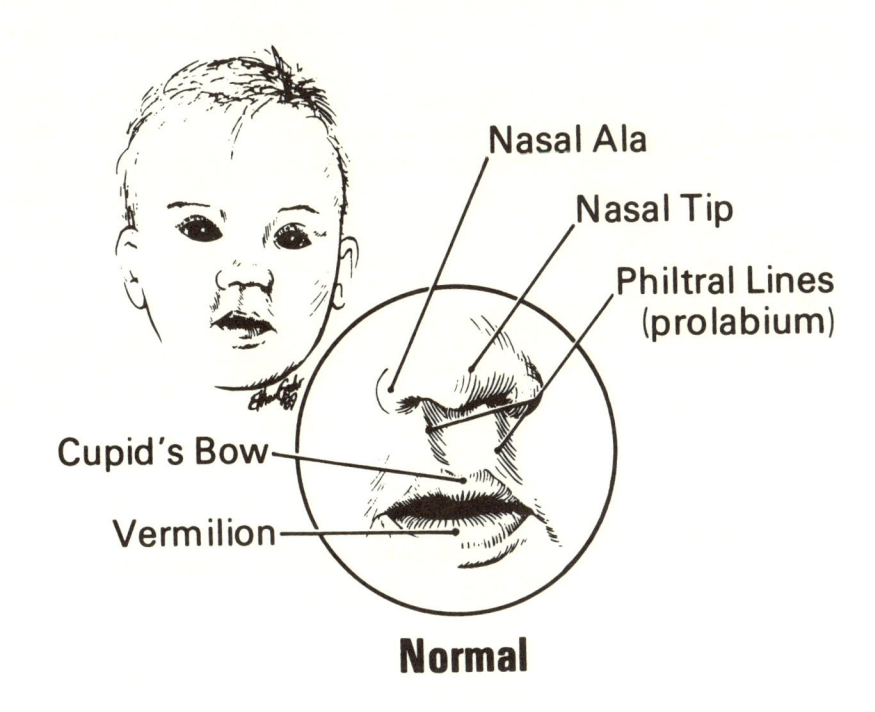

Figure 30.1.

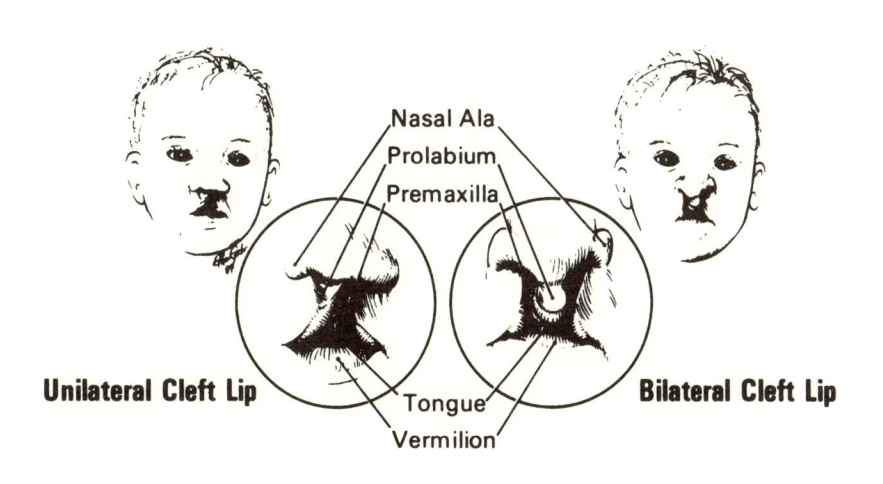

Figure 30.2.

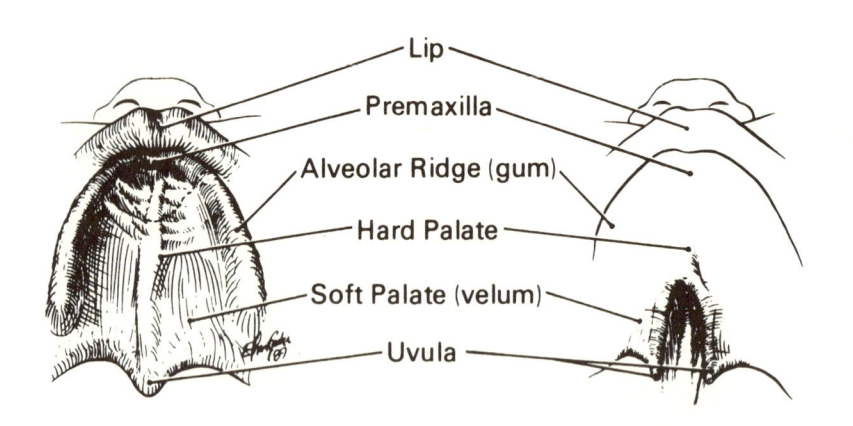

Normal Palate   **Incomplete Cleft Palate**

Figure 30.3.

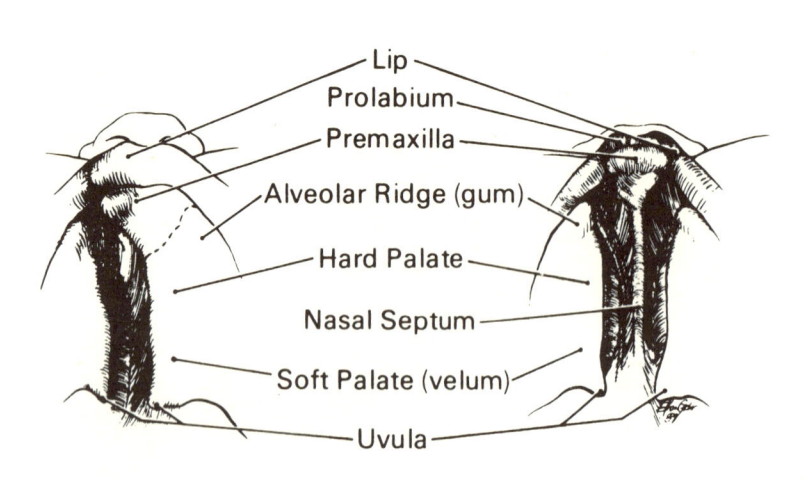

Unilateral Cleft Palate (Lip Repaired)   **Bilateral Cleft Palate**

Figure 30.4.

Cleft Lip and Cleft Palate

The Care of an Infant and Young Child with a Cleft

The first and primary concern is that your infant thrive and remain healthy. Your pediatrician and other specialists will work with you to insure your infant's good health and development. A baby with a cleft needs the same love and care required by any other baby; however, there are some aspects of care that differ and these will be discussed.

Feeding an Infant with a Cleft

Infants with an isolated cleft of the lip or of the soft palate seldom have significant feeding problems. They can usually be fed like any other infant. However, infants with a cleft of the hard palate often have difficulty creating adequate pressure on the nipple because of the opening in the roof of their mouth. All of these infants need proper nourishment and a pleasurable, gratifying feeding experience. For infants with any type of cleft, as for noncleft infants, the two primary choices are breast feeding and bottle feeding.

While there are differences of opinion about breast feeding an infant with a cleft, health care professionals agree that breast milk is the best food. Breast feeding an infant with a cleft requires adjustments in technique and considerable patience. Feeding may need to be facilitated by using a breast pump. If a mother chooses to breast feed, her physician or a local La Leche League nursing coach may help her establish an effective nursing pattern. If these attempts fail, the mother should provide alternate feeding. Prolonged frustration with feeding may impair both the infant's nourishment and mother-infant bonding.

The alternative to breast feeding is bottle feeding. The nutritional composition of the formula will be decided by the infant's doctor. A variety of nipples and bottles are available for an infant with a cleft. The use of a regular bottle or a compressible feeder and a soft, premature (premie) nipple with an enlarged opening usually works successfully. The larger opening allows the milk to flow more freely. The nipple should be angled away from the cleft, and the infant will feed better if held in a semi-upright position. Some doctors recommend the use of a feeding appliance, which is a small, acrylic (plastic) plate made by a dental specialist, which fits in the roof of the mouth and acts as an "artificial" palate during feeding.

Although feeding an infant with a cleft may take extra time at first, the time needed for each feeding should steadily decrease. If your infant requires 45 minutes or longer per feeding, he/she may be working too hard and burning up calories required for weight gain. In this case, your physician should be consulted. As your baby develops and grows you will introduce various other foods although it may be necessary to keep these foods somewhat more liquid than usual.

A final word of advice about infant feeding—be flexible. Try several techniques before you decide which is best for you and your baby. The Cleft Palate Foundation has a booklet on *Feeding An Infant with a Cleft* which provides more detailed information. Remember that whatever method of feeding you use, that method is successful if your baby is receiving adequate nourishment and if you are comfortable when feeding your baby.

Telling Family and Friends about the Cleft

At the time of your infant's birth it is sometimes hard to find the right words to explain to others about the cleft. As you learn more about cleft conditions you will find it easier. Professionals and support groups for parents can answer your questions. The better informed your family and friends are the easier it will be for everyone to see your baby as a normal child with a physical difference which will require surgery, dental work and possibly speech therapy to correct.

Simple, matter-of-fact answers to questions from children or adults about your child's cleft help to establish an attitude of normality toward your child. For example: "He/she was born with a hole in his/her mouth, but the doctors will fix it soon," or "He/she was born with a separation in his/her lip but the doctors will fix it in a few weeks." Children, and even some adults, need reassurance that the "hole" doesn't hurt the baby. Answering questions honestly and openly in front of your child as he/she begins to understand language will help him/her to feel confident.

Taking pictures is usually an important event following the birth of a baby. The cleft is a part of your new baby and you do not want to deny that fact. The pictures you take do not need to be like the clinical poses the professionals need. You should take pictures of this child just as you would any child. Most children enjoy reviewing their own baby pictures and by taking pictures from infancy onward you have a means of reviewing with your child his/her stages of development. From the approach you take, your child will realize that although he/

Cleft Lip and Cleft Palate

she was born with a cleft, that is only a part of the total person. This approach seems to foster the child's self-awareness and self-esteem.

Cleft Palate—Craniofacial Anomalies Teams

One of the more important decisions parents will make regarding their child's care is the selection of the surgeon who does the initial surgery. Thus, very early in their child's life, parents should be aware of Cleft Lip and Palate and Craniofacial Anomalies Teams. Such teams consist of groups of specialists who are primarily interested in the care of children who have clefts and craniofacial anomalies. Most teams include representatives from many of the following specialties: plastic surgery, pediatrics, dentistry (pedodontics, orthodontics, prosthodontics oral surgery), speech and language pathology, social work, audiology, otolaryngology, psychology, nursing, and genetics. The Cleft Palate Foundation suggests that parents choose a team based upon the experience of both the team and the individual specialists serving on the team. The advantage of the team approach is that the child's treatment and care can be systematically and comprehensively planned. After examining a child, the team members meet together and recommend a program for the child's treatment. The team coordinator then forwards the recommended outline of treatment to the family and also to local doctors and specialists who may also participate in the child's care. Parents can locate teams by asking their local physician, other health care provider or by contacting The Cleft Palate Foundation.

Surgical Repair of the Cleft

The object of surgery on the lip is to close the cleft so that scarring will be minimal, appearance is pleasing, and the face develops normally. The goal of palate surgery is to close the cleft so that the palate can function normally during eating and drinking and can provide sufficient length and movement of the palate to insure normal speech production. There are wide variations in both the timing and the technique of surgical repair. It is important that you be comfortable with your baby's surgeon and feel confident about his/her skills, experience, and credentials. Ask lots of questions!

Surgical closure of the lip is usually scheduled around three months of age. At this time the infant is big enough, has been shown to be free of other problems, and has sufficient blood volume to insure a safe procedure and uncomplicated healing. The repair may be accomplished in one procedure; but sometimes it is done in two stages.

Lip surgery usually requires a hospital stay of one or two days to allow the baby time to begin drinking sufficient liquids so that intravenous fluids can be stopped. In some cases the procedure may be performed as an out-patient. The lip scar begins to look paler and more flexible within several months although it will always be visible. After surgery the baby's hands may be restrained with stiff material to keep them away from the mouth and lips. Postoperative care will be discussed by your surgeon.

Palatal closure may involve more than one surgical procedure. Generally, the palate is closed between twelve and eighteen months of age; but timing of closure depends on a variety of factors. Occasionally, a blood transfusion is necessary during palatal surgery. Ask your surgeon how to plan for a safe transfusion, should it be necessary. Sometimes a child will be fitted with an acrylic (plastic), removable palatal appliance to be worn between various surgical procedures. Palatal surgery usually involves a hospital stay of three to five days. Once again there may be special care used to feed your baby. Foods need to be liquified and the baby may need to drink from a cup for a few weeks. So if your baby still drinks exclusively from a bottle, it is helpful to familiarize him/her with drinking from a cup before surgery. The baby's hands are usually restrained for several days after surgery. These changes do not seem to upset most babies for the brief time they are necessary. Your doctors will discuss postoperative care in detail with you.

Before your baby is admitted to the hospital, there are a number of questions parents need to ask about accommodations for themselves, arrangements for their own meals, and the routine for the baby's care. Parents need to check what the hospital provides such as diapers, formula, etc., and what they need to bring from home. It is often helpful to bring the baby's "security blanket" or favorite toy.

Additional surgery will very likely be necessary as your child grows and matures. Some of the areas which often require further surgery are the lip, nose, gum, and palate. Surgical timing and techniques are planned to allow the best facial growth and development (particularly the jaw and the nose) and to promote normal appearance and speech. For example, final surgery on the nose is often postponed until the teenage years when the face has reached full growth. Sometimes it is necessary to complete certain phases of dental or orthodontic correction prior to surgical procedures. The surgical plans are coordinated with other aspects of the child's development, such as tooth eruption

Cleft Lip and Cleft Palate

and speech, as well as with schedules for school and other important extracurricular activities.

Care of the Ears

Children with clefts of the palate have an increased risk of having ear infections early in life. These problems are the result of inadequate function of some of the palatal muscles. These muscles are needed to open the eustachian tubes (small tubes connecting the throat to the middle ear). When the eustachian tubes do not open effectively then air is prevented from entering the middle ear. This lack of ventilation causes fluid to form and eventually accumulate in the middle ear. This condition is called otitis media. The fluid can then become infected and the child experiences a fever and painful earache.

Because of the frequency of this problem children with clefts of the palate should be examined by an otolaryngologist (an Ear, Nose, and Throat or "ENT" specialist) within the first few months of life. If that specialist determines that fluid is present in the middle ear, medication may be prescribed to "dry up" the fluid or when lip surgery is scheduled (usually around three months of age), a minor surgical procedure called a myringotomy may be scheduled. This procedure consists of making a small slit in the eardrum to drain the fluid. Following drainage, tiny tubes may be inserted (called PE tubes) in the slits to allow air to enter the middle ear and prevent fluid from reforming. Once the tubes are out, these small slits heal readily and they do not usually result in any permanent damage to the eardrum.

Parents need to realize that fluid in the middle ears does not always result in symptoms like earaches that are easy to detect. However, constant fluid in the middle ear creates a risk that the ear drum may be permanently deformed. In addition, children with persistent middle ear disease are more likely to have some loss of hearing and this loss adversely affects speech development. Consequently, children with clefts of the palate should have frequent ear examinations. The first one should be scheduled no later than three to six months after birth. Thereafter the child should be re-examined on a routine basis.

Hearing Testing

Because of problems with ear infections, children with clefts of the palate may experience some hearing loss which changes over time. Consequently, it is important that parents make sure that their child's hearing is tested regularly during his/her early years. Preferably this testing should be done by an audiologist who has the specialized training and audiometric equipment to test very young children.

Parents often wonder how babies and very young children can have their hearing tested. Audiologists have a variety of techniques for testing the hearing of even newborn babies. These same tests can be used with infants and toddlers until they are mature enough to participate in other types of tests. For these children, tests called ABR (Auditory Brainstem Response) or BSER (Brainstem Evoked Response) can evaluate the brain's response to sound for each ear. This is a quick test and if a baby should fail an ABR screening, then a longer, full ABR test can be conducted. Results of this test can determine if a hearing loss is present. Depending on how the test is done, results may be able to specify whether the problem is in the middle ear or the inner ear.

Once a baby is between 4 and 7 months of age testing called behavioral audiometry can be done. In this test, the baby is placed in a sound-treated, quiet room with the parent. Sounds are fed into the room through speakers and the baby's response to sound is observed by the audiologist. Responses like turning toward the source of the sound (localization) make it obvious when the baby hears the sound. Some audiologists also utilize toys that light up when the baby localizes the sound correctly and this technique is also very effective. Once the baby is several months of age a test called impedance audiometry is very valuable. This test can measure whether there is pressure (often indicating fluid) at the ear drum.

When a child reaches 2½ to 3 years of age, a technique called play audiometry can be used. In this test earphones are put on the child and the child is trained to do something whenever a sound is heard (for example, the child might drop a block into a container whenever he/she hears a sound). By the age of 4½ to 5 years, children can respond to the tests routinely utilized with adults.

A young child who experiences some degree of hearing loss is at risk for other problems. A hearing loss may cause problems with speech and language development. In addition, a loss in hearing may result in a habit of inattention which could lead to future language or learning problems. Consequently, frequent checking of hearing is important for young children with clefts of the palate.

Speech Development

The parents of an infant with a cleft often ask how well their baby will talk. Speech-language pathologists have studied the speech

Cleft Lip and Cleft Palate

development of many children with clefts and their findings may be used as a guide. If a child has an isolated cleft of the lip, and no other problems, then speech should be normal or close to normal. Approximately 80% of children with a cleft of the palate develop normal speech once their palate is closed. The others may require further surgery, speech therapy, or a prosthetic speech aid to improve their speech. A major goal of palatal surgery is to ensure good speech quality at the earliest age. The speech-language pathologist may consult with the surgeon and other specialists in planning the type of palatal surgery and the best age to schedule the surgery.

Children with clefts of the palate tend to develop speech and language a bit more slowly than other children. Their articulation and resonance will be abnormal until palatal surgery is performed but they tend to "catch up" after the palatal surgery has been completed. This "catch-up" process often continues for four or five years and speech therapy may be necessary during some of these years. Children with clefts are also at increased risk for some type of language disorder. For these reasons periodic evaluations by a speech-language pathologist knowledgeable about cleft lip and palate is important. The first evaluation should be scheduled by 3 to 6 months of age with follow up testing scheduled every 6 to 12 months during the first three to four years.

Parents sometimes wonder how a baby's speech and language can be evaluated before the infant even begins to speak. From birth onward babies follow a well documented course of speech and language development. The sucking, blowing, and chewing activities that all babies engage in involve the oral muscles eventually used to speak and the proficiency of these activities can be charted. Months before babies say their first word, they already make many cooing and babbling sounds and they can communicate a variety of things to their parents and caretakers. The rate and order of this development can be recorded. Once the child begins to talk the individual speech sounds and the words the child understands and uses can be measured and compared to norms. Use of these developmental milestones allows speech-language pathologists to recognize problems that may require intervention before the child begins school.

Parents have a crucial role to play in their child's speech development. We know that the interactions between parents and their small children are codependent. Each influences and is influenced by the other. One easy way to stimulate a child's speech development is for the parent to follow the child's lead. When the baby makes a sound, the parent can imitate that sound, then wait for the child to respond (count to ten silently) before repeating the sound. Once this "game" is established, the parent may change the sound and see if the child will follow the parent's lead. When a child is imitating sounds, words usually follow.

Parents need to interact with their child with a cleft just as they would with any child who is learning to talk. Encourage and respond to the child's intended meaning even if these first words sound different or have a nasal quality. Parents who talk with their child about what is happening, play little nursery games with them, and read to them are providing good speech and language stimulation.

A final question parents have is whether speech therapy is always necessary. Some children may need to be involved with their parents in a program of speech and language stimulation, others may need therapy during the "catch up" period, while still others may not require any therapy during the preschool years. However, all children need to be evaluated routinely to determine their individual needs.

Dental Care

Children with clefts of the lip and palate have the same dental problems as noncleft children. In addition, they may have special problems associated with the cleft. A cleft may affect the alveolar ridge (upper gum containing the teeth). Consequently, some teeth may be incorrectly shaped, out of correct position, or even entirely missing. The teeth most commonly affected are the upper incisors and cuspids on the side of the cleft (see Figure 30.5).

The dental treatment of cleft children may best be coordinated among several dental specialists interacting on a team that begins to follow the baby at birth. The dental specialties may include pediatric dentistry, orthodontics, oral surgery, and prosthodontics. These specialists are all concerned with the size and shape of the jaws, the position of the teeth within the jaws, and the prevention of decay. To assist in planning treatment for the child with a cleft, comprehensive dental records will need to be obtained. These records will include study models, x-rays, and photographs.

The pediatric dentist is trained to care for the dental needs of the very young child. These needs may include fillings, cleaning the teeth, space maintenance, and all other types of routine care.

Special dental appliances (prostheses) may be placed in the mouths of some infants with cleft palates to assist them in feeding. At later ages, obturators (speech appliances) may be used to close palatal openings and to provide assistance in obtaining better speech. A prosthodontic

Cleft Lip and Cleft Palate

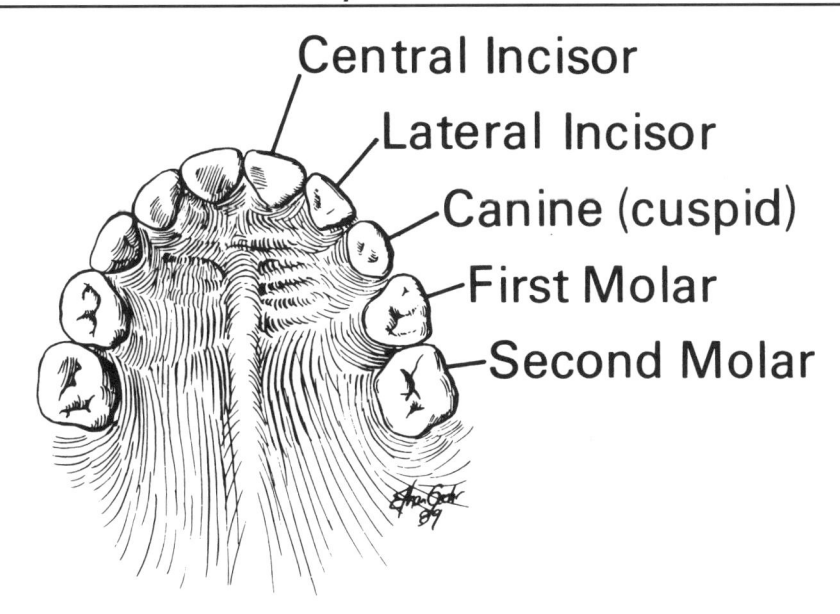

Central Incisor
Lateral Incisor
Canine (cuspid)
First Molar
Second Molar

Figure 30.5. Primary teeth

specialist generally places this appliance in the child's mouth after consultation with other specialists on the team.

The orthodontist may treat a child with a cleft in two distinct phases. Phase I may begin at approximately age 8, but in some children can begin much earlier. Treatment is aimed at correcting extreme irregularities and crossbites (where the top teeth are inside of the bottom teeth). This may be accomplished by using a palatal expansion appliance. Phase II may begin at about 10 to 12 years of age when most of the permanent teeth have erupted. At this time the teeth may be repositioned using braces.

The maxillofacial or oral surgeon may be involved during the earlier surgeries when he/she utilizes a bone graft to stabilize expansion of the palate and to provide bone for the erupting teeth. During the teen years when facial growth is complete, this specialist may recommend surgery to the upper and/or lower jaw to improve tooth and jaw relationships and to improve facial appearance.

Psychological Aspects

Clinical psychologists and other mental health professionals serve on cleft palate-craniofacial teams. Sometimes parents feel that seeing a mental health professional means there is something seriously "wrong" with them or with their child. This is not true. Most people need some help adjusting to having or being a child with a birth defect. The mental health professional is on the team to provide that help. Some teams routinely provide clinic services from a mental health professional. These services usually include an interview to help identify concerns or problems. Other teams may provide these services only when they are requested.

Parents, children, or both may need the help of a mental health professional. Parents can experience intense shock, anger, guilt, depression and confusion following the birth of an infant with a cleft. They may also have to deal with the stresses of hospitalizing their child for surgery, coping with financial strains, and juggling child care and work schedules. Brothers and sisters of the child with a cleft may have mixed feelings about this new family member. Parents may be faced with new problems involving child management and discipline. The team mental health professional can assist parents in coping with these new problems.

Children with clefts as young as 2 years may have adjustment problems of a psychological nature. They may have concerns about the way other people react to their speech or appearance. Psychologists can provide guidance to help children develop their self-confidence and deal appropriately with teasing. By 3 years of age, children can learn to answer simple questions about their appearance or speech. They can say, "I was born with a split here (pointing). The doctor fixed it." or "My mama says I'll talk better soon." Children ages 2-4 can also experience fears about the hospital and surgery. They may cry and get upset when they have to go to the hospital. Sometimes children try to cope with these problems by acting "shy" or avoiding people. Other times they may become more dependent on their parents or act immature for their age. Parents can help their children with these problems by requesting play therapy for the child or counseling education for themselves.

The clinical psychologist also participates with other team members in assessing the child's overall developmental level. This information is especially important when parents are planning for school placement. Being able to compete successfully in school immediately increases a child's self-esteem.

A cleft lip and/or palate poses several expected adjustment problems for both the child with a cleft and his/her family. The role of the psychologist or mental health professional is to assist the child and the family in coping with these problems.

Cleft Lip and Cleft Palate

Preschool Education

Services for children with special problems and for their parents are expanding and improving within the educational system. In 1986 Public Law 99-457 was signed requiring the development of services for children from birth to two years of age with identifiable handicaps. The full implementation of this law is on a progressive year by year basis and will not be fully in operation for approximately five years. In the meantime your state education department has a plan which has been submitted to the federal government to meet the requirements of the law. Parents may contact the governor's office to obtain more specific information regarding the implementation of PL 99-457 in their own state.

The services that may be provided by the public schools include an assessment and a written Individualized Family Service Plan (IFSP) developed by a multidisciplinary team and the parents. Case management services must be provided for the child and parents. Special educational services may include: special education, speech and language pathology, audiology, psychological services, parent training, and medical services for diagnostic purposes and to enable the child to benefit from early intervention.

Even if children with clefts may not require the specialized services mandated by PL 99-457, parents still wonder about part-time or full-time preschool. For all children the preschool experience presents many advantages and perhaps some disadvantages that parents should consider. However, the advantages and disadvantages relate more to the type of preschool chosen than to the concept of preschool in general. In order for a preschool experience to be good for any child, the teachers, aides, and other caregivers must be caring people who understand child development. Preschools should capitalize on the fact that young children learn through play. They need to learn through pleasurable, exciting, first hand experiences with other children and adults, and with new play materials. They need time to explore, reflect, share, listen, and discover. The preschool experience gives children the opportunity to relate to adults outside of the home and become a part of a group with a daily routine. The child can experience a feeling of being "special" outside of the family and look forward to going to a place where people are waiting and excited to see him/her. When all of this is present, the advantages of a preschool can be tremendous.

The preschool experience provides some advantages for the parents as well as the child. Parents can observe their child in a group of other children and can see not only how their child operates but also how other children of the same age function. Parents can observe other adults relating to their child and they can get advice from professionals trained to understand preschool children. Not to be minimized, preschool gives parents a time to get other work accomplished or have individual time with other children in the family who may be feeling "left out" because of the attention focused on the child with a cleft. Knowing their child is in a good preschool can allow both parents to work without feeling that they are cheating their child.

Before a parent enrolls a child in any preschool, check the school thoroughly. Make certain the atmosphere and activities are pleasurable and enriching for your child. Meet and find out about the teachers and other caregivers who will actually interact with your child. Are these persons interested in understanding your child and do they appear excited about the possibility of having him/her as a student? Do the other children appear relaxed and happy in their play in contrast to the rigid classrooms where preschoolers are expected to behave like children in grade school? Do other parents appear satisfied with the preschool? If these answers are positive, then enroll your child on a trial basis. When you find the right preschool, this experience can foster the development of good communication skills, socialization with peers and learning through play.

Sources of Support for Parents

Parent/Patient Support Groups

Many parents who have a baby with a cleft lip, cleft palate, or both feel isolated and alone. They often say that it is very helpful to be able to talk to other parents of children with clefts. In many parts of the country there are local parent groups. These are organizations of parents of children with clefts and adults with clefts who meet to share common concerns and ideas. Because these individuals share similar experiences, they prove to be a continuing source of support for each other. The Parent-Patient Liaison Committee of the Cleft Palate Foundation produces a newsletter for parents and patients and there is also a national group (the National Cleft Palate Association) which meets in conjunction with the annual meeting of the American Cleft Palate–Craniofacial Association (an organization of professionals who care for children with clefts and other craniofacial defects). Members of your local cleft palate team, your local health

Cleft Lip and Cleft Palate

care providers, or The Cleft Palate Foundation can put you in touch with parent support groups in your area.

Funding for Treatment

Financial resources to help pay all or part of the costs of treating a child with cleft lip and/or palate fall into three general categories. Your own private or group health insurance will usually cover a portion of the cost of treatment after a certain deductible is met. When buying future insurance be sure to check if the coverage applies only to surgery or if it includes such crucial aspects as dental care and services such as hearing testing, speech and language testing and treatment, and psychological testing and/or counselling. There are also federal and state programs such as Champus, Medicaid, and Children's Special Health Services (formerly called the Crippled Children's Program). Some private and non-profit agencies such as the Easter Seal Society, the March of Dimes Birth Defect Foundation, the Grottos of America and the National Association for the Craniofacially Handicapped may all provide funds or special services to meet some aspects of your child's needs. The social worker or team coordinator should also be able to provide you with information regarding funding.

Parents recommend that if a private company initially rejects a bill, you discuss the case with the company. If the bill was rejected because they did not understand the problem of clefting and the habilitation procedures required, a discussion could result in the company paying the bill.

Mental Health Professionals

As the parent of a child with a cleft lip, cleft palate, or both, you already understand the shock of being told that your child has a birth defect that will require treatment possibly over a period of years. In addition you must still make all the adjustments required of any new parent. The first step in coping successfully is learning to acknowledge and accept the unfamiliar and painful feelings that may seem overwhelming during the first few years. These feelings are not unusual and will not go away unless you learn to deal with them. Parents need to take time during the first year to begin to learn acceptance of the problem and to give their feelings a chance to surface and heal.

Initially parents may seek comfort and support from their family and friends. They can also speak to other parents who have already faced the same situation. Knowing that someone else has faced what you are facing is often both informative and comforting. However, if the emotional pain is not reduced after the first six months of your child's life, or if it significantly interferes with your ability to function at home, at work, or in your relationships, you may want to speak to a qualified mental health professional. Your cleft palate-craniofacial team or your physician may be able to recommend someone. If paying for such help is a problem, then the team coordinator or your physician may be able to refer you to a mental health facility that accepts fee reductions or third party payments. The emotional health of the parents is essential to their ability to help their child.

The Cleft Palate Foundation

This foundation is associated with the American Cleft Palate–Craniofacial Association, a group of various specialists including surgeons, dentists, speech-language pathologists, psychologists, nurses, and others who have a major interest in the care of children with clefts and craniofacial defects. The Foundation produced this material as well as other publications and free Information Sheets.

In addition, the Foundation operates a toll-free Cleftline to provide information to anyone who has questions about clefting. The number is:

1-800-24-CLEFT (Voice/TDD)

You may also write to the Foundation at their national office. The address is:

The Cleft Palate Foundation
1218 Grandview Avenue
Pittsburgh, PA 15211
(412) 481-1376

Selected Bibliography for Parents of Children with Cleft Lip/Palate

The following list of publications for parents of children with cleft lip/palate was compiled by the Parent-Patient Liaison Committee of the Cleft Palate Foundation. The sources of the publications are reported. The committee stresses that not one of the pamphlets is appropriate in its entirety for any given child. Please consult with the professional people who are caring for your child for a better understanding of the written material as it applies to your child's specific needs.

Cleft Palate Foundation Publications

Multiple orders require postage & handling fees. CPF offers discounts for bulk orders. Call for details. Prices are subject to change.

Booklets

For Parents of Newborn Babies with Cleft Lip/Palate, 1980. Pp. 4. $.20.

A los Padres de los Bebes Recien Nacidos con Labio Leporino/Paladar Hendido, 1988. Pp. 4. $.20.

Cleft Lip and Cleft Palate: The First Four Years, 1989. Pp. 16. $2.00.

Labio Hendido y Paladar Hendido: Los Cuatro Primeros Anos, 1989. Pp. 18. $2.00.

Cleft Lip and Cleft Palate: The School-Aged Child, 1996. $2.00.

Information for the Teenager Born with a Cleft Lip and/or Palate, 1980. Pp. 12. $2.00.

Feeding an Infant with a Cleft, 1992. Pp. 20. $2.00.

Como Alimentar a un Bebe con Paladar Hendido, 1993. Pp. 20. $2.00.

The Genetics of Cleft Lip and Palate: Information for Families, 1996. Pp. 6. $2.00.

Free Information

- Information about Choosing a Cleft Palate or Craniofacial Team
- Information about Crouzon's Disease
- Information about Dental Care
- Information about Financial Assistance

- Information about Pierre Robin Malformation Sequence
- Information about Submucous Cleft
- Information about Treacher Collins Syndrome
- Information about Treatment for Adults with Cleft Lip and Palate

Information Published by Other Sources

Order directly from these sources.

AboutFace, *AboutFace Newsletter*. AboutFace, U.S.A., P.O. Box 737, Warrington, PA 18976. Call (800)225-FACE. Or AboutFace International, 99 Crowns Lane, 3rd Floor, Toronto, Ontario M5R 3P4 Canada. Call (800)665-FACE. Minimum $20.00 donation requested.

Berkowitz, S., *The Cleft Palate Story*, 1994. Quintessence Publishing Company, Inc., 551 North Kimberly Drive, Carol Stream, IL 60188-1881. Telephone (800)621-0387 or (708)682-3223.

Childbirth Graphics Ltd., *Nursing Your Baby with Cleft Palate or Cleft Lip*. Childbirth Graphics, P.O. Box 21207, Waco, TX 76702-1207. Phone: (800)299-3366. $.59

The Craniofacial Center, *Feeding Your Special Baby*, 1982. Attn: Marcia Aduss, University of Illinois at Chicago, M/C 588, 808 So. Wood Street, Chicago, IL 60612. $1.75. Contact for bulk order discounts.

Easter Seal Society, *Un Futuro Prometedor: Para Su Nino con Labio Hendido y Paladar Hendido*, National Easter Seal Society, 230 West Monroe, Suite 1800, Chicago, IL 60606. $2.50.

Elms, L., Minerva, A., and Starr, P., *Our Child with a Cleft Lip and Palate*, 1978. Lancaster Cleft Palate Clinic, 223 North Lime Street, Lancaster, PA 17602. Pp. 9. $2.00.

Georgiade, N., Clifford, E., and Massengill, R., *The Child with Cleft Lip or Palate*. National Foundation/March of Dimes, Box 2000, White Plains, NY 10602. Pp. 21. Free.

MacDonald, S., *Caring for Your Newborn*. Prescription Parents, Inc., P.O. Box 161, West Roxbury, MA 02132. Pp. 10. $1.95.

Cleft Lip and Cleft Palate

MacDonald, S., *Hearing and Behavior in Children with Cleft Lip and Palate*. Prescription Parents, Inc., P.O. Box 161. West Roxbury. MA 02132. Pp. 15. $1.95.

McDonald, E., *Bright Promise*, National Easter Seal Society, 230 West Monroe, Suite 1800, Chicago, IL 60606. Pp. 21. $2.50. Available in Spanish.

Mead Johnson, *Looking Forward, Guide for Parents of the Child with Cleft Lip and Palate*, Mead Johnson and Company, Evansville, IN 47721. Pp. 37. Free.

Moller, K., Starr, C., Johnson, S., *A Parent's Guide to Cleft Lip and Palate*, 1990. University of Minnesota Press, 2037 University Avenue S.E., Minneapolis, MN 55414. Pp. 131. $14.95 cloth plus $3.00 shipping & handling. Prepayment, VISA or MasterCard accepted, call (800)388-3863.

Peckinpah, Sandra Lee, *Rosey...the Imperfect Angel*, 1991. Scholars Press, hardbound, 32 pages, $15.95 distributed through B. Dalton/Barnes & Noble/Walden Books, or Dasan Productions at (800)348-4401 or in California (818)597-8380.

Shadyside Maxillofacial and Cleft Palate Prosthetics Center, *Cleft Palate Reflections* (Newsletter). Shadyside Maxillofacial and Cleft Palate Prosthetics Center, Shadyside Medical Center, 5230 Centre Avenue, Suite 207, Pittsburgh. PA 15232. $10.00/year.

Starr, P., *Cleft Lip and/or Palate: Will It Affect My Child?*, 1978. Lancaster Cleft Palate Clinic, 223 North Lime Street, Lancaster, PA 17602. Pp. 43. $2.00.

Wicka, D., and Falk, M., *Advice to Parents of a Cleft Palate Child*, 1982, 2nd Edition. Charles Thomas Publisher, 2600 So. 1st Street, Springfield, IL 62704. Pp. 80. $ 19.25 + $4.00 shipping/handling.

Wide Smiles, *Wide Smiles Newsletter*. Wide Smiles, P.O. Box 5153, Stockton, CA 95205-0153. $18.00/year.

Wynn, S., *Team Approach to the Cleft Lip and Palate Child*. Children's Hospital of Wisconsin, 9000 West Wisconsin Avenue, MS #747, Cleft Palate Clinic, Box 1997, Milwaukee, WI 53201. Pp. 12.

Glossary

Alveolar Ridge: The bony ridge of the maxilla and mandible containing the teeth.

Articulation: The process of forming speech sounds.

Articulation Test: An evaluation which provides information about how speech sounds are formed.

Audiogram: A standard graph used to record hearing levels or sensitivity.

Audiologist: A person with a degree, license, and certification in audiology (science of hearing) who measures hearing, identifies hearing loss, and participates in rehabilitation of hearing impairment.

Cineradiography: Motion picture recording of physiological activity often used to diagnose velopharyngeal competence.

Columella: The central, lower portion of the nose which divides the nostrils.

Communication Disorder: An interference with a person's ability to comprehend others or express themselves (usually in verbal form).

Comprehension: Knowledge or understanding of spoken or written language.

Congenital: A disease, deformity, or deficiency existing at the time of birth.

Crossbite: A dental condition where the upper teeth are behind the lower teeth rather than in front of them.

Denasality: The quality of voice that lacks normal nasal resonance for /m/n/ng.

Dental Arch: The curved structure formed by the teeth in their normal position.

Cleft Lip and Cleft Palate

Eardrum: Tympanic membrane which vibrates and transmits sound to the middle ear.

E.N.T.: The abbreviation for ear, nose, and throat.

Eustachian Tube: The air duct which connects the nasopharynx (back of the throat) with the middle ear; usually closed at one end, opens with yawning and swallowing; allows ventilation of the middle ear cavity and equalization of pressure on two sides of the eardrum.

Evaluation: Assessment. Test.

Expressive Language: Communication of one's ideas, desires, or intentions to others usually through speech or printed words.

Fistula: An abnormal opening.

Genetics: The science of heredity.

Hare Lip: An outdated term referring to cleft lip; so-called because of the resemblance to that of a rabbit.

Hearing Impairment: A loss in hearing which may range from mild loss to complete deafness.

Heredity: The total of the physical characteristics, abilities, and potentialities genetically derived from one's ancestors.

Hypernasality: Greater than normal nasal resonance or vocal tone heard during speech.

Hyponasality: Denasality. A lack of normal nasal resonance during speech.

Language Disorder or Impairment: Inability to communicate normally and effectively due to problems with comprehension or expression of language.

Malocclusion: A deviation from normal occlusion or incorrect positioning of the upper teeth in relation to the lower teeth.

Mandible: The lower jaw.

Maxilla: The upper jaw.

Middle Ear: The portion of the ear behind the eardrum. It contains three small bones which transfer sound from the eardrum to the inner ear.

Myringotomy: A minor surgical procedure in which a small slit is made in the eardrum to allow fluid to drain from the middle ear.

Nasal Emission or Nasal Escape: An abnormal flow of air through the nose during speech. Usually indicative of an incomplete seal between oral and nasal cavities.

Nasopharyngoscope: A lighted telescopic instrument used for examining the passages in the back of the throat. Useful in assessing velopharyngeal closure.

Occlusion: Relationship between upper and lower teeth when they are in contact. Refers to the alignment of teeth as well as relationship of dental arches.

Oral Cavity: The mouth bounded by the teeth in front and the soft palate at the back.

Orofacial: Relating to the mouth and face.

Orthodontics: The specialty of dentistry concerned with the correction and prevention of irregularities and malocclusion of the teeth and jaws.

Otitis Media: Inflammation of the middle ear with accumulation of thick, mucous fluid.

Otolaryngologist: A physician specializing in the diagnosis of the ear and larynx and in treatment of problems diagnosed.

Palatal Insufficiency: A lack or shortness of tissue preventing the velum from contacting the back of the throat (pharynx).

Cleft Lip and Cleft Palate

Palate: The roof of the mouth including the front portion or hard palate and the posterior portion or the soft palate also called the velum.

Pediatric Dentistry: The specialty of dentistry concerned with the care of children's teeth.

Pediatrician: A physician specializing in treatment of children.

Pharyngeal Flap: A surgical procedure in which a flap of skin is used to close most of the opening between the velum and the nasopharynx.

Plastic Surgery: The medical specialty dealing with the restoration and repair of various external defects.

Premaxilla: The small bone in the upper jaw which contains the upper four front teeth. Connects with the lateral segments of the upper jaw or maxilla.

Prosthesis: An artificial substitute for a missing body part.

Prosthetic Speech Aid: A removable acrylic appliance which provides a structural means of achieving velopharyngeal closure.

Prosthodontist: A dentist who specializes in providing prosthetic appliances for oral structures.

Psychologist: An individual with the necessary academic training and experience to be licensed to practice psychology as a profession.

Radiography: Photographic film or plate depicting images of internal body parts. X-ray.

Resonance: Vocal quality associated with the vibration of air in the oral and nasal cavities.

Soft Palate: The velum.

Speech-Language Pathologist: An individual with the necessary academic training and experience to be certified or licensed to diagnose and treat disorders of speech, language, and communication.

Speech Defect: Deviation of speech from the range of normal.

Uvula: Small, cone-shaped muscular process hanging at the back of the soft palate.

Velopharyngeal Closure: The closing of the nasal cavity from the oral cavity which directs air used in speech through the mouth rather than the nose. It requires interaction of the muscles in the palate and back of the throat.

Velopharyngeal Incompetence: Inability to achieve adequate velopharyngeal closure despite structures that may appear normal.

Velopharyngeal Insufficiency: A structural or functional disorder resulting in the inability to achieve adequate separation of the nasal and oral cavities.

Velum: The soft palate.

Chapter 31

Sturge-Weber Syndrome

Introduction

Sturge-Weber syndrome (encephalotrigeminal angiomatosis) is a congenital, non-familial disorder of unknown incidence and cause. It is characterized by a congenital facial birthmark and neurological abnormalities. Other symptoms associated with Sturge-Weber can include eye and internal organ irregularities. Each case of Sturge-Weber syndrome is unique and exhibits the characterizing findings to varying degrees.

Facial Birthmark

The most apparent indication of Sturge-Weber syndrome is a facial birthmark or "port wine stain" present at birth and typically involving at least one upper eyelid and the forehead. Much variation in the size of the stain has been reported and may be limited to one side of the face or may involve both sides. The stain, varying from light pink to deep purple, is due to an overabundance of capillaries just beneath the surface of the involved skin. In persons with dark pigmentation, the stain may be difficult to recognize. In rare instances, there is an absence of a port wine stain.

This chapter contains two undated documents produced by the Sturge-Weber Foundation: "Sturge-Weber Syndrome," and "The Laymen's Guide to Sturge-Weber Medical Terminology;" reprinted with permission.

Neurological Abnormalities

Neurological concerns relate to the development of excessive blood vessel growth on the surface of the brain (angiomas). These are located typically on the back (occipital) region of the brain on the same side as the port wine stain. These angiomas create abnormal conditions for brain function in the region. Seizure activity is the most common early problem, often starting by one year of age. The convulsions usually appear on the opposite side of the body from the port wine stain and vary in severity. Vigorous attempts are made to control the seizures with medication. A weakening or loss of use of one side of the body (hemiparesis), may develop opposite to the port wine stain. Developmental delay of motor and cognitive skills may also occur to varying degrees.

Other Features

Increased pressure within the eye (glaucoma) is another condition which can be present at birth or develop later. The incidence of glaucoma in patients with Sturge-Weber is approximately 30%. The glaucoma is usually restricted to the eye which has the stain involvement. Enlarging of the eye (buphthalmos) can also occur in the eye which has been affected by the stain.

Multiple other body organs can rarely be affected in Sturge-Weber syndrome. Infants with Sturge-Weber syndrome are often followed medically by a pediatrician, neurologist, ophthalmologist, and dermatologist.

Therapy

Laser treatment is available to lighten and/or remove port wine stains in children as young as one month of age. Anti-convulsants are used to control the seizures. Surgery and/or eyedrops are used to control the glaucoma.

The Sturge-Weber Foundation

The Sturge-Weber Foundation was incorporated in 1987 as a non-profit organization for parents, professionals and others concerned with Sturge-Weber syndrome (SWS). In 1993, the Foundation expanded

Sturge-Weber Syndrome

its outreach to include Klippel-Trenaunay Weber (KTW) and Port Wine Stains. As the cause of these syndromes are not known, research is needed. Join us in our efforts to obtain research so that the families of a child with SWS, KTW or a Port Wine Stain may have a brighter future.

Sturge-Weber Foundation
PO Box 418
Mt. Freedom, NJ 07970
(201) 895-4445
(800) 627-5482

The Laymen's Guide to Sturge-Weber Medical Terminology

Amblyopia: Poor vision due to non-use of an eye caused by underdevelopment of the visual pathway to the brain.

Angiogram: X-ray test to outline the blood vessels of an organ such as the brain. Uses a dye which is injected into a blood vessel (arteries) in the arm or groin. The dye shows up on the X-ray and therefore outlines all the blood vessels.

Angioid Streaks: Lines resembling blood vessels.

Angioma: Any malformation made up of blood vessels. These could be veins or a combination of arteries and veins (arteriovenous malformations or AVMs).

Anticonvulsant: Any medication that counteracts *seizures*.

Arteriogram: Same as *angiogram*.

Astigmatism: Unequal curve of the refractive surfaces of the eye, leading to a blurry image on the retina when the astigmatism is of significant degree.

Babinski's Reflex: A reflex named after Prof. Babinski. Stroking the sole of the foot should normally cause the big toe to point downwards. A Babinski sign is when it points up instead, and the other toes fan out. Implies spasticity. A Babinski reflex is considered normal in the immature nervous system, such as in a baby.

Bilateral: Both sides, as opposed to *unilateral* (one side).

Buphthalmos: Enlarged size of the eye. Caused by *glaucoma* occurring in infancy.

CAT Scan: (Computed Axial Tomography) X-ray test of any organ, including the brain that uses computer reconstruction of multiple images at different planes.

Cataract: An opacity in the lens of the eye. May obstruct vision.

Congenital: Occurring from the time of birth.

Contralateral: On the opposite side.

Convulsion: *Seizure.* Abnormal electrical discharge of the brain causing a motor, sensory, or behavioral disturbance.

Corpus Callosum: White matter connecting the left and right hemispheres (halves) of the brain.

Cutaneous Lesions: Skin lesions.

Dermatologist: Skin doctor.

EEG (Electroencephalogram): A recording of brain electrical activity.

Focal Seizure: *Seizure* confined to one part of the body i.e., eyes.

Forme Fruste: An aborted form of disease arrested before running its course. Thus the disease appears in an atypical and indefinite form.

Frontal Lobe: Most forward lobe of the brain. Deals with higher cognitive function i.e., planning, organizing, etc.

Generalized Seizure: *Seizure* involving loss of consciousness.

Glaucoma: Increased pressure in the eye causing damage. May lead to blindness if not treated.

Sturge-Weber Syndrome

Hemangioma: Cluster of blood vessels.

Hemiparesis: Weakness of one side of the body.

Hemispherectomy: Operation where one half of the brain is removed.

Hemiplegia: The extreme of *hemiparesis*, where one side of the body is completely paralyzed.

Homonymous Hemianopsia: Visual impairment of one half of one's visual field i.e., left half of each visual field in each eye (not one eye).

Intracranial Calcification: Calcium deposits in the brain.

Intractable Seizure: *Seizure* that cannot be controlled.

Ipsilateral: On the same side (as opposed to *contralateral*).

Lobectomy: Operation to remove one lobe of the brain. There are four lobes on each side of the brain (frontal lobe, temporal lobe, parietal lobe, occipital lobe).

MRI (Magnetic Resonance Imaging): A scan of the brain (or other organ) which does not use radiation, but uses magnetic energy.

Neurologist: A doctor who specializes in diseases of the brain, spinal cord, nerves and muscles.

Neurosurgeon: A doctor who specializes in operations of the brain, spinal cord, and nerves.

Occipital Lobe: The lobe at the most posterior (back) part of the brain. Deals with vision.

Occupational Therapist: A professional specialist in development of fine motor skills.

Ophthalmologist: A doctor with a medial degree, who specializes in diseases of the eye.

Parietal Lobe: Just in front of the *occipital lobe*. Deals with sensory functions.

PET Scan (Positron Emission Tomography): A scan that looks at function, rather than structure of an organ, including the brain.

Physical Therapist: A professional specialist in development of gross motor skills and physical activities.

Port Wine Stain: Characteristic birthmark of SWS. Usually on the face, but can extend to other parts of the body, particularly the neck and trunk. A port wine stain by itself does not necessarily constitute SWS.

Prognosis: Predicted outcome.

Seizure: Often used synonymously with *convulsion*.

Stroke: In common usage, this refers to a part of the brain being suddenly deprived of its blood supply, leading to weakness or other symptoms.

Temporal Lobe: The lobes on either side of the brain, slightly above and in front of the ears. Deals with emotions, memory, speech.

Thrombosis: Blood clot.

Trabeculectomy: A type of glaucoma surgery to lower the pressure in a glaucomatous eye.

Unilateral: On one side.

Chapter 32

Hemangiomas

There has been a great deal of confusion in the terms used to describe different types of vascular lesions or birthmarks. In the past, the word hemangioma has been used to describe a variety of lesions with differing origins and characteristics. A new classification system was published in 1982 by Mulliken and Glowacki, designed to simplify the nomenclature based on cellular biology with diagnostic applicability to the natural progression of these birthmarks. In this system, vascular birthmarks are divided into two major categories: hemangiomas and malformations. Hemangiomas are the vascular tumors that demonstrate rapid cell turnover or proliferation. Malformations are all other vascular tumors which have a normal endothelial cell turnover or cycle. This article discusses the diagnosis, clinical course and treatment of hemangiomas.

Diagnosis

Hemangiomas are the most common tumors found in infants. Of all newborns, approximately 1% to 3% have hemangiomas. Most hemangiomas are not noted at birth but do appear several weeks later with an incidence of 10% to 12% by 1 year of age. Females are more commonly affected than males by a ratio of 3 to 1. Of the infants diagnosed with a hemangioma 15% to 20% will have multiple lesions.

From *Faces*, Summer 1996; a publication of The National Association for the Craniofacially Handicapped, P.O. Box 11082, Chattanooga, TN 37401, Phone 1-800-332-2373; reprinted with permission.

The first sign of a hemangioma is an erythematous patch or small telangiectasia surrounded by a pale halo. The most common area on the body appears to be the head and neck region.

Clinical Course

Hemangiomas characteristically go through stages of rapid proliferation followed by spontaneous slow involution. These may begin as a "herald spot", which is a small, well demarcated pale patch, an erythematous macular patch, or a small area of telangiectasia surrounded by a pale halo. Hemangiomas usually go through their growth phase the first 8 months of life. The exact time of involution is variable but may start by 18 months of age. Large series of hemangiomas that have been reported show that by age 5, 50% have totally resolved and by age 7, 75% to 90% have disappeared. The size nor the site of the hemangioma has any effect on the time or degree of involution. The lesions that have the best results are ones that have significantly involuted by the age of 5. One of the first signs of involution is the changing of the bright red color to a darker red. They may be followed by a gray appearance to the surface with small white spots appearing. The skin becomes less tense with wrinkling as the lesion involutes.

Treatment

The majority of hemangiomas will involute and should be permitted to regress spontaneously. However, even with total involution of the hemangioma, return of the skin to normal is rare. Some hemangiomas can cause problems with function and should then be evaluated for active or early treatment. A lesion that results in blockage of the airway, visual fields, or ear canal should receive immediate treatment. Other problems such as massive growth of a facial lesion, large ulceration and bleeding, or multiple hemangiomas causing congestive heart failure should be considered for treatment. The most common forms of treatment involves steroid therapy or operative excision. Reported studies have shown that oral steroids may accelerate the start of involution in hemangiomas that are rapidly expanding. Good to excellent results have been achieved by authors in 50% to 90% with oral steroids. Infants less than 6 months of age tend to be more responsive than older patients. When we feel treatment of a hemangioma is indicated, we give an oral dose of Prednisone at 3-5 mg/kg/

day for 6-8 weeks. A response should be noted during this time period. In our experience, complications from such treatment are rare.

Operative treatment is usually limited to contouring of the skin after the lesion has involuted. The psychological impact of a hemangioma on the face may become a factor in the child starting school. We therefore feel that in certain patients, excision of the hemangioma may be indicated or beneficial. Hemangiomas of the tip of the nose may be such lesions. Larger lesions that have not involuted by the time the child starts school should also be considered for excision. The type and extent of excision is based on judgement and experience with careful placement of scars and consideration of long term aesthetic results.

— by Larry A. Sargent, M.D.

Dr. Sargent is Professor of Plastic Surgery, Chattanooga Unit, University of Tennessee College of Medicine, Medical Director, Tennessee Craniofacial Center, Chattanooga, Tennessee.

Part Six

Chemicals, Medications, and Infectious Organisms Linked to Congenital Disorders

Chapter 33

Chemicals and Birth Defects

Popular Solvent, TCE, Seems to Cause Serious Birth Defects in Animals, Humans

#267—January 8, 1992.

The solvent trichloroethylene or TCE is the contaminant found most often at hazardous waste dumps and in groundwater (underground water supplies). The federal government has found TCE at 614 (47%) of the nation's 1300 official Superfund sites.[1] [Reference numbers refer to references at the end of each section.] TCE causes leukemia and liver cancer ln laboratory animals and it may cause leukemia in humans, though the studies showing this have been challenged.[2]

There is substantial recent evidence that TCE causes birth defects in newborn animals and is associated with similar defects in humans; specifically, TCE exposure causes heart defects in baby chickens and rats[5], and is associated with similar defects in human newborns[6]. Heart defects are the fastest-growing type of birth defects in the U.S. population[3].

This chapter contains reprints of six articles from *RACHEL's* [Remote Access Chemical Hazards Electronic Library] *Environment and Health Weekly* (formerly *RACHEL's Hazardous Waste News*) 1992-1994, produced by the Environmental Research Foundation, P.O. Box 5036, Annapolis MD 21403-7036; phone (410) 263-1584; fax (410) 263-8944; e-mail erf@rachel.clark.net.

363

TCE is mainly used as a degreasing solvent in the metal products and automotive industries, though it can also be found in some typewriter correction fluids, paint removers/strippers, adhesives, spot removers, and rug-cleaning fluids.[1]

Humans invented TCE; it does not occur in nature, so the human body has not had an opportunity to develop detoxifying or other protective mechanisms specific to TCE. In 1990 only two U.S. companies manufactured trichloroethylene (Dow Chemical in Freeport, TX, and PPG Industries at Lake Charles, LA) but each of the 50 states has large industrial users of TCE—some 878 major users in all[1], plus countless smaller users. Total U.S. estimated use of TCE exceeded 200 million pounds in 1990. All 200 million pounds entered the general environment sooner or later.

When it gets loose, TCE has a strong tendency to enter the atmosphere. Average air concentrations for TCE range from 0.04 ppb [parts per billion] in Portland, Oregon in 1984, to 0.29 ppb in Philadelphia in 1983-84, and 0.1 to 0.225 ppb in 10 major cities across the country in 1980-81. The air over six landfills in New Jersey ranges from 0.08 to 2.43 ppb TCE (maximum: 12.3 ppb). But even remote, unspoiled areas have TCE in their air; in the Arctic in 1982-83 air averaged 0.008 to 0.009 ppb TCE. In other words, the whole atmosphere is contaminated with TCE at low concentrations.

Any particular molecule of TCE only remains in the atmosphere a few days. Rain brings TCE back to the ground where it then moves into streams, rivers, lakes, and oceans. Once it enters water, much of it moves back into the atmosphere quickly, but some of it enters plants, then small animals, then fish. Fish from various waterways contain TCE in the range of 10 to 100 ppb. Clams and oysters in Louisiana contain TCE (0.8 to 5.7 ppb). Snow in Alaska contains TCE (0.03 to 0.039 ppb). Rain contains TCE. So naturally, fresh tomatoes, potatoes, apples and pears contain TCE (1.7, 0-3, 5 and 4 ppb, respectively).[1]

It helps to understand that EPA (U.S. Environmental Protection Agency) has set 5 ppb as the maximum allowable concentration in drinking water—so finding 5 ppb in a fresh apple should give us pause. Many processed foods contain TCE because they are often made with water contaminated with TCE. The federal Agency for Toxic Substances and Disease Registry [ATSDR] reports: Chinese-style sauce (28 ppb), quince jelly (40 ppb), chocolate sauce (50 ppb), grape jelly (20 ppb). Fresh bread contains 7 ppb, various brands of margarine contain 440 to 3600 ppb. These are not national averages, so the foodstuffs in your refrigerator may contain less or more than these values.

Chemicals and Birth Defects

In sum, we industrial humans have managed to spread TCE everywhere.

Humans ingest TCE by drinking fluids, by breathing, and through their skin. In 133 American cities, TCE averaged 0.47 ppb in water samples at the tap. If you take a shower in such water, you inhale considerable TCE but you also absorb an equal amount through your skin.[2]

All of this explains why Americans have measurable amounts of TCE on their breath.

There is no doubt that TCE causes leukemia in animals. But the evidence for leukemia in humans is not so clear. People at Woburn, Massachusetts, drinking a TCE-contaminated water supply, did get leukemia in unusually high numbers but some people in the community also got leukemia even though they had a different water supply, so the picture is not crystal clear.[1]

In 1990, two studies were published linking TCE to heart defects. A large group of people in Tucson, Arizona, drank TCE-contaminated water for up to a decade. A careful study of children born to these families revealed an unusually large number of birth defects of the heart. Among these children, the chances of being born with a heart defect were three times the normal chances of having such a defect.[6] Earlier studies of baby chicks, and in 1990 of baby rats[5] revealed that TCE causes heart defects in these species. Although cause-and-effect has not been shown to a scientific certainty by the Tucson study, after reading the available evidence, pregnant women will almost certainly want to minimize their exposure to TCE. The families in Tucson were drinking water that contained from 6 to 200 ppb of TCE.

Another long-term effect of TCE exposure was revealed in a 1988 study of nerve function in people in Woburn, Massachusetts who had been drinking water contaminated with TCE (118 to 267 ppb). The people had stopped drinking the contaminated water six years prior to the test, yet there was unmistakable evidence of damage to their cranial (brain) nerves.[4]

In addition, there is now a growing body of medical and scientific literature showing associations between exposure of men to solvents (including TCE) in the workplace, and birth defects and cancers in their children.[8,9] Damage to the men's sperm is the suspected mechanism for effects in the children.

TCE evaporates easily and is difficult to control. It is representative of a large number of chlorinated chemicals that now appear to be more dangerous than we previously knew. Subtle but important health effects, which were never looked for during previous decades, are now being discovered. The more we look the more bad news we learn.

References

1. Agency for Toxic Substances and Disease Registry [ATSDR]. *Draft Toxicological Profile for Trichloroethylene*. Atlanta, GA: Agency for Toxic Substances and Disease Registry [Division of Toxicology, Mail Stop E-29, Atlanta, GA 30333], October, 1991. Free as long as supplies last but requests must be in writing.

2. Anthony B. Miller and others, *Environmental Epidemiology Vol 1; Public Health and Hazardous Wastes* (Washington, DC: National Academy Press, 1991).

3. Larry D. Edmonds and Levy M. James, "Temporal Trends in the Prevalence of Congenital Malformations at Birth Based on the Birth Defects Monitoring Program, United States, 1979-1987," *MMWR [Morbidity and Mortality Weekly Report] CDC [Centers for Disease Control] Surveillance Summaries* Vol. 39 No. SS-4 (December, 1990), pgs. 19-23.

4. Robert G. Feldman and others, "Blink Reflex Latency after Exposure to Trichloroethylene in Well Water," *Archives of Environmental Health* Vol 43, No. 2 (March/April, 1988), pgs. 143-148.

5. Brenda V. Dawson and others, "Cardiac Teratogenesis of Trichloroethylene and Dichloroethylene in a Mammalian Model," *Journal of the American College of Cardiology* Vol. 16, No. 5 (November 1, 1990), pgs. 1304-1309.

6. Stanley J. Goldberg "An Association of Human Congenital Cardiac Malformations and Drinking Water Contaminants," *Journal of the American College of Cardiology* Vol. 16, No. 1 (July, 1990), pgs. 155-164.

7. M.K. Smith and others, "Development Effects of Dichloroacetic Acid in Long-Evans Rats," *Teratology* Vol. 39 (1989), pg. 482.

8. John M. Peters and others, "Brain Tumors in Children and Occupational Exposure of Parents," *Science* Vol. 213 (July 10, 1981), pgs. 235-236.

9. Helena Taskinen and others, "Spontaneous abortions and congenital malformations among the wives of men occupationally exposed to organic solvents," *Scandinavian Journal of Work Environment and Health* Vol. 15 (1989), pgs. 345-352.

Children Born to Women Living Near Old Dumps Have Higher Risk of Birth Defects

#313—November 25, 1992.

Pregnant women who live near hazardous waste sites have an increased risk of bearing children with major birth defects, a new study has concluded.[1]

Researchers at the Yale University School of Medicine and the New York State Department of Health (NYDOH) studied 27,115 births and concluded that, overall, women living within a mile of an inactive dump have a 12% greater chance of bearing a child with a major birth defect, compared to women living further than a mile from a dump.

The researchers looked at 590 inactive dump sites in 20 northern New York Counties. Among the 590 sites studied, 90 were ranked as "high risk" sites because there was documented evidence that chemicals had migrated off the sites. The study found that women living within a mile of any of these 90 sites had a 63% greater chance of bearing a child with a major birth defect, compared to women living further than a mile from all of the 90 sites.

The study posed four questions: first, is residential proximity (closeness) to dumps associated with major birth defects? Second, are particular types of birth defects associated with proximity to dumps? Third, do particular characteristics of dumps (for example, documented off-site migration of chemicals) increase a waste site's risk to neighbors' health? Fourth, are specific chemical groups (such as pesticides or metals) associated with particular birth defects as previous studies have shown (for example, pesticides and cleft palate)? The answers to all four questions turned out to be yes.

The Yale/NYDOH study began by examining the New York State Congenital Malformation Registry; they found records of 9,313 infants born in 20 northern New York counties during the two-year period 1983-1984 with major birth defects of the nervous system, muscle and skeletal system, and skin. They omitted New York City.

The researchers then selected 17,802 normal infants from the same 20 counties born during the same time-period, to serve as controls.

The residential locations of the mothers of all 27,115 infants were then converted into latitude and longitude, so they could be plotted on a map, and the distance to the nearest dump was calculated for each residence. (Residential location was determined to be accurate within 200 feet in 80% of the cases, and within 1300 feet in the remaining 20 percent of cases.) Then a comparison was made between the infants born to women who lived within a mile of a dump, versus infants born to women who lived more than a mile from any dump. Infants whose mothers lived a mile or less from a dump had a 12 percent greater chance of being born with a major birth defect.

During the second part of the study, each of the 590 dumps was assigned a numerical hazard score, based on criteria developed by EPA (U.S. Environmental Protection Agency) and modified by NYDOH. Dumps considered most likely to produce toxic exposures of any kind (through breathing, ingestion, or skin contact, via air, water, or soil) received the highest scores. Then each individual woman in the study was assigned an "exposure risk"—a number that combined her proximity to a dump with the hazard score for that dump. Then the women were split into two groups—those with a "high exposure risk" (greater than 30) and those with a "low exposure risk" (less than 30).

Further analysis revealed that specific kinds of birth defects are associated with proximity to dumps, particularly birth defects of the nervous system (29 percent more likely), musculoskeletal system (16 percent more likely), and the skin (also known as the body's integument system) (32 percent more likely). Birth defects of the digestive system and oral clefts were not significantly associated with proximity to dumps.

The danger of birth defects is especially high near dumps where off-site migration of wastes has been documented. Near the 90 dumps with documented off-site migration, birth defects are 63% more likely to occur, compared to dumps where off-site migration has not been documented.

Lastly, the study revealed that dumps containing specific kinds of toxins were associated with specific kinds of birth defects, thus

Chemicals and Birth Defects

confirming associations that have been noted in previous studies. For example, pesticides were associated with cleft palate in the Yale/NYDOH study. Pesticides and birth defects of the muscular system were also associated. Metals and solvents were each associated with nervous system birth defects. Plastics were associated with chromosome anomalies.

Strengths of This Study

Previous studies have found a connection between a mother's exposure to chemicals and birth defects in her offspring,[2] but the Yale/NYDOH study is the first to examine such a large number of births, and thus is far more convincing than previous studies. This study also did not rely upon information provided by individuals about themselves, so "recall bias" (errors or distortions caused by faulty memory) was eliminated from this study. A previous study[3] of residents near the Stringfellow Acid Pits had shown that people near the Stringfellow dump reported excessive occurrences of ear infections, bronchitis, asthma, angina pectoris (heart-related chest pains), skin rashes, blurred vision, pain in the ears, daily cough for more than a month, nausea, frequent diarrhea, unsteady gait when walking, and frequent urination. However, the Stringfellow researchers were unable to rule out the effects of "recall bias" because they relied entirely on people telling them about their symptoms, so skeptics remained unconvinced that the study revealed anything about real diseases caused by the nearby dump.

As the authors of the Yale/NYDOH study said, their results in this study do not prove a cause-and-effect relationship between birth defects and proximity to dumps, but their results "do exhibit many characteristics of causal associations." Each of the four types of analysis (the four questions discussed previously) showed increased rates of birth defects associated with proximity to dumps. As the analysis became more specific, the associations between dumps and disease remained similar or became even stronger. Rates for certain birth defects associated with chemical exposures in previous scientific studies were statistically elevated, while other defects, with little or no previous data to suggest a relationship with chemical exposure, showed no increases. Finally, a kind of dose-response relationship was apparent between proximity to higher-risk dumps and birth defects. In other words, the closer a woman lived to a high-risk dump, the greater were her chances of bearing a child with a major birth defect.

Limitations of This Study

This study may underestimate the number of defective births associated with proximity to dumps for two reasons: The study did not examine spontaneous abortions and fetal deaths—both of which are known to be associated with human exposures to chemicals. Furthermore, there is evidence that about 20 percent of women move their residence during pregnancy. If this were true, it would result in misclassification of subjects, which would weaken the ability of the Yale/NYDOH study to discern the full effect of living near dumps.

Lastly, the Yale/NYDOH study does not prove conclusively that chemicals in the dumps *caused* the birth defects because no actual chemical exposures of women were measured. Proximity to dumps was used as a surrogate (substitute) for exposure to chemicals. Since no chemical exposures were actually measured, chemicals cannot be definitely fingered as the cause of the birth defects. Furthermore the Yale/NYDOH study did not take into account possible differences in lifestyle (for example, tobacco and alcohol use), occupational exposures to chemicals, and possible exposures to chemicals from nearby industrial operations. Thus the Yale/NYDOH study is "highly suggestive" but is not sufficient, by itself, to prove cause and effect.

Further studies are now underway to try to remedy the shortcomings of the Yale/NYDOH study. Unfortunately, it will be several years, perhaps a decade, before results of these follow-up studies will be published. In the meantime, does the Yale/NYDOH study give us reason to be concerned about pregnant women living within a mile of a dump? In our opinion, definitely yes. We believe any pregnant woman who can avoid living within a mile of a dump would be well-advised to do so. The further away from industrial poisons, the better.

The authors of the Yale/NYDOH study said their study revealed a "small additional risk" of bearing a child with a major birth defect. To them, a 12 percent increase is "small." But look at it this way: the authors say the "normal" occurrence of major birth defects in the 20 counties they studied in New York is 30 defects per 1000 live births. Among women living within a mile of a dump, the occurrence is 34 defects per 1000 live births—a 12 percent increase. In the period they studied, 1983-1984, there were 506,183 live births in the 20 counties. If *none* of these women lived within a mile of a dump, the number of spontaneous birth defects would be 15,186. On the other hand, if *all* the women lived within a mile of a dump, there would be 17,210 babies with major birth defects born during the 2-year period, or 17,210-15,186=2024 excess (dump-related) birth defects in a two-year period in the 20-county area, or about 1000 excess (dump-related) major birth defects each year in the 20-county area.

References

1. Sandra A. Geschwind and others, "Risk of Congenital Malformations Associated with Proximity to Hazardous Waste Sites," *American Journal of Epidemiology* Vol. 135 (1992), pgs 1197-1207.

2. For discussion of additional studies, see Anthony B. Miller and others, *Environmental Epidemiology; Public Health and Hazardous Wastes* (Washington, D.C.: National Academy Press, 1991).

3. Dean B. Baker and others, "A Health Study of Two Communities [sic] Near the Stringfellow Waste Disposal Site," *Archives of Environmental Health* Vol. 43 (Sept./Oct., 1988), pgs. 325-334.

America Learns about Teratogens

#322—January 27, 1993.

In 1954, enterprising German chemists created a new drug, which they named thalidomide.[1] It seemed to be an ideal sleeping pill and tranquilizer, and after three years of animal tests thalidomide was judged so safe that it was approved for over-the-counter (non-prescription) sale throughout Germany. By 1960, thalidomide was Germany's most popular sleeping pill and tranquilizer. It was a huge financial success, marketed under 50 different trade names in 24 countries.

In 1960 the Merrell pharmaceutical company of Cincinnati applied to the U.S. Food and Drug Administration (FDA) for permission to market thalidomide in the U.S. The application was assigned to FDA staff member Frances O. Kelsey who had 60 days to consider the application.

To the Merrell Company's distress, Dr. Kelsey asked for more data; she was concerned that thalidomide acted differently in animals than it did in humans (it wasn't a sedative in animals). The Merrell Company sent officials to Washington to complain that Dr. Kelsey was holding up progress, but FDA officials held firm.

During this time a single report appeared in a British medical journal, indicating that some long-time users of thalidomide had developed nerve damage in their hands and feet. The Merrell company proposed to put a warning label on the package, but Dr. Kelsey replied that Merrell would need to conduct studies to show that thalidomide could be safely taken by pregnant women without harming the fetus. Merrell officials were appalled that this "stubborn bureaucrat" could derail their plans for marketing a sure-fire best-seller. However Dr. Kelsey held firm, and so did her supervisors at FDA.

Long before Merrell could complete its tests, news filtered across the Atlantic from Germany of an out-break of phocomelia (literally "seal limbs")—a terrible deformity in which babies are born with tiny flipper-like stumps instead of arms and hands. In November, 1961, Dr. Widuking Lenz in Germany and Dr. W. G. McBride in Australia, almost simultaneously, observed that the mothers of several babies with phocomelia had one thing in common—they had taken thalidomide in the first 20 to 40 days of pregnancy.

In September, 1962, the extent of the disaster in West Germany was officially confirmed. Since 1957, when the pill was first approved for over-the-counter sales, thalidomide has caused 10,000 cases of birth malformations in West Germany. Nearly a thousand other cases were reported in England. So far as we know, no one has ever tallied the damage in the 22 other countries where thalidomide was sold—in western Europe and Japan, and throughout South America.

Interestingly enough, the thalidomide story was told in several places—in *Science* magazine (5/25/62), and in the *New York Times* (4/12/62)—back on page 37—but it drew no real attention until Morton Mintz of the *Washington Post* told the story on page 1 (7/15/62) about Dr. Kelsey, who had single-handedly held firm against great pressure and abuse, thus averting an American thalidomide tragedy. (Seventeen American babies were born with phocomelia because, as was allowed at the time, Merrell gave free samples to physicians as soon as the company applied to FDA for permission to sell the drug.) The heroism of Dr. Kelsey caught the public imagination, and then the thalidomide story spread rapidly. President Kennedy eventually awarded Dr. Kelsey a medal for Distinguished Civilian Service.

Congress responded to thalidomide by passing the Kefauver-Harris drug law, which the President signed in October, 1962. This law, for the first time, gave FDA the power to require specific procedures for testing new drugs for safety and effectiveness.

Chemicals and Birth Defects

But a much broader change began to occur as a result of the thalidomide disaster. Up until this time, some Americans had been concerned about cancer from chemicals, but thalidomide brought home the dangers of teratogens and mutagens. Teratogens cause birth defects and mutagens cause inheritable genetic changes.

As a result, Americans in general became a little less eager to try the latest drug for every new ailment. And they gained new respect for the great damage a small amount of a chemical might do.

The next developments in our consciousness of chemicals occurred in the workplace. Workers have always been the people exposed first to new chemicals, and exposed most heavily. Up until 1970, when Congress passed the Occupational Safety and Health Act, workers were not protected in any systematic way from chemicals. There were no federal standards for exposure and no legal protections except a patchwork quilt of conflicting state statutes. Naturally, management had some appreciation of acute toxic effects from chemicals (sick workers can't be productive, and they might sue), but the only long-term consequence that anyone talked about was cancer. Although the systematic medical literature on occupational health reaches back to the year 1700, concern about teratogens and mutagens is almost brand new. Even as recently as 1969, the "standard" work on occupational safety and health, Donald Hunter's *Diseases of Occupations*, in its fourth edition contained no references to either teratogens or mutagens.

However, the thalidomide disaster prompted a great deal of research on reproductive health and chemicals, and by the mid-1970s articles began to appear in the medical literature linking chemical exposures of both men and women to miscarriages, infertility, and other reproductive disorders.[2]

However, as knowledge of teratogens and mutagens developed, measures to protect workers took a peculiar turn.

Although the early studies clearly showed that chemical exposures of both women *and men* could damage offspring, corporate management tended to ignore the evidence about male exposures and developed policies aimed only at "protection" of women.

The issue came to the forefront in the late 1970s when it became widely publicized that the American Cyanamid Company had established a policy barring all fertile women from numerous high-paying jobs at its Willow Island, West Virginia, plant, claiming the prohibition was necessary to avoid the possibility of birth defects in the offspring of exposed workers. The American Cyanamid case was particularly troublesome because five women workers at the plant "voluntarily" underwent surgical sterilization so they could keep their jobs.[3] Despite the ugly cast of these measures to "protect" women, such policies spread rapidly throughout American industry. Rather than clean up the workplace, management found it expedient to exclude female workers on the specious grounds that their reproductive systems were sensitive to chemicals, whereas men's were not. (As a sidelight, it is interesting to recall that the "right to know" movement has its origins in this same period; rather than clean up work places, authorities began to agree to allow workers to learn the names and some of the characteristics of the chemicals they were being exposed to.)

Throughout the 1980s, the "protection" issue continued to fester. For many women, it was a simple matter of rights; they did not want to be told they had to choose between having a child and having a job. Federal courts decided half a dozen cases involving "fetal protection" policies (cases involving Olin Corp., General Motors, B.F. Goodrich, and several hospitals). In no instance was a company's discriminatory policy struck down. The best-known case was that of Johnson Controls, the nation's largest manufacturer of automotive batteries. A coalition of labor and women's rights activists challenged Johnson's policy of excluding women from jobs involving exposure to lead. (To keep her job on the production line at any Johnson Controls' battery factory, a woman had to offer medical proof that she was sterile.)

In October, 1989, a panel of judges on the federal Court of Appeals for the 7th Circuit in Chicago ruled that Johnson had the right to exclude fertile women from jobs involving exposure to lead, even women who said they had no intention of getting pregnant. One judge on the 7th Circuit bench, who dissented in the Johnson Controls case, estimated that 15 to 20 million women would be excluded from high-paying jobs by the majority's decision.[4]

However, a broad coalition of labor and women's rights organizations pursued the case into the U.S. Supreme Court and on March 20, 1991, the court ruled unanimously that employers had no right (under the Civil Rights Act of 1964) to discriminate against women even to "protect" them or their fetuses.[5]

With that argument settled, scientists and medical researchers have begun to recognize, and to confirm, what the older literature had showed 20 years ago.[6] They are finding that toxic chemicals can cause men to father defective children.

References

1. Edward W. Lawless, *Technology and Social Shock* (New Brunswick, NJ.: Rutgers University Press, 1977), pgs. 140-147.

2. For example, I. V. Sanotskii, "Aspects of the Toxicology of Chloroprene: Immediate and Long-Term Effects," *Environmental Health Perspectives* Vol. 17 (1976), pgs. 85-93. And: Peter F, Infante and Others, "Genetic Risks of Vinyl Chloride," *The Lancet* (April 3, 1976), pgs. 734-735.

3. Joan E. Bertin, "People Protection Not 'Fetal Protection,'" *New Solutions* (Summer 1991), pgs. 5-9.

4. William E. Schmidt, "Risk to Fetus Ruled as Barring Women from Jobs," *New York Times* October 3, 1989, pg. A16.

5. Linda Greenhouse, "Court Backs Right of Women to Jobs With Health Risks," *New York Times* March 21, 1991, pgs. 1, B12.

6. Sandra Blakeslee, "Research on Birth Defects Turns to Flaws in Sperm," *New York Times* Jan. 1, 1991, pgs. 1, 36.

Male Reproductive System is Harmed by Toxic Exposures, Causing Birth Defects, Sterility

#323—February 3, 1993 (Revised).

The ancient Greeks observed that men heavily exposed to lead became sterile. But this knowledge was not passed to the Romans, who stored their drinking water and their wine in lead-lined containers. Romans also added lead to some of their drinks as a sweetener. Based on examination of lead in Roman bones, some historians conclude that the Roman upper classes probably couldn't reproduce themselves, contributing to the fall of Rome.[1]

Until very recently, scientists paid little attention to the effects of environmental agents on human reproduction. The modern period began in 1941 when blindness, deafness and death were reported among the offspring of pregnant women exposed to rubella (German measles). The thalidomide catastrophe in 1954-1961 brought home the potential dangers of chemicals, in this case a prescription drug. The birth of nearly 20,000 defective children following a Rubella epidemic in the early 1960s confirmed the association of environmental factors and birth defects.[2]

As recently as the early 1970s, few state governments were maintaining records of birth defects. In 1974 the federal government established the first national register of birth defects, monitoring hospital records that account for about 15% of all births.[3] Even today this program monitors only birth defects observed in newborns, which probably represent only about a sixth of the total defects that actually occur because many defects do not become apparent for several years.[2]

As of 1980, approximately 200,000 birth defects were estimated to have occurred in the U.S., accounting for about 7 percent of all live births. In addition, more than 560,000 infant deaths, spontaneous abortions, stillbirths and miscarriages were recorded due to defective fetal development.[2]

In 1990, the federal Centers for Disease Control (CDC) reported trends in birth defects between 1979 and 1987 in the U.S. They looked at 38 specific defects and found that 29 of the 38 had increased, two had decreased and 7 had remained stable.[3] The largest increases (29 percent and 20.2 percent) occurred in defects of the heart; no doubt some of this increase is due to better detection methods. However, there was also a 9.6 percent increase in eye defects and a 2.7 percent increase in cleft lip, so it seems likely that real increases are occurring.

The traditional view of birth defects highlights the role of women and disregards the role of men, even when there is good evidence showing men exposed to toxic chemicals father defective children. The traditional reason for ignoring such research is that, until recently, there has been no satisfactory theory to explain how male exposures could affect offspring, so a cause-and-effect relationship could not be established. The argument was that women are born with all the eggs they will ever have, so each egg can be exposed to toxins over a long period. Men on the other hand, produce new sperm constantly, so any individual sperm has only a brief opportunity to be exposed to toxins.

Another reason for ignoring the effect of toxins on male reproduction was the "macho sperm" theory, which said that only the fittest sperm were hardy enough to go the distance necessary to fertilize an egg.[4] According to this theory, defective sperm could never reach an

Chemicals and Birth Defects

egg to fertilize it, so men couldn't be responsible for producing defective children. Now research has shown that the female reproductive tract has ways of moving sperms along whether they are healthy or defective.

Researchers used to believe that there was an effective barrier between blood vessels and the tissues where sperm originates in the testes. It is now known that the barrier is not effective against many chemicals.

Then of course there's a cultural bias, reaching back to the Salem witch trials, to blame women for trouble. "You don't have to be Sigmund Freud to figure out that there are cultural factors to say why we have paid so much attention to the female and so little to the male," says Dr. Devra Lee Davis, an epidemiologist with the National Research Council.

Research during the past decade has shown that there are two basic ways that chemicals can affect male reproduction.[5,6] Chemicals can directly affect the testes, where sperm originates. The numbers of sperm can be diminished, or some sperm can be damaged, or sperm may even carry toxins directly into the egg. Alternatively, toxins can attack the male nervous system, or endocrine system, affecting the flow of hormones that act as messengers regulating the complex chemical processes that must all work well for conception to occur.

No matter what the mechanism of damage may be, there is a growing body of evidence showing that male exposure to toxins can produce defective children. Here is a sampling:

- A nationwide study of 99,186 pregnancies in Finland showed an increased likelihood of spontaneous abortion if the father was occupationally exposed to rubber chemicals, solvents used in the manufacture of rubber products, solvents used in oil refineries, or ethylene oxide.[7]

- A study of 22,192 children born with birth defects in British Columbia showed that paternal occupation as a fire fighter was related to the occurrence of heart defects. Fire fighters are often heavily exposed to carbon monoxide and to polycyclic aromatic hydrocarbons (PAHs)—the nasty chemicals in smoke and soot.[8]

- A study of paternal occupation among 149 patients with Wilm's tumor (a childhood cancer of the kidney) showed that a significantly greater number of the fathers were exposed to lead on the job, compared to fathers of a control group of children without the disease.[9]

- A study of 6000 men in Finland showed that paternal exposure to organic solvents nearly tripled the likelihood of spontaneous abortion as a pregnancy outcome, compared to controls not exposed to organic solvents. Painters, wood workers (for example, carpenters in the construction, furniture industry and the boat industry) were found to be at risk. The solvent toluene stood out as a particularly bad actor in his study.[10]

- A study of anesthetists in the West Midlands region of England (half men, half women) showed that, during a 20 year period, 9.3% of their children were born with defects, and 31% of the anesthetists reported having trouble begetting children. Furthermore nearly all the children were born underweight. The gender of the anesthetists did not affect the likelihood of problems in their children, but female children seemed to suffer greater birth defects.[11]

- A recent review of several studies of paternal occupational exposures in relation to childhood cancer in the offspring showed consistently that work in hydrocarbon-related occupations (the petroleum and chemical industries), especially exposure to paint, is associated with brain cancer. Male exposure to paint is also linked to leukemias in offspring.[12]

What does all this evidence mean? It means neither men nor women can be safely exposed to toxic chemicals.

References

1. S.C. Gilfillan, "Lead Poisoning and the Fall of Rome," *Journal of Occupational Medicine* Vol. 7 (Feb. 1965), pgs. 53-60.

2. Raymond D. Harbison, "Teratogens," in John Doull and others, editors, *Casarett and Doull's Toxicology* 2nd edition (N.Y.: Macmillan, 1980), pgs. 158-175.

3. Larry D. Edmonds and Levy M. James, "Temporal Trends in the Prevalence of Congenital Malformations at Birth Based on the

Birth Defects Monitoring Program, United States, 1979-1987." *Morbidity and Mortality Weekly Reports CDC Surveillance Summaries* Vol. 39, No. SS-4 (December, 1990), pgs. 19-23.

4. Sandra Blakeslee, "Research on Birth Defects Turns to Flaws in Sperm," *New York Times* (January 1, 1991), pgs. 1, 36.

5. Lowell Sever and Nancy A. Hessol, "Toxic Effects of Occupational and Environmental Chemicals on the Testes," in J.A. Thomas and others, editors, *Endocrine Toxicology* (N.Y.: Raven Press, 1985), pgs. 211-248.

6. Harold Zenick, "Mechanisms of Environmental Agents by Class Associated with Adverse Male Reproductive Outcomes," in *Reproduction: The New Frontier in Occupational and Environmental Health Research* (N.Y.: Alan R. Liss, Inc., 1984), pgs. 335-361.

7. Marja-Lusa Lindbohm and others, "Effects of Paternal Occupational Exposure in Spontaneous Abortions," *American Journal of Public Health* (August, 1991), pgs. 1029-1033.

8. Andrew F. Olshan and others, "Birth Defects Among Offspring of Firemen," *American Journal of Epidemiology* Vol. 131 (1990), pgs. 312-321.

9. Arlene F. Kantor and others, "Occupations of fathers of patients with Wilm's tumour," *Journal of Epidemiology and Community Health* Vol. 33 (1979), pgs. 253-256.

10. Helena Taskinen and others, "Spontaneous abortions and congenital malformations among the wives of men occupationally exposed to organic solvents," *Scandinavian Journal of Work, Environment and Health* Vol. 15 (1989), pgs. 345-352.

11. P. J. Tomlin, "Health problems of anesthetists and their families in the West Midlands," *British Medical Journal* (24 March, 1979), pgs. 779-784.

12. David A. Savitz and Jianjua Chen, "Parental Occupation and Childhood Cancer: Review of Epidemiological Studies," *Environmental Health Perspectives* Vol. 88 (1990), pgs. 325-337.

Birth Defects

#410—October 6, 1994.

The Birth Defects Monitoring Program (BDMP) is a U.S. government effort to monitor birth defects (congenital malformations) using data collected when newborn infants are discharged from the hospital.[1] The BDMP was initiated by the federal Centers for Disease Control (CDC) in 1974. The current BDMP database includes information on roughly 15 million births that have occurred at 1200 predominantly mid-sized community hospitals in the U.S. during the past 20 years.

The BDMP database is not comprehensive (it does not include information on every birth that occurs in the U.S.). Neither does it represent a randomly-selected sample of all U.S. births; therefore data from the BDMP cannot be considered representative of the entire "universe" of all U.S. newborns. In 1987 the BDMP received information on 15% of all U.S. births, which gives an idea of how comprehensive the coverage is. Because the data are mostly from mid-sized hospitals, we might expect that some of the largest hospitals in the largest cities are under-represented. Nevertheless, as the CDC says, the BDMP "represents the largest single set of uniformly collected and coded discharge data on congenital malformations in the United States." It is simply the best information available on birth defects in the U.S.

CDC says that the BDMP "functions primarily as an early warning system; however it can be useful also for correlating incidence [occurrence] patterns with such trends as the temporal [time-related] and geographic distribution of drugs, chemicals, and other possible human teratogens." A teratogen (from the Greek words meaning "monster producing") is anything that causes birth defects. Examples of teratogens are diseases such as German measles; infections; inherited genetic defects; radiation; and certain chemicals.

In 1990, researchers looked for trends in the BDMP database, examining records for 38 types of birth defects from 1979-80 through 1986-87. During this 7-year period, of the 38 types of birth defects, 29 increased; 2 decreased; and 7 remained stable (meaning they changed less than 2% per year during the 7-year period.)

Table 33.1 shows the annual percent change for 30 types of birth defects. All of them increased during the 7-year period (though some increased at a rate less than 2% per year, and are thus classified as "stable" by the CDC).

Chemicals and Birth Defects

Defect type	Number of defects per 10,000 births 1979-80	Number of defects per 10,000 births 1986-87	Percent change in occurrence, 1979-80 to 1986-87
CENTRAL NERVOUS SYSTEM			
Hydrocephalus without spina bifida (fluid in the skull)	4.34	5.84	4.3
Encephalocele (gap in the skull)	1.10	1.16	0.8
Microcephalus (small head)	2.12	2.61	3.0
EYES			
Anophthalmos (absence of eyes)	0.57	0.68	2.6
Congenital cataract (eye cataracts at birth)	0.71	1.02	5.3
Coloboma of eye (eye parts missing)	0.21	0.40	9.6
Aniridia (absence of the iris)	0.07	0.10	5.2
HEART			
Common truncus (undeveloped main arteries)	0.19	0.40	11.2
Transposition of great arteries (reversal of main arteries)	0.87	1.45	7.6
Tetralogy of Fallot (4 common defects simultaneously)	0.73	1.82	13.9
Ventricular septal defect (opening between lower chambers)	11.34	20.49	8.8
Atrial septal defect (opening between upper chambers)	1.16	3.69	18.0
Endocardial cushion defect	0.34	0.95	15.8
Pulmonary valve atresia and stenosis (obstructed blood flow)	0.58	3.44	29.0
Tricuspid valve atresia and stenosis (obstructed blood flow)	0.16	0.36	12.3
Aortic valve stenosis and atresia (obstructed blood flow)	0.22	0.79	20.0
Hypoplastic left heart syndrome (undeveloped left side)	0.56	1.25	12.2
Patent ductus arteriosus (pulmonary artery open to aorta)	17.87	35.43	10.3
Coarctation of aorta (constriction of the aorta)	0.74	1.15	6.5
Pulmonary artery anomaly	1.12	2.66	13.2
Lung agenesis and hypoplasia (undeveloped lungs)	1.66	3.84	12.7
FACIAL CLEFTS			
Cleft palate without cleft lip	5.05	5.33	0.8
Cleft lip	7.76	9.35	2.7
GASTROINTESTINAL			
Tracheoesophageal anomalies (upper airway problems)	1.86	2.49	4.3
Rectal and intestinal atresia (blockage)	3.23	3.80	2.3
GENITOURINARY			
Renal agenesis and hypoplasia (one kidney or small kidneys)	1.23	2.34	9.6
Bladder exstrophy (gap in abdomen, revealing bladder)	0.29	0.33	1.9
MUSCULOSKELETAL			
Reduction deformity, upper limbs (arms short or missing)	1.53	1.58	0.5
Reduction deformity, lower limbs (legs short or missing)	0.78	0.83	0.9
Congenital arthrogryposis (contracted or bent limbs)	1.33	1.93	5.5

Figure 33.1. Birth Defects: Annual Percent Change in Occurrence During 7-year Period, 1979-80 to 1986-87. (Source: Larry D. Edmonds and others, "Temporal Trends in the Prevalence of Congenital Malformations at Birth Based on the Birth Defects Monitoring Program, United States, 1979-1987," Morbidity and Mortality Weekly Report, CDC Surveillance Summaries, *Vol. 39, No. SS-4 (December 1990), pg. 22.*)

Table 33.1 contains 3 columns of numbers. The first two columns show the actual number of birth defects per 10,000 births; the first column shows data for the earlier period, 1979-80, the second column shows the later period, 1986-87. The third column shows the yearly percentage increase during the 7-year period.

Some of these increases are explained by better health care and better diagnosis. For example, some of the heart defects listed in Table 33.1 are so serious that an infant might not have survived such a defect 10 years ago but might survive it today. Likewise, some of the heart defects might be revealed by high-tech medical diagnostic machines today, whereas they might have gone unnoticed 10 years ago.

However, many of the increases in birth defects in Table 33.1 cannot be explained by better health care or better diagnosis. If a child were born 10 years ago with the iris missing from one or both of its eyes, chances are good that the mother or her doctor or a nurse would see it. (The iris is the part of the eye that makes blue eyes blue and brown eyes brown.) So the 5.2% *annual increase* in "aniridia" (absence of an iris) is very likely a real increase.

The same can be said for birth defects of the central nervous system, facial clefts, musculoskeletal defects and some of the gastrointestinal and genitourinary defects. Most of these defects are so obvious that they would have been noticed as easily 10 years ago as today. Therefore, increases in these defects are very likely real increases.

Some of the increases shown in Table 33.1 are surprisingly large. For example, coloboma of the eye increased 9.6% each year during the 7-year period; this means the occurrence of this defect doubled during the study period. (Coloboma of the eye means a wedge-shaped piece is missing from the iris, or some other part of the eye is missing.) Other eye disorders (congenital cataract, for example) are increasing about 5% each year, thus doubling every 14 years.

Are most birth defects caused by the parents' genetic characteristics, or by something in the environment?

In July 1994 an important study of birth defects in Norway appeared in the *New England Journal of Medicine*.[2] It indicated that environmental factors may be more important than previously thought.

Norway has maintained a Medical Birth Registry since 1967; the registry now contains data on 1.5 million births. Norwegian and American researchers examined records of 371,933 women who had given birth to first and second children in Norway between 1967 and 1989. For the 9192 women whose first infant had a birth defect, they examined the risk of similar or dissimilar effects in the second infant. And they examined the risk of a birth defect in the second child among mothers who lived in the same municipality during both pregnancies vs. mothers who moved to a new municipality before the second child was born. (The control group was the 362,741 women whose first infant did not have a birth defect.)

The researchers found that 2.5% of all infants born in Norway have a birth defect. Examining 23 different kinds of birth defects, they found that in every category, mothers whose first infant had a defect were more likely to have a second infant with a defect, as would be expected if birth defects are genetic in origin. What was "surprising" to the researchers was that women who moved to a new city between pregnancies were only half as likely to have a second child with a birth defect. Mothers whose first child had a defect were 11.6 times as likely to have a second child with a defect (compared to mothers whose first child did not have a defect), but if a mother moved to a new municipality between pregnancies she was only 5.1 times as likely to have a second child with a defect. The researchers concluded, "...[W]e find strong if indirect, evidence... suggesting that important environmental teratogens have yet to be discovered."

References

1. Larry D. Edmonds, "Temporal Trends in the Prevalence of Congenital Malformations at Birth Based on the Birth Defects Monitoring Program, United States, 1979-1987," *Morbidity and Mortality Weekly Report, CDC Surveillance Summaries* Vol. 39, No. SS-4 (Dec., 1990), pgs. 19-23.

2. Rolv Terje Lie and others, "A Population-Based Study of the Risk of Recurrence of Birth Defects," *New England Journal of Medicine* Vol. 331, No. 1 (July 7, 1994), pgs. 1-4.

Why Birth Defects Will Continue to Rise

#411—October 13, 1994.

In the previous section we saw that 30 types of birth defects are increasing steadily in the United States, some increasingly rapidly, others more slowly. Some of these increases are due to better diagnosis; however, many of the increases are real. This section will examine 10 reasons why birth defects are rising and will almost certainly continue to rise.

There is abundant scientific evidence that birth defects in laboratory animals and in humans have occurred as a result of exposure to four classes of pollutants: radiation;[1-2] pesticides;[3-9] metals (including mercury, cadmium, lead, and others);[10-14] solvents;[15-23] and dioxin-like chemicals including PCBs [polychlorinatedbiphenyls].[24-27] From studies of pharmaceutical drugs found to cause birth defects, it is certain that other chemicals are teratogens (causing birth defects) as well.[28]

Because municipal landfills and toxic waste dumps are laced with pesticides, toxic metals, solvents, dioxin-like compounds, and sometimes even radioactive materials, at least seven studies have now reported finding unusually high numbers of birth defects in children born to parents residing near dumps.[29-35]

- The main reason why birth defects will continue to increase is that more than 500 new chemicals are introduced into commercial use each year. There will never be enough money available for independent scientists to conduct definitive (or even adequate) studies of all these chemicals to see if they cause birth defects in laboratory animals. For ethical reasons, chemicals cannot be tested in any organized way on humans (though, contrarily, most Americans don't object to the experimental exposures that occur routinely in the workplace, and in the home via consumer products). In addition to 500 new chemicals appearing each year, more than 50,000 chemicals already in commercial use have never been tested for their ability to cause birth defects.

- The prevailing American philosophy is that chemicals are innocent until proven guilty. Therefore, when new chemicals are released into the environment, the burden of proof rests on the general public to show that damage has occurred before scientific studies are undertaken to describe the damage in detail. This philosophy guarantees that people *must be harmed* before study can begin.

- Scientific studies can take years to complete. Even when an effect is grossly obvious, pinning down the cause can take a decade or longer. For example, mercury poisoned dozens of babies in the womb at Minamata, Japan, in 1955 but scientists did not clearly establish the cause for 15 to 18 years.[11]

- After research scientists are convinced, there is a long delay before the general public learns the facts, if it ever does. (As an anti-environmental viewpoint comes to dominate major media, such as the *New York Times*, *Los Angeles Times*, and *20/20* on ABC-TV, in many cases new information simply never gets widely disseminated).

- Furthermore, the results of studies may not be clear-cut, for many reasons: it is difficult to measure exposure so usually a "surrogate" for exposure is used, such as place of residence, or occupation; many birth defect studies rely upon mothers recalling what chemical exposures occurred during their early months of pregnancy and all such recollections are dubious; therefore it is difficult to absolutely rule out many possible causes of an observed effect.

- A society that demands scientific certainty before it will restrict the use of suspected teratogens, guarantees that the rate of birth defects will continue rising. Scientific certainty about anything involving humans is, and will remain, elusive and rare.

- Given the philosophical climate, public health officials are reluctant to raise an alarm on less-than-100%-certain data. As a practical matter, an official will get in much more trouble for raising a false alarm about a suspected chemical than for making the opposite error (which allows birth defects to continue). In the present philosophical climate (requiring scientific certainty), even well-justified alarm based on less-than-certain data draws an angry response from powerful monied interests. On the other hand, allowing birth defects to continue will only affect one family at a time. Individual, unorganized victims do not threaten a public health official's job security.[36]

- When studies reveal that a particular chemical probably causes birth defects, the producers and users of the chemical typically conduct a lengthy campaign to deny and obscure what is known. For example, the lead industry has known for at least 100 years that lead causes reproductive and developmental disorders in humans. But starting in 1925 medical doctors hired by the lead industry argued that lead occurs naturally in the human body and, therefore, the dangers of lead in gasoline were not worth worrying about, much less studying. This strategy was persuasive to the public health community for 40 years.[37]

- The public health community relies almost exclusively on a decision-making technique that cannot take into account multiple exposures and cumulative effects, a technique called "risk assessment." At its best, risk assessment can provide a ballpark guesstimate of a few of the many hazards created by a single toxic chemical. However in real life we are all exposed to multiple chemicals all the time, and risk assessment cannot account for cumulative effects and multiple interactions. Heavy reliance upon such an unrealistic tool for decision-making leads to decisions that harm public health.

- Finally, even the knowledgeable environmental community fails to fully adopt the clear requirements of a public health policy based on prevention of disease: persistent toxic pollutants must be banned. Recently when Environmental Defense Fund (EDF) and Physicians for Social Responsibility (PSR), followed separately by Greenpeace, published their recommendations for public policy on dioxin, they all argued that U.S. dioxin policy should be modeled on U.S. Environmental Protection Agency's lead policy.[36] (Greenpeace set a goal of zero dioxins, but recommended the lead policy as a way to get there.) Over the last 20 years EPA's lead policy has forced a mere 8% reduction in total U.S. "consumption" of lead. At this rate it will take 3500 years for lead "consumption" to fall below 1000 pounds per year and thus disappear as a public health problem.

References

1. Niel Wald, "Evaluation of Human Exposure Data," in K.Z. Morgan and J.E. Turner, editors, *Principles of Radiation Protection: A Textbook of Health Physics* (Huntington, N.Y.: Robert E. Krieger Publishing, 1973), pgs. 448-496.

2. John W. Gofman, *Radiation and Human Health* (San Francisco: Sierra Club, 1981); see chapter 21.

3. Anne Kricker and others, "Women and the environment: a study of congenital limb anomalies," *Community Health Studies* Vol. 10, No. 1 (1986), pgs. 1-11.

4. M. Restrepo and others, "Prevalence of adverse reproductive outcomes in a population occupationally exposed to pesticides in Colombia," *Scandinavian Journal of Work, Environment and Health* Vol. 16 (1990), pgs. 232-238.

5. P. Rita and others, "Monitoring of Workers Occupationally Exposed to Pesticides in Grape Gardens of Andhra Pradesh," *Environmental Research* Vol. 44 (1987), pgs. 1-5.

6. David A. Schwartz and others, "Congenital Limb Reduction Defects in the Agricultural Setting," *American Journal of Public Health* Vol. 78, No. 6 (June 1988) pgs. 654-658.

7. D.A. Schwartz and others, "Parental occupation and birth outcomes in an agricultural community," *Scandinavian Journal of Work, Environment and Health* Vol. 12 No. 1 (February 1986), pgs. 51-54.

8. T.E. Taha and R.H. Gray, "Agricultural pesticide exposure and perinatal mortality in central Sudan," *Bulletin of the World Health Organization* Vol. 71 (1993), pgs. 317-321.

9. Jun Zhang and others, "Occupational Hazards and Pregnancy Outcomes," *American Journal of Industrial Medicine* Vol. 21 (1992), pgs. 397-408.

10. Thomas W. Clarkson and others, "Reproductive and developmental toxicity of metals," *Scandinavian Journal of Work, Environment and Health* Vol. 11 (1985), pgs. 145-154.

11. Masazumi Harada, "Congenital Minamata Disease: Intrauterine Methylmercury Poisoning," *Teratology* Vol. 18 (1978), pgs. 285-288.

12. H.A. Ragan and T.J. Mast, "Cadmium Inhalation and Male Reproductive Toxicity," *Reviews of Environmental Contamination and Toxicology* Vol. 114 (1990), pgs. 1-22.

13. Petter Kristensen and others, "Perinatal Outcome among Children of Men Exposed to Lead and Organic Solvents in the Printing Industry," *American Journal of Epidemiology* Vol. 137, No. 2 (1993), pgs. 134-144.

14. D.G. Wibberley and others, "Lead levels in human placentae from normal and malformed births," *Medical Genetics,* Vol. 14, No. 5 (October 1977), pgs. 339-345.

15. Jorma Tikkanen and Olli P. Heinonen, "Cardiovascular Malformations and Organic Solvent Exposure During Pregnancy in Finland," *American Journal of Industrial Medicine* Vol. 14 (1988), pgs. 1-8.

16. Gary M. Shaw, "Maternal Workplace Exposures to Organic Solvents and Congenital Cardiac Anomalies," *Journal of Occupational Medicine and Toxicology*, Vol. 1, No. 4 (1992), pgs. 371-376.

17. Andrew F. Olshan and others, "Paternal Occupation and Congenital Anomalies in Offspring," *American Journal of Industrial Medicine* Vol. 20 (October 1991), pgs. 447-475.

18. C. Loffredo and others, "Organic solvents and cardiovascular malformations in the Baltimore-Washington Infant Study [abstract]," *Teratology* Vol. 43 (May 1991), pg. 450.

19. Evert Hansson and others, "Pregnancy outcome in women working in laboratories in some of the pharmaceutical industries in Sweden," *Scandinavian Journal of Work, Environment and Health* Vol. 6 (1980), pgs. 131-134.

20. Stanley J. Goldberg and others, "An Association of Human Congenital Cardiac Malformations and Drinking Water Contaminants," *Journal of the American College of Cardiology* Vol. 16, No. 1 (July, 1990), pgs. 155-164.

21. Anders Ericson and others, "Delivery Outcome of Women Working in Laboratories During Pregnancy," *Archives of Environmental Health* Vol. 39, No. 1 (1984), pgs. 5-10.

22. Sylvaine Cordier and others, "Maternal occupational exposure and congenital malformations," *Scandinavian Journal of Work, Environment and Health* Vol. 18, No. 1 (February 1992), Pgs. 11-17.

23. Urban Blomqvist and others, "Delivery outcome for women working in the pulp and paper industry," *Scandinavian Journal of Work, Environment and Health* Vol. 7, No. 2 (1981), pgs. 114-118.

24. Hugh A. Tilson and others, "Polychlorinated Biphenyls and the Developing Nervous System: Cross-Species Comparisons," *Neurotoxicology and Teratology* Vol. 12 (1990), pgs. 239-248.

25. Joseph L. Jacobson and others, "Effects of in utero exposure to polychlorinated biphenyls and related contaminants on cognitive

functioning in young children," *Journal of Pediatrics* Vol. 116 (January, 1990), pgs. 38-45.

26. Joseph L. Jacobson and others, "Effects of Exposure to PCBs and Related Compounds on Growth and Activity in Children," *Neurotoxicology and Teratology* Vol. 12 (1990), Pgs. 319-326.

27. Richard A. Albanese, *United States Air Force Personnel and Exposure to Herbicide Orange, Interim Report for Period March 1984-February 1988* (United States Air Force: Brooks Air Force Base, Texas, Feb., 1988).

28. Muin J. Khoury "Epidemiology of Birth Defects," *Epidemiologic Reviews* Vol. 11 (1989), pgs. 244-248.

29. L. Goulet and M. Goldberg, "Reproductive Outcomes among Women Living Near a Sanitary Landfill Site in Montreal, Quebec, Canada, 1979-1989 [abstract]." *American Journal of Epidemiology* Vol. 138, No. 8 (1993), Pg. 587.

30. G. Shaw and others, "Congenital Malformations and Birthweight in Areas with Potential Environmental Contamination," *Archives of Environmental Health* Vol. 47, No. 2 (March/April 1992), pgs. 147-154.

31. Agency for Toxic Substances and Disease Registry, U.S. Public Health Service, U.S. Department of Health and Human Services, *California: Birth Defects Study* (Atlanta, Ga.: Agency for Toxic Substances and Disease Registry, 1990).

32. G. Reza Najem and Lisa K. Voyce, "Health Effects of a Thorium Waste Disposal Site," *American Journal of Public Health* Vol. 80, (April 1990), pgs. 478-480.

33. Nicholas Vianna and Adele Polan, "Incidence of Low Birth Weight Among Love Canal Residents," *Science* Vol. 226, No. 4679 (December 7, 1984), pgs. 1217-1219.

34. Lynn R. Goldman and others, "Low Birth Weight, Prematurity and Birth Defects in Children Living Near the Hazardous Waste Site, Love Canal," *Hazardous Waste & Hazardous Materials* Vol. 2 No. 2 (1985), pgs. 209-223.

35. Lawrence Budnick, and others, "Cancer and Birth Defects Near the Drake Superfund Site, Pennsylvania," *Archives of Environmental Health,* Vol. 39, No. 6 (November/December, 1984), pgs. 409-413.

36. David Ozonoff and Leslie I. Boden, "Truth and Consequences: Health Agency Responses to Environmental Health Problems," *Science, Technology & Human Values* Vol. 12 Nos. 3 & 4 (Summer/Fall 1987), pgs. 70-77. In statistical terms, public health officials will get in less trouble for making a Type I error than a Type II error. Therefore, experiments are often designed to favor avoidance of Type I errors rather than Type II errors.

37. Alan Loeb, "The First Federal Environmental Review: Its Long-Term Consequences," *International Society of Exposure Analysis Newsletter* (Fall 1993), pg. 3.

38. Julia Moore and others, *Putting the Lid on Dioxins* (Washington, D.C.: Physicians for Social Responsibility, (1994); Joe Thornton, *Achieving Zero Dioxin* (Washington, D.C.: Greenpeace, 1994). PSR and EDF failed to call for real prevention; instead they advocated that the major source of dioxin emissions (incinerators) be operated "at optimal conditions" rather than be shut down or phased out.

Chapter 34

The Thalidomide Tragedy

A "miracle" drug, they called it, unlike any other in chemical structure and in its ability to provide quick, calm sleep with none of the hangover and overdose dangers of barbiturates. A "wonder" drug, they said, so safe that you could take handfuls without killing yourself.

With these superlatives, with these striking claims, the drug thalidomide went on the market in Canada, Great Britain, and other European countries, beginning in West Germany in 1958.

It was so safe, West German officials determined, that it could be sold there without prescription, like aspirin.

But the celebrated debut of thalidomide was soon to become a nightmare.

In 1959, a dozen grossly deformed infants were born in various parts of West Germany. Photos and X-rays of two of the infants were shown at a medical meeting in the fall of 1960 because of the previous rarity of the condition, known as phocomelia, combining the Greek words for seal and limb. Malformed fingers or toes appeared at the ends of very foreshortened limbs—making them look like flippers. Even a pediatrician with a long interest in birth defects exclaimed that he had never, in his practice or training, seen this condition before. Otherwise, the exhibit got little attention, and a distinguished American pediatrician attending the meeting lamented that she had missed seeing it. No connection was made with drug use, much less the use of any specific drug. Nor was any connection soon in coming. After all, weren't most such abnormalities spontaneous and unexplained?

FDA Consumer, February 1987.

Wasn't the placenta a marvelous protection for the fetus? Didn't it prevent harmful substances in a mother's blood from reaching the unborn child?

These popular perceptions would soon be shattered. But meanwhile, an application to sell thalidomide in the United States had been submitted to the Food and Drug Administration by the century-old William S. Merrell Co. of Cincinnati. The studies submitted in support of the drug's safety filled four volumes the size of metropolitan telephone books.

In September 1960 the marketing application for thalidomide was given to a new FDA employee, Dr. Frances Kelsey. "It was deemed to be a simple application, and since I had just reported to work, it was assigned to me," Kelsey recalled. But, though new to FDA, Kelsey was not a novice on drugs and their side effects. She was both a physician and a pharmacologist—an expert in the science of drugs. (And even as a student she had been part of a group helping to track down the cause of 107 deaths from a then-new sulfa elixir in 1937-38. The deaths, most of them in children, helped prompt Congress to require companies to submit to FDA proof that drugs were safe, if not necessarily effective, and win FDA's approval before marketing the products.)

Under the law at the time, Kelsey had 60 days to review the thalidomide application, though deadlines could be extended if additional information was needed.

Kelsey was alerted to the unusual nature of thalidomide not only by the claims that it was free of barbiturate-like side effects, but by an oddity: It acted differently in people than in animals. "I was bothered by the fact that thalidomide would not put some of the test animals to sleep," she said. "Why would it induce sleep in human beings and not in animals? It was a very unusual kind of drug and we had no idea how it worked."

She and the other reviewers—a chemist and another pharmacologist—asked Merrell for additional information—and then asked for still more. "All reviewers found deficiencies," Kelsey says in her no-nonsense way, "and the company was so informed."

Meanwhile, West German pediatric clinics that had seen no phocomelia cases in the previous five years now reported 83 in 1960. Still, no specific cause was suspected.

In the United States, Kelsey notes, FDA and the American Academy of Pediatrics were increasingly aware that fetuses could respond differently to drugs than adults did. As a result, they were working to develop guidelines for better drug testing. Kelsey herself, with her

The Thalidomide Tragedy

husband, F. Ellis Kelsey, had done research showing that embryos developed the capacity to produce various enzymes for breaking down certain chemicals at various stages in their growth. Thus, if a certain enzyme hadn't been produced yet, the unborn child could not process certain chemicals that an adult or a more mature fetus could.

In February 1961, Kelsey saw a letter in a British medical journal noting a tingling nerve inflammation in the fingers of patients who had taken thalidomide for a long time. (This link, soon confirmed by other physicians, led West Germany to make thalidomide a prescription drug.)

For Kelsey, the question arising from this association was whether this painful tingling and numbness of the extremities in an adult might have a parallel in the fetus...."whether harm might come to the fetus if the mother took the drug during pregnancy," she said.

Thalidomide's marketing application provided case reports assuring that its use in pregnancy did not hurt the unborn child, but the cases cited involved the drug's use late in pregnancy.

So the new FDA employee again asked the company for further information. Some of the company's representatives made no secret of their displeasure over the resulting delay of a drug that, they pointed out, had been safely used in Europe for years.

For similar reasons, Kelsey said, the company at first resisted a suggestion that the drug's labeling warn against use during pregnancy.

Meanwhile, phocomelia was becoming an unexplained European epidemic. Some infants had no legs at all, just toes sprouting from their hips, along with foreshortened, flipper-like arms. Some people blamed radioactive fallout from atom bomb testing, which concerned many citizens at the time. Others thought abnormal chromosomes might be to blame, or X-rays of the mother while she was pregnant. Food ingredients, various contaminants, blood incompatibilities between parents—all these were among the causes that were suspected, checked and discarded.

Finally, in Hamburg, West Germany, a pediatrician, Dr. Widukind Lenz, began to make a tentative connection. Questioning showed that about 20 percent of the mothers bringing deformed infants to his clinic had taken Contergan, the German trade name for thalidomide. But, of course, this might be coincidence. Many people took thalidomide. It had become a very commonly used drug.

With great care, in early November 1961, Lenz requestioned his patients. Now the percentage of mothers saying they had used thalidomide rose to 50 percent. (Many said they hadn't thought to mention the common drug when first asked.)

Lenz' work was quickly confirmed in Australia where a physician reported that the mothers of six phocomelia victims had taken Distaval, as thalidomide was called there. A similar report came from Scotland.

Thalidomide was withdrawn in Germany and elsewhere at the end of November. The William S. Merrell Co. notified FDA of the phocomelia reports. Soon thereafter the company withdrew its drug application.

All this happened without many Americans, even physicians, knowing about it. Not until the next year, in April of 1962, did Dr. Helen B. Taussig, professor of pediatrics at Johns Hopkins University, bring the situation home to physicians. After learning of the situation abroad in January 1962, she had visited European pediatric clinics to observe the phocomelia epidemic. Now, returning to the United States, she told stunned physicians that thousands of deformed babies had been born abroad. She described how a link had finally been established between the malformations and thalidomide.

Taussig was renowned as the heart specialist who developed the "blue-baby" operation for a deadly congenital heart defect. A dispatch from Philadelphia in *The New York Times* said that Taussig warned fellow physicians in a special meeting at the annual American College of Physicians gathering, "This compound [thalidomide] could have passed our present drug laws. There is no question we need to strengthen our food and drug regulations to include routine testing of new compounds on pregnant animals."

But it took a *Washington Post* story, two months later on July 15, 1962, to ignite the public.

"This is the story of how the skepticism and stubbornness of a government physician prevented what could have been an appalling American tragedy, the birth of hundreds or indeed thousands of armless and legless children...." *Post* reporter Morton Mintz began his story.

"She saw her duty in sternly simple terms, and she carried it out, living the while with insinuations that she was a bureaucratic nitpicker, unreasonable—even, she said, stupid."

The story was immediately relayed on the wire services. Bestirred and horrified, Americans watched as the toll rose to some 5,000 deformed infants in Germany alone. Britain had several hundred. Many pregnant women, having already taken thalidomide, carried their infants to term in great fear.

The Thalidomide Tragedy

You could not turn the pages of a newspaper, a newsmagazine or picture magazine—nor even *Scientific American*—without these powerless, limbless infants staring up at you. One woman's drama made daily headlines: Sherri Finkbine, an American who had taken thalidomide that her husband had obtained overseas, was refused an abortion in Arizona—and fled abroad. There were many other, unpublicized abortions.

FDA discovered that the drug had been distributed to more than 3,000 women in the United States—a marketing promotion in the guise of a clinical test. But there was nothing illegal about this at that time. At least nine deformed infants were eventually linked to such distributions.

There were other occurrences in those days that might seem irregular today—and began to look irregular then, too, in the light of thalidomide. For example, FDA Commissioner George P. Larrick announced that the agency had discovered that some research submitted to get drugs approved appeared to have been misreported—or perhaps not even done at all!

Larrick later reported that a major drug firm had "accumulated reports of jaundice and death....for....over five years before it reported them to us." The drug responsible was Flexin, a muscle relaxant.

In 1961, President Eisenhower's Secretary of Health, Education and Welfare, Arthur W. Fleming, had called for a strengthened drug law, but a bill written by Sen. Estes Kefauver of Tennessee was held up in committee.

But at last the story of thalidomide carried the day in Congress. And what the *Journal of the American Medical Association* called a "landmark" drug law was passed in 1962. The law tightened the safety requirements for testing new prescription drugs on human subjects and stipulated that patients be told if they are getting an experimental drug. The law required that drug companies report adverse effects during clinical tests and after marketing; that a new drug be proved effective, as well as safe; that a drug label carry the common or generic name of the product, as well as its commercial brand name; and that prescription drug advertising to doctors list side effects along with the benefits of the drug.

President Kennedy signed the legislation and, with great ceremony, gave Kelsey a medal, the Distinguished Federal Civilian Service Award. "Through high ability and steadfast confidence in her professional decision," the award said, "she has made an outstanding contribution to the protection of the health of the American people."

Many people today can hardly believe the story of thalidomide. In particular, young mothers schooled to avoid alcohol, cigarettes and drugs may find it hard to believe that just 25 years ago, the science of birth defects—teratology—was so new and unformed that thalidomide could and did happen....and that an estimated 10,000 infants were born with gross limb defects as a result.

Today, physicians and informed women use drugs in pregnancy only when absolutely necessary. Even the most innocuous-seeming nonprescription drugs, if they circulate inside the body, now carry a warning against their use in pregnancy.

Each new drug must be tested in at least two species of pregnant animals to examine any effects on the fetus. Information on these studies, plus any experience in humans, is provided to physicians and pharmacists. If a particularly useful drug may potentially cause harm to the unborn, information for physicians (and, sometimes, directly for patients) is developed to prevent the drug's inappropriate or accidental use in pregnancy.

Except under the most unusual circumstances, patients today are not given experimental drugs without their informed and written consent. And women who could be, or become, pregnant do not receive a drug until animal testing for fetal effects has been completed. Also, a strong system for collecting data on the unexpected side effects of marketed drugs has been developed at FDA.

The 1962 law also gave FDA stronger authority for drug factory inspection and required manufacturers to perform specific tests and maintain records of them. Drug labeling and advertising requirements were also tightened.

No one can say there will never be another thalidomide, Dr. Kelsey says, in part because so little is known about how most drugs work. "However," she adds, "the reforms set in motion by thalidomide should lead to much earlier detection—hopefully in early animal tests, but certainly much sooner in a drug's commercial distribution" of any side effects.

Since animal studies are not always reliable predictors of a drug's action in people, and since pregnant women generally are not used as research subjects, caution continues to be needed in the use of any drug, particularly a new drug, during pregnancy.

Editor's Note [in original text]: Today, thalidomide has a limited use in the treatment of leprosy. Frances Kelsey still works for FDA, heading a staff of investigators who check on drug research to make sure

The Thalidomide Tragedy

it is done properly and its results are correctly reported. The *Post*'s Morton Mintz has written extensively on thalidomide and on faulty and fraudulent drug research.

—by William Grigg

William Grigg is the director of FDA's press relations staff. He reported on the thalidomide tragedy 25 years ago as a reporter for *The Washington Star*.

Chapter 35

Accutane

Some likened the decision asked of FDA to that required of the biblical Solomon when two women seemed to have equal claim to being mother of the same child.

The issue before FDA, however, was not one of parentage, but whether a drug that has the ability to clear a very severe and disfiguring form of acne should be taken off the market because it also carries a high risk of causing a deformed baby or miscarriage if taken by a pregnant woman.

The name of the drug is Accutane (generically called isotretinoin). The issues surrounding it could serve as a basis for a course in medical ethics. Summarized, these issues are:

- A relative of vitamin A, Accutane was known to cause birth defects in animals and suspected of causing them in humans even before it was approved by FDA in 1983. Although the labeling has always forbidden use of the drug during pregnancy, such use has nevertheless occurred. Marketing experience with the drug indicates that Accutane causes birth defects in about one out of every four exposed fetuses.

- The condition for which the drug was approved, severe recalcitrant cystic acne unresponsive to other therapy, is much more common in males than in females. Yet 40 percent of the prescriptions are written for women, virtually all of whom are of

FDA Consumer, October 1988.

childbearing age. The primary reason given for this is that women seek treatment for this condition more often than men.

- Accutane is the only drug that can clear this severe and disfiguring form of acne. Other drugs approved to treat the same condition must be taken for extended periods and, when stopped, the condition usually reappears. But with Accutane, most patients need to take the drug for only a few months. When the drug is discontinued, the acne usually does not return.

- Birth defects continued to occur despite repeated revisions of the labeling, letters to physicians from the manufacturer, Hoffmann-La Roche, and articles in the *FDA Drug Bulletin* (a publication sent to more than 1 million health professionals) that the drug should not be used by women of childbearing age unless they were using an effective form of contraception. Miscarriages (technically called spontaneous abortions when occurring in the first three months of pregnancy) also continued to occur at a rate substantially higher than in the general population. In addition, there has been an increased rate of elective abortion among women taking Accutane, apparently resulting from the wish to avoid giving birth to a deformed child.

To publicly consider these issues, FDA convened a meeting last April of its Dermatologic Drugs Advisory Committee, a panel of experts from outside the agency. Highly knowledgeable and respected scientists lined up on both sides of the issue. Representatives from the federal Centers for Disease Control (part of the Public Health Service) and the American Academy of Pediatrics recommended that the drug be withdrawn from the market. Consumer advocates proposed severe restrictions. Spokespersons from the American Academy of Dermatology, representing skin specialists (who write 90 percent of all Accutane prescriptions), emphasized its therapeutic value and the physical and psychological scarring, along with the social ostracism, that patients with severe cystic acne often endure. They recommended continued marketing with a number of restrictions.

Proponents of keeping the drug on the market showed slides of patients with disfiguring acne, not only on the face but also on the shoulders, arms, back, and chest.

Proponents of severely restricting or totally banning the drug showed slides of babies with the birth defect syndrome known to be associated with the drug: misshapen head, lack of ears or ears placed low next to a too-small jaw, and cleft palate. They also described the defects of the brain and heart and explained that the drug does the most damage to the fetus in the early weeks of pregnancy, often before a woman realizes she is pregnant.

How was FDA to choose between protecting the unborn and healing patients with a disfiguring physical problem?

Should the agency allow a drug to remain on the market that continued to be a cause of birth defects despite warnings that it not be used in women who were pregnant or who might become pregnant?

On the other hand, could FDA ethically remove from the market a drug that had the capacity to clear up a disfiguring condition when no other marketed drug was as effective?

Fortunately, FDA had a solution available to it that was not available to Solomon: compromise.

Taking into account advice from consumer and professional organizations, the agency and Hoffmann-La Roche have been hammering out further restrictions and unprecedented labeling warnings in the expectation that these will insure the appropriate use of the drug and, thus, the elimination of birth defects associated with its use.

One aspect of this plan is the inclusion, in the patient information labeling, of a drawing of a baby with the syndrome of deformities associated with Accutane use. The drawing is meant as an attention-getter and as a deterrent to women who might otherwise take lightly the warning not to take the drug unless they are using an effective form of contraception.

The patient labeling will also state that there is at least a one in four chance that a woman who becomes pregnant while taking Accutane will give birth to a deformed baby. The patient consent form, which the woman and her physician must sign, will include a discussion of the potential for birth defects. To prevent starting the drug when a pregnancy has begun but is not yet recognized, the patient leaflet will instruct the woman that the drug should be started only on the second or third day after the start of a normal menstrual period. A phone number will be given for women to call if they think they may be pregnant and want additional information.

The "don't use in pregnancy" symbol (a pregnant woman within a bisected circle, the international symbol for "not" or "don't") will be displayed both on each page of the patient leaflet and on each panel of the new blister-pack packaging. The blister pack will include a tear-off prepaid postcard addressed to Hoffmann-La Roche on which the patient can inform the company of her name, phone number, and address, and grant permission to the company to contact her for follow-up studies to determine whether women taking Accutane are continuing to become pregnant.

The physician labeling, which will also display the "don't use in pregnancy" symbol, will be extensively revised to more strongly emphasize the risk of birth defects. The print size for the boxed pregnancy contraindication will be doubled. The boxed warning will forbid Accutane's use in women of childbearing age unless *all* of the following conditions are met:

- The patient has severe, disfiguring cystic acne that does not respond to other therapies.

- She is reliable in understanding and carrying out instructions.

- She is capable of complying with mandatory contraceptive measures.

- She has received both verbal and written warnings of the hazards of pregnancy, the risks of contraceptive failure, and has acknowledged these in writing.

- Within two weeks before starting the drug, the patient has had a negative pregnancy test, performed in a physician's office or by a licensed laboratory.

The physician labeling will also contain instructions that Accutane should be prescribed only by physicians, such as dermatologists, who have special competence in the diagnosis and treatment of severe, recalcitrant cystic acne, and who understand the risk of birth defects.

In addition to the labeling changes, Hoffmann-La Roche has agreed to extensive professional educational and follow-up efforts. The firm will report to FDA all cases in which a woman using Accutane becomes pregnant, whether or not a birth defect or other adverse reaction occurs. It also will undertake research into the reasons why, despite warnings, pregnancies have occurred in the past. Data concerning the use of the drug, including information about age and sex of patients, will be supplied to FDA quarterly. The company is also designing studies using lower doses of the drug, and using higher doses for a shorter period.

Accutane

In conjunction with the labeling changes, the American Academy of Dermatology has developed guidelines for the appropriate use of Accutane.

This program is a bold example of what can be accomplished when a manufacturer, professional organizations, and FDA cooperate in finding ways to minimize the risks of a drug while preserving its availability to those who can greatly benefit from it. Only time will tell whether the responsible use of Accutane will make the decision to keep it on the market with increased warnings and restrictions a decision worthy of the wisdom of Solomon.

Vitamin A and Birth Defects

It is no secret that high doses of vitamin A may cause birth defects when taken by a pregnant woman. Although data on its effects in humans are sparse, studies in animals have conclusively shown it to be a teratogen—a cause of birth defects.

It was, therefore, no surprise when Accutane, a synthetic derivative of vitamin A, caused human birth defects. From the time the drug first went on the market, it was placed in "Pregnancy Category X," meaning that it should not be used in pregnant women or in those likely to become pregnant. Originally this categorization was based on animal studies, but it took only a few months on the market for it to become evident that it was a potent teratogen in humans as well.

On the heels of the problems with Accutane, concern has arisen about two other drugs that also are vitamin A derivatives: Retin-A (tretinoin), a topical cream and lotion used to treat acne and recently ballyhooed in the press for easing wrinkles, and Tegison (etretinate), an oral medication for the treatment of severe psoriasis unresponsive to other treatments.

Because Retin-A is a topical product and not absorbed a great deal into the body, all evidence to date seems to be reassuring that there is not an increased danger of birth defects to the fetuses of women who may become pregnant while using it. The drug is in Pregnancy Category B, which means that it should be used in pregnancy only when clearly needed.

Tegison, however, is another story. A more potent teratogen than even Accutane, like Accutane it is in Pregnancy Category X. Its teratogenic effect may persist longer than Accutane's; Tegison's labeling warns that it is not known exactly how long this effect lasts after a woman stops taking the drug. Therefore, the labeling requires that a woman taking Tegison use an effective form of contraception one month before starting, during, and for an indefinite period after stopping therapy. Possibly because people suffering from psoriasis are usually older than those with acne (use of Tegison in women of childbearing age is only 5 percent that of Accutane's use in that group), there have been no reports of birth defects associated with Tegison's use in this country since it was approved in late 1986. However, a report from Brazil of a baby born with a syndrome of birth defects similar to that seen with Accutane serves as a warning. In that particular case, that baby was conceived 11 months after the mother stopped taking Tegison.

Regarding vitamin A itself, data from animal studies clearly show it to be a teratogen whose effect, similar to Tegison's, persists for some time after use is discontinued. But it is not yet known at what dosage level it becomes a threat to the developing human fetus. For one thing, because it can be purchased over the counter as a dietary supplement, the extent of its use by pregnant women is unknown, and data on its effects are hard to come by. Further, because it is known to cause birth defects in animals, as do Accutane and Tegison, controlled trials in pregnant women would be unethical. FDA scientists are presently trying to collect more data on vitamin A. But until more definitive studies are completed, women who are pregnant or planning to become pregnant would be wise to avoid taking supplements with more than a total of 8,000 International Units of vitamin A per day. There is no known benefit to anyone, including pregnant women, in taking more than this amount, but there are potential dangers.

— by Judith Willis

Judith Willis is the editor of the *FDA Drug Bulletin*, a publication for health professionals.

Chapter 36

ACE Inhibitors and Birth Defects

Levels of angiotensin II are normally elevated during pregnancy, but women are resistant to its pressor effects. Some women lose this resistance quite a while before the due date—sometimes as early in pregnancy as week 23—and within a few weeks hypertension develops. Angiotensin-converting enzyme (ACE) inhibitors would seem a logical choice for hypertension of pregnancy, and they have been used for this indication for more than a decade. However, there have been numerous reports of severe fetal and neonatal morbidity and mortality in women who received ACE inhibitors for hypertension during pregnancy. As early as 1980, studies with rabbits, sheep, and goats showed that ACE inhibitors administered during the second and third trimesters can cause substantial fetal and perinatal mortality. In rabbits, fetal death rate was 86% in captopril-treated animals compared with 1% in placebo-treated animals, and 100% in enalapril-treated animals (single oral doses, 30 mg/kg, given late in pregnancy). In women, captopril and enalapril cross the placenta (plasma levels are similar in maternal and umbilical blood, and plasma renin activity is significantly elevated in neonates). Using these agents during pregnancy often results in neonatal hypotension and respiratory distress. Prolonged hypotension occurs in 10% of the infants, and respiratory complications in 14%. Other adverse effects observed include fetal and neonatal renal failure, oligohydramnios (due to fetal renal failure),

From *Medical Sciences Bulletin*, August 1994, Volume No. 16, Issue # 12; reprinted with permission of Pharmaceutical Information Associates, Ltd. (PIA), 2761 Trenton Road, Levittown, PA 19506, phone: (215) 949-0490.

intrauterine growth retardation, premature labor, bony malformations, limb contractures, persistent patent ductus arteriosus, pulmonary hypoplasia, respiratory distress syndrome, and neonatal death.

ACE inhibitors may also be teratogenic. One infant exposed to captopril had an enlarged fontanelle with decreased skull ossification, deviation of the nasal septum, horizontal chin crease, glabellar crease, a bell-shaped chest, contractures of knees and elbows, and positional deformities of the hands. The infant had severe hypotension and respiratory and renal failure; death occurred 25 hours after delivery. Other anuric, hypoxic, acidotic infants have been described, often with defective skulls and/or defective limbs. While hypertension itself can have adverse effects on the fetus, the distinct constellation of symptoms and abnormalities observed in neonates after ACE inhibitor exposure in utero—prolonged anuria, hypotension, and skull ossification defects—are not commonly associated with maternal hypertension or its treatment and may be caused by the ACE inhibitor itself.

While captopril and enalapril are the ACE inhibitors most commonly implicated in fetal and neonatal morbidity and mortality, it is likely that other drugs in this category are equally dangerous. The FDA has officially warned against the use of ACE inhibitors during the second and third trimesters of pregnancy, but first trimester use may also be hazardous to the fetus. (Shotan A et al. *Am J Med*. 1994; 96:451-456.)

Chapter 37

Outcomes of Pregnancy Associated with Antiepileptic Drugs

Exposure to antiepileptic drugs (AEDs) during pregnancy is associated with increased risk of congenital anomalies in the offspring. All anticonvulsant drugs have been implicated.[1,2] It has been suggested, until recently, that phenobarbital and carbamazepine are less likely to produce anomalies.[3] However, recent reports have documented congenital anomalies, cognitive delay, and neural tube defects in the offspring of women taking carbamazepine during pregnancy.[4] We prospectively studied 211 women with epilepsy to ascertain the relative risks of the major AEDs in a busy high-risk obstetric clinic. Herein, we document the outcome of the pregnancies during the years 1987 through 1990.

About This Study

Objective. To determine whether exposure to antiepileptic drugs during pregnancy is associated with poor fetal outcomes (anomalies and death) and to assess the relative risks with phenobarbital, phenytoin sodium, and carbamazepine.

Design. The design was a prospective case-control cohort study of pregnant women with epilepsy and their offspring. Outcomes were compared with those of a control group of 355 healthy women and their offspring.

From *Archives of Neurology*, March 1994, Volume 51, pp. 250-53; copyright 1994, American Medical Association;.reprinted with permission.

Setting. The obstetrics service at Los Angeles County/University of Southern California Medical Center, Los Angeles, a large, inner-city, teaching hospital.

Patients. Two hundred eleven subjects who were pregnant during the years 1987 through 1990, 174 of whom were delivered of infants, were available for analysis. A control group of 355 healthy women and their offspring from the same hospital were randomly selected from a computerized database.

Interventions. None.

Main Outcome Measure. Anomalies and fetal death were the primary outcomes measures.

Results. Offspring of women with epilepsy who were exposed to antiepileptic drugs had a higher rate of fetal death and anomalies than did the control population ($P=.001$). Abnormal outcomes were associated with the three major antiepileptic drugs (carbamazepine, phenytoin, and phenobarbital). In terms of abnormal outcome (death and anomalies), phenobarbital was associated with the highest relative risk, phenytoin with intermediate relative risk, and carbamazepine with the lowest relative risk ($P=.019$). Numbers were insufficient for assessment of risk associated with valproic acid.

Conclusion. All three major antiepileptic drugs (phenobarbital, phenytoin, and carbamazepine) are associated with an increased risk of fetal death and anomalies. We found phenobarbital to be most associated with poor pregnancy outcome.

Study Subjects and Methods

From 1987 through March 1990, 211 women were followed up in our high-risk obstetric clinic in which pregnant women with epilepsy and other neurologic disorders are treated. These women were referred by outside clinics or from the routine neurology clinic at Los Angeles County/University of Southern California (LAC/USC) Medical Center, Los Angeles. Our population consisted of poor, inner-city, predominantly Hispanic patients. Although this is a population of poor women, all are medically insured (state insurance) during pregnancy to ensure adequate prenatal monitoring. Both the women with epilepsy

Outcomes of Pregnancy Associated with Antiepileptic Drugs

and control groups are drawn from the same socioeconomic group and geographic location. Patients received standard obstetric care at the clinic, but an attending neurologist took a history, performed an examination, and monitored the administration of AEDs throughout the pregnancy. In all cases, the AED treatment was initiated by the referring physician. In some cases, AEDs were not used at all owing to infrequent seizures or unwillingness of the patient to take medications during pregnancy. All data were documented at each visit on a standard form that included medications, drug levels, and seizure frequency.

Antiepileptic drugs were added or treatment was adjusted, as clinically necessary, by the attending neurologist. All women who were exposed to an AED during the first trimester were noted. The majority of these women gave birth at the LAC/USC Medical Center. At the time of delivery, the infants underwent a standardized examination by a physician and/or nurse clinician trained to recognize major and minor anomalies. Minor anomalies were defined as unusual morphologic features with no serious medical or cosmetic consequence, while major anomalies were defined as identifiable structural defects in organs associated with significant functional abnormality.[6]

Data from the obstetric clinic and the infants' delivery charts were entered into a database (dBASE IV, Borland International, Scotts Valley, Calif.) and included mother's age, parity, gestational age, complications of delivery, medications taken, number of seizures during pregnancy, total number of seizures during lifetime, pregnancy outcome, birth weight, Apgar scores, head circumference, and any abnormal outcome. We defined abnormal outcome as any congenital anomaly in or death of the infant.

A control population of 355 patients was selected from a computer-generated list of all women who gave birth in the same facility during this period. Every third woman was selected, and the infants' charts were examined. The control group represented mothers from various clinics in the hospital. Mothers who abused alcohol and other drugs were excluded from both the patient and control groups. The epileptic mothers and the control group were similar in age (mean ± SD, 27.1 ± 5.3 and 25.9 ± 6.1 years, respectively).

Statistical Analysis

Percentages of anomalies in the epileptic and control groups were compared by χ^2 analysis and Fisher's Exact Test: (1) for all drugs combined; and, (2) for each of the three drugs and the polytherapy group separately. The .05 level of significance for rejection of the null hypothesis was corrected for multiple comparisons to .0125 (Bonferroni's correction). This analysis was repeated with the epileptic group composed only of those who received a drug during the first trimester. Differences for birth weight, head circumference, and length between the two groups were evaluated with use of a t test.

Percentages of anomalies associated with each drug in the first trimester were compared with use of Fisher's Exact Test. The ages of mothers receiving each drug were compared with one-way analysis of variance.

Explanation of Study Results

Of the 211 pregnancies, data from 174 were available for analysis (see Table 37.1). Thirty-seven of these pregnancies were not included owing to therapeutic abortions (n=4) or delivery at other hospitals (n=7) or because the patient moved or the records could not be found (n=26).

Of the 174 pregnancies included in the analysis, 159 women were exposed to AEDs during pregnancy. No abnormal pregnancy outcomes were detected in the 15 pregnancies in which there was no exposure to AEDs. In the remaining 159 pregnancies, 17 (10.7%) abnormal outcomes were found compared with 12 (3.4%) abnormal outcomes in 355 control pregnancies ($P=.001$). Abnormal outcomes included death and congenital anomalies (major and minor). Head circumference (34.5 ± 1.3 vs 34.7 ± 2.1 cm) and birth weight (3.40 ± 0.60 vs 3.38 ± 0.60 g) were identical in the two populations of infants born to epileptic and nonepileptic mothers, respectively (Table 37.1).

Table 37.2 lists the congenital anomalies, the AED taken, the gestational age, and other contributing factors. Congenital anomalies are divided into major, minor, and mixed categories. All three AEDs were associated with anomalies. Six deaths occurred in the epileptic group compared with two in the control group ($P=.01$). No cause of death could be found in three cases, and three autopsies were performed (Table 3). In one case, sclerosis of the placental villi was believed to be the primary cause of death and the infection (chorionitis) the secondary cause of death, resulting in fetal amniotic fluid aspiration and death. Another fetal death was attributed to infection, and the last was believed to be due to unknown natural causes.

Of the 159 patients treated with AEDs, 115 were exposed during the first trimester. Thirteen (11.3%) abnormal outcomes (deaths and anomalies) occurred in the population of 115 women exposed to AEDs during the first trimester (Table 37.4). Five cases were not included in the monotherapy medication group, as exposure to unknown AEDs acquired from a foreign country (n=4) and clonazepam (n=1) occurred. Deaths (n=5) were significantly increased in infants of women with epilepsy exposed to AEDs compared with controls ($P=.009$). Only phenobarbital ($P=.001$ was significantly associated with abnormal outcomes compared with controls. The analysis of the percentages of anomalies associated with the three drugs revealed a borderline significant result ($P=.057$) as determined with Fisher's Exact Test. The observed percentages were as follows: 3.0% for carbamazepine, 10.7% for phenytoin, and 23.8% for phenobarbital. A post hoc test for linear trend revealed a significant increasing trend in the percentages of abnormal outcomes across the three drug groups ($P=.019$). With use of analysis of variance, no significant difference was noted between mothers' ages for exposure to the three major AEDs ($P=.42$).

It has been suggested that seizures may cause congenital anomalies in the offspring.[7] We analyzed seizure frequency during pregnancy and found no correlation between seizure frequency and outcome, but our data were incomplete, as information regarding seizure frequency was not available for all patients.

Comment

Our study demonstrates that the three major AEDs—phenobarbital, phenytoin, and carbamazepine—are associated with an increased risk of abnormal pregnancy outcomes (deaths and anomalies). Of the three drugs, phenobarbital was most likely to result in a major anomaly in or death of the offspring. Trend analysis also reveals the lowest risk with carbamazepine, intermediate risk with phenytoin, and greatest risk with phenobarbital.

Our study focused on major anomalies. It is possible that some of the more subtle craniofacial abnormalities documented in a previous study of patients taking carbamazepine may have been overlooked. As epicanthal folds have been noted in 28% to 59%[8] of offspring of epileptic mothers, our documentation of only one such case suggests that we are not recognizing some of the minor abnormalities on routine perinatal examinations. If our ascertainment is low, this presumably would be consistent across all drug groups. We also recognize that failure to match patients and controls for parity or previous pregnancy outcome or to prospectively randomize the choice of AED among our subjects are further limitations.

Table 37.1. Summary of Data for Study Group and Controls*

	Epileptic	Control	P
All pregnant women	211	355	...
Pregnancy outcomes unavailable	33	...	...
Induced abortion	4	...	...
Delivered infants available for analysis	174	355	...
Mean age of mothers, y	27.1±5.3	25.9±6.1	NS
No. of infants exposed to AEDs	159/174(91.4)	...	...
Abnormal outcomes (deaths and anomalies)	17/159(10.7)	12/355(3.4)	.001
No. of infants exposed to AEDs during first trimester	115/159(72.3)	...	...
Mean birth weight, kg	3.4±0.6	3.38±0.6	NS
Mean head circumference, cm	34.6±1.5	34.7±2.1	NS
Abnormal outcomes (deaths and anomalies)	13/115(11.3)	12/355(3.4)	.002

*NS indicates not significant; AEDs, antiepileptic drugs. Values are number or number affected/total number (percent) unless otherwise stated.

Outcomes of Pregnancy Associated with Antiepileptic Drugs

Table 37.2. Congenital Anomalies Found in Infants Exposed to Antiepileptic Drugs at Any Time During Pregnancy*

Congenital Anomaly	Gestational Medication	Other Age, wk	Factors
Major			
Gastroschisis	Phenytoin sodium	38	...
Meningomyelocele/ patent ductus arteriosus	Phenobarbital	37	...
VSD	Phenobarbital	39	Seizures
VSD	Valproic acid/ phenobarbital/ phenytoin (after 11 wk)	33	Seizures
Minor			
Broad nasal bridge	Phenytoin	40	Maternal chickenpox
Foot defect	Phenytoin	40	...
Club foot	Carbamazepine	34	...
Dilated right ventricle	Phenytoin/ carbamazepine (after 30 wk)	38	Seizures
epicanthal folds	Carbamazepine	39	Seizures
Mixed			
Supernumerary nipple/thin upper lip/ long philtrum	Valproic acid/ phenobarbital/ thioridazine	38	Seizures
Abnormal feet/ asymmetric face/ murmur	Phenytoin/ diazepam	38	Seizures

*There were 11 total anomalies among 159 women exposed. VSD indicates ventricular septal defect.

Table 37.3. Deaths in Infants Exposed to Antiepileptic Drugs.

Intrauterine Pregnancy, wk	Autopsy	Medications	Other Factors
11	...	Phenytoin sodium	...
21	...	Phenobarbital	...
22	...	Clonazepam	Malpresentation (double footling breech)
35	Sclerosis of placental villi, chorionitis, moderate-severe amniotic fluid aspiration, blood culture yielded *Enterococcus*	Phenobarbital	...
38	Intrauterine infection; acute amnionitis; blood culture yielded *Escherichia coli, Enterococcus*	Phenobarbital	Seizures
40	Unknown natural causes; membrane: meconium staining	Carbamazepine (6 wk before death only)	Seizures, anemia elevated liver function tests

*Six infant deaths occurred among 159 exposed.

Outcomes of Pregnancy Associated with Antiepileptic Drugs

Table 37.4. Abnormal Outcomes in Infants Exposed to Phenytoin, Carbamazepine, Phenobarbital Monotherapy, or Multiple Antiepileptic Drugs (AEDs)*

	Phenytoin Sodium	Carba-mazepine	Pheno-barbital	Multiple AEDs†
No. of abnormal outcomes	3	1	5	3
Total No. exposed during first trimester	28	33	21	28
% of abnormal outcomes	10.7	3	23.8	10.7
P compared with controls	.09	.69	.001	.09

*Excludes infants exposed to unknown AEDs (n=4) administered in a foreign country. Excludes one death at 22 weeks' gestation (double footling breech with exposure to clonazepam).
†Multiple AEDs were valproic acid/phenobarbital (n=2) and phenytoin/diazepam (n=1).

In our study, one neural tube defect was recognized in association with phenobarbital use. Given the infrequency of this defect and the size of our study, it is not surprising that we did not see this defect in association with other AEDs. A recent study[5] documented three cases of spina bifida (a neural tube defect) in 107 women taking carbamazepine. On further analysis, these women were also exposed to valproic acid (n=1), phenytoin, barbiturates, or primidone (n=2). These authors[5] argued that independently, phenytoin, barbiturates, or primidone were not associated with spina bifida and therefore were unlikely to confound the carbamazepine results. Our only case of a neural tube defect was detected in a woman who was exposed to phenobarbital alone during the first trimester of pregnancy. Therefore, we cannot support these authors' conclusions.

Neural tube defects have been associated with all of the most commonly prescribed AEDs.[9] It has been documented and studied most frequently with valproic acid, but our clinic population rarely uses this AED. We report no cases of prenatally detected neural tube defects resulting in therapeutic abortion.

We see no greater percentage of poor outcomes than reported in other published studies. The death rate is twofold to threefold higher in infants born to women with epilepsy compared with controls, and this rate is described in other studies.[10] Yet, there are statistically significant differences between the rates of anomalies and death in the two populations. Three of the infant deaths could be considered spontaneous abortions, which, by definition, were not included in the control population of live births. The remaining three infants who died underwent autopsy, and it cannot be determined whether the AEDs had any impact on these outcomes.

We were unable to separate the major and minor anomalies for each AED and statistically analyze this, as the numbers of these anomalies were too small in each group. This is an argument for large multicenter studies, as no center can study enough infants to determine which AED is safest during pregnancy.

Acknowledgements

The report of this study was accepted for publication April 15, 1993.

This project was partially supported by an educational grant from Ciba-Geigy, Summit, NJ, to the USC Department of Neurology.

Presented in part at the American Epilepsy Society Meeting, San Diego, CA, November 11, 1990; the American Neurological Association Meeting, Seattle, Wash, October 1, 1991; and the American Pediatric Society Meeting, Baltimore, MD, May 5, 1992.

We wish to thank Paul Wu, MD, Department of Pediatrics, LAC/USC Medical Center, for reviewing the manuscript; Stanley Azen, PhD, Division of Biometry, Department of Preventive Medicine, University of Southern California, for statistical review; Regina Olivas-Ho, RN, for data entry; and Lou Mallory and Patricia De La Cruz for preparation of the manuscript.

Reprint requests to the Department of Neurology, University of Southern California, 1510 San Pablo St, Suite 615, Los Angeles, CA 90033 (Dr. Waters).

References

1. Nakane Y, Okuma T, Takashashi R, et al. Multi-institutional study on the teratogenicity and fetal toxicity of antiepileptic drug: a report of a collaborative study group in Japan. *Epilepsia* 1980;21:663-680.

2. Bertollini R, Kallen B, Mastroiacovo P, Robert E. Anticonvulsant drugs in monotherapy. *Eur J Epidemiol* 1987;3:164-171.

3. Saunders M. Epilepsy in women of childbearing age. *BMJ* 1989;299:581.

4. Jones KL, Lacro RV, Johnson KA, Adams J. Patten of malformations in children of women treated with carbamazepine during pregnancy. *N Engl J Med* 1989;320:1661-1666.

5. Rosa FW. Spina bifida in infants of women treated with carbamazepine during pregnancy. *N Engl J Med* 1991; 324:674-677.

6. Jones KL, ed. *Smith's Recognizable Patterns of Human Malformations*. Philadelphia, Pa: WB Saunders Co; 1988:662-681.

7. Annegers JF, Elvebeck LR, Hauser WA, Kurland LT. Do anticonvulsants have teratogenic effects? *Arch Neurol* 1974; 31:364-373.

8. Gaily E, Granstrom ML, Hiilesmaa V, Bard A. Minor anomalies in offspring of epileptic mothers. *J Pediatr* 1988;112:520-529.

9. Dansky L, Andermann E, Andermann F. Major congenital malformations in the offspring of epileptic patients: genetic and environmental risk factors. In: Janz D, Dam M, Richens A, Boss L, Helge H, Schmidt D, eds. *Epilepsy, Pregnancy, and the Child*. New York, NY: Raven Press; 1982:223-234.

10. Hiilesmaa VK. Pregnancy and birth in women with epilepsy. *Neurology* 1992;42(suppl 5):8-11.

— by Cheryl H. Waters, MD, FRCPC; Yitzak Belai, MD; Peggy S. Gott, PhD; Perry Shen, MD; Christopher M. De Giorgio, MD

From the Department of Neurology, University of Southern California, School of Medicine (Drs. Waters, Gott, Shen, and De Giorgio), and the Department of Obstetrics and Gynecology, Los Angeles County/University of Southern California Medical Center (Dr. Belai), Los Angeles.

Chapter 38

Rubella

Twenty-five years ago, rubella was one of the common viral diseases affecting many thousands of children in the United States. Since the introduction of rubella vaccine in 1969, reported cases of rubella in the U.S. dropped from 60,000 to fewer than 400 in 1989. Rubella—also known as the German measles or the three-day measles—is only moderately contagious, and many people who are exposed to rubella as children do not become infected.

Although usually a mild disease in children, rubella is a devastating infection in a developing fetus. A baby born to a woman who was infected with rubella virus early in her pregnancy has a very high risk of being born with major congenital defects, known as congenital rubella syndrome (CRS). In addition, rubella infection can cause fetal and neonatal death. Today, as a result of widespread vaccination of children and young adults in the U.S., virtually no babies are born with the syndrome.

Rubella Symptoms

Children with rubella generally develop only a mild rash, but young adults commonly develop generalized symptoms such as headache and body aches, eye inflammation, low fever, and swollen glands a week or so before the rash appears. The rash usually begins on the face and spreads over the rest of the body. It usually disappears after three to

---

Prepared by the NIAID Office of Communications, National Institutes of Health, Bethesda, MD, July 1991.

five days. However, as many as half of those infected with rubella virus never develop noticeable symptoms at all.

Rubella virus is spread through airborne droplets or through direct contact with respiratory secretions from an infected person. It is contagious for a week before symptoms appear and for up to two weeks after the rash appears.

Occasionally, complications occur following rubella infection. In nearly one-third of adult women with rubella, joint problems develop at the same time or shortly after the rash. Joint pain can be mild, lasting for a few days, or severe with swelling and redness of the joints, most commonly affecting the fingers, wrists, and knees. Rubella arthritis usually disappears within a few weeks, although it can sometimes persist for several months.

Neurologic complications are extremely rare but very serious. In an estimated 1 in 6000 cases, a child will develop a high fever, convulsions, and other symptoms of encephalitis. Nearly one in five of these children die, but those who recover usually do so completely.

Other rare complications include bleeding disorders and inflammation of the heart and liver.

Congenital Rubella Syndrome

CRS is a constellation of deformities that may include malformations of major organ systems such as the heart, as well as deafness, cataracts, glaucoma, mental retardation, slow growth, and bone disease. Although most of these abnormalities are evident early in life, older children and young adults who were born with CRS have a high incidence of autoimmune disorders such as diabetes mellitus and thyroid disease.

It is estimated that the average cost for health care of a single patient with CRS is more than $200,000. At the time the vaccine became available, there were 60-70 cases of CRS reported each year in the United States. In 1989, there were only three reported cases of CRS.

Prevention by Rubella Vaccine

Three live, attenuated (weakened) rubella virus vaccines became available in the U.S. during 1969 and 1970. Since 1979, only one rubella vaccine—made from virus grown in human diploid cell culture and then weakened—has been distributed in the United States.

Rubella

The Centers for Disease Control (CDC) recommends that all children receive rubella vaccine, usually at 15 months of age in a combination vaccine that also protects against measles and mumps. In addition, older children who have never been vaccinated against rubella should receive the vaccine even if they are thought to have had rubella infection. It is particularly important for women of childbearing age to have received the vaccine, but they should not become pregnant for three months after vaccination because the rubella virus can cross the placenta. Although the virus used in the vaccine is weakened, there is a potential risk that the vaccine could cause fetal infection. However, no cases of CRS have been reported among babies whose mothers received rubella vaccine during pregnancy.

As with any vaccine, rubella vaccine can cause minor side effects that include low-grade fever, rash, and swollen lymph glands. In addition, an estimated 15 percent of adult female vaccinees experience joint pain, stiffness, swelling and redness one to three weeks after vaccination. These symptoms, which occur at rates that are much lower than following natural infection, generally last for a few days to weeks, but some women have reported chronic joint symptoms. Studies are under way to learn why infection with rubella virus is sometimes associated with chronic arthralgia or arthritis. Armed with that knowledge, it should be possible to design rubella vaccines in the future that will not cause these adverse effects.

Research on Rubella

The routine use of rubella vaccine in the U.S. has led to a dramatic decline in the number of rubella cases in this country; most important, it has virtually eliminated congenital rubella syndrome, resulting in more productive and healthy lives for hundreds of thousands of children who might otherwise have been infected with rubella virus before birth. Despite this success, however, there are concerns about the adverse effects of this vaccine in adult women and about the possibility of adversely affecting the developing fetuses of pregnant women who are vaccinated.

The National Institute of Allergy and Infectious Diseases (NIAID) is supporting research aimed at developing an improved rubella vaccine. Specifically, NIAID-supported scientists hope to identify both the components of rubella virus that are necessary for producing long-term immunity and the components associated with adverse effects. In addition, scientists are studying the genetic sequences of these components, which would enable them to construct a genetically engineered vaccine that would be effective, cause fewer adverse reactions and unable to infect the fetus during maternal immunization.

Chapter 39

Streptococcus B Infection of the Newborn

The U.S. Public Health Service Centers for Disease Control and Prevention (the CDC) has issued guidelines recommending that all pregnant women be screened for Streptococcus B Infection (Strep B).

Strep B is a very serious bacterial infection threatening the health of 7,500 newborn babies each year in the USA. Six percent of the infected babies die, often in the first week of life; of those infants who survive, 20% have brain damage, hearing loss or blindness. The infection is the most common cause in the newborn of sepsis (infection in the blood) and meningitis (infection of membranes covering the brain). The infant becomes infected during delivery, getting the infection from an unsuspecting mother who is often symptom free.

10 to 30% of pregnant women have a Strep B infection but have no symptoms. The infection spreads to the baby via amniotic fluid during labor and delivery. Risk of infection is highest among: babies whose mothers have a history of having had a Strep B infection in a previous baby; infants whose mothers are less than 20 years of age; and babies who are born 18 hours after the amniotic fluid breaks (the "water breaks"). African-American infants appear to be at much higher risk of infection then others.

The CDC recommends that all pregnant women be screened for Strep B infection between 35-37 weeks of pregnancy (7-8 months) and if found to be positive, be offered treatment with antibiotics.

Research Fact Sheet, United Cerebral Palsy Research and Educational Foundation, © October 1996; reprinted with permission

Recommendations are also made for the treatment of women who are in labor and are: less than 37 weeks pregnant and have not been tested; or if their water breaks and they do not deliver within 18 hours; or have a fever of 100.4 F° degree or more.

Comment

The consequences of Strep B infection of the newborn can be disastrous. Pregnant women need to be aware of this and discuss with their doctors the need for screening for infection, the treatment of infection, and treatment during delivery if they have not been screened. An ounce of prevention is surely better than a pound of cure—particularly if there is no "cure" for the brain injured infant.

Since vaginal infection is a cause of premature labor, another issue is under study: the routine testing of all pregnant women for vaginal infections of any type (e.g.: bacterial; trichomonas, etc.). There is important debate among experts about the usefulness of testing all pregnant women for vaginal infections in order to help prevent premature delivery. A research study is being conducted to learn if routine testing is effective for all pregnant women or should be considered only for pregnant women with other risk factors of delivering prematurely.

For More Information

This *Research Fact Sheet* was prepared by the United Cerebral Palsy Research and Educational Foundation (UCP). To contact UCP call or write:

United Cerebral Palsy Research and Educational Foundation
1600 L Street, NW
Suite 700
Washington, DC 20036
1-800-USA-5UCP
(202) 776-0406
TDD (202) 973-7197
FAX (202) 776-0414

Chapter 40

Toxoplasmosis

Why Be Concerned about Toxoplasmosis?

Although up to 50 percent of the U.S. adult population has been infected with the parasite that causes toxoplasmosis, most people have no clue that their bodies are home to the parasite. However, for the baby of a woman who acquires the infection during pregnancy, the disease can cause stillbirth, neurologic problems, and blindness. And in immune-deficiency patients, the illness can be life-threatening.

The main sources of infection for people are cat feces and raw or poorly cooked meat. Without realizing it, people touch these materials and then carry the microscopic parasites from their hands to their mouths. Simple precautions can reduce the risk of contact during pregnancy:

- Avoid kitty-litter boxes (cat droppings also contaminate soil and sandboxes)

- Cook meat thoroughly

- Wash hands regularly, especially after touching raw meat

National Institute of Allergy and Infectious Diseases (NIAID), National Institutes of Health, Public Health Service, U.S. Department of Health and Human Services, July 1992.

Background

Toxoplasmosis is a parasitic disease that is found throughout the world. It is caused by a single-celled organism, a protozoan, called *Toxoplasma gondii*. This parasite was first discovered more than 80 years ago in a small African rodent, the gondi, from which it derives its name. It has since been found that any warm-blooded animal, and many reptiles, can be infected with the parasite.

Symptoms

In a newly acquired infection in otherwise healthy persons, the disease usually runs a mild, self-limited course, with few or no symptoms. Among people who do have signs of infection (about 10 percent of the cases), the symptoms resemble those of infectious mononucleosis, where patients typically experience swollen glands and fatigue. The other common symptoms are malaise, muscle pain, a fluctuating low fever, rash, headache, and sore throat. Eye inflammation, with blurred vision, occurs in about one percent of persons with acquired infection. In rare instances, the lungs, heart, brain, and liver may be affected.

Generally, the symptoms appear a week or two after infection and then subside gradually over a period of two weeks to several months. The parasite itself goes into a dormant state, although it never leaves the body.

The parasite, however, can become active again if the immune system is suppressed—for example, by drugs given to treat cancer or to prevent rejection of transplanted organs. Reactivated toxoplasmosis in patients with acquired immunodeficiency syndrome (AIDS) can be fatal.

Toxoplasmosis in Pregnancy and the Newborn

An estimated 10 to 20 percent of women of childbearing age in the United States have been infected with *T. gondii* and, therefore, harbor the organism in their bodies. If these women become pregnant, there is no threat to the fetus because the parasite is dormant in the mother's body. But if the woman contracts the parasite for the first time while she is pregnant, the fetus may also become infected. The disease can severely damage an unborn child while being mild or symptomless in the mother.

Toxoplasmosis

If a pregnant woman becomes infected during her first trimester of pregnancy, there is only a small chance that the fetus will become infected, but if it does, it is probable that the consequences to the fetus will be severe. Spontaneous abortion, stillbirth, or delivery of a premature or full-term infant with congenital disease may result.

Symptoms at Birth

Generalized illness or significant damage to the central nervous system and eyes is apparent at birth in about 30 percent of infants born with toxoplasmosis. Among the first symptoms apparent at birth are hydrocephalus (fluid in the skull) and neurologic symptoms such as convulsions and seizures.

The number of babies born with toxoplasmosis has not been determined. Some estimates are as high as one per 1,000 live births, while other studies indicate an infection rate of only one per 10,000.

Late-Developing Symptoms

In cases where a woman first becomes infected with *T. gondii* during her third trimester of pregnancy, the chances that the infant will be infected are greatly increased. Although such infants appear to be normal at birth, they may develop severe symptoms later in life, including blindness, epilepsy, and mental retardation. Increasingly, there are reports of eye damage that does not become evident until the person reaches adulthood or late maturity.

Diagnosis

The primary method for diagnosing toxoplasmosis is a blood test that detects *Toxoplasma* antibodies, proteins our bodies produce to defend against the parasite. A positive test result indicates only that the patient has been infected with the parasite at some point in the past. Determining whether it is a newly acquired infection—which is crucial if a woman is pregnant—may require a combination of tests that must be carefully interpreted. At present, researchers are working to make the tests more accurate.

Pre-Pregnancy Screening

Ideally, every woman who might become pregnant should undergo systematic toxoplasmosis screening—starting before she becomes pregnant. However, until more is known about the number of babies affected, the cost effectiveness of this approach is not clear. A woman who tests positive before pregnancy can be reasonably sure that she has already been exposed to the parasite, that she has developed protective antibodies, and that there is little, if any, risk to the fetus.

Testing During Pregnancy

In cases where a newly pregnant patient develops symptoms suggestive of toxoplasmosis, her doctor will start screening for potential infection as early as possible, beginning in the first trimester, with follow-up testing in the second and the third trimesters. If any of the tests comes out positive, the woman is retested three weeks later. Generally, a significant rise in antibody level in the second testing confirms the diagnosis of recently acquired infection.

Testing the Fetus

When the tests indicate that the fetus is at risk, the doctor may request a prenatal ultrasound examination to detect possible physical abnormalities in the fetus. In a new diagnostic technique, samples of amniotic fluid or umbilical blood, which are drawn through the uterine wall with a syringe, can be cultured to detect *Toxoplasma* antibodies. If fetal infection is confirmed, the patient and her doctor can discuss medical options.

Treatment

Most individuals with toxoplasmosis do not require treatment. However, pregnant women who acquire their infection during gestation, infected newborns, and immune-deficient patients with new or reactivated infection should undergo therapy. Of the women who become infected during pregnancy—and do not receive treatment—50 percent will give birth to infected infants.

The standard treatment in the United States is a combination of pyrimethamine (an antimalarial drug) with sulfadiazine or triple-sulfa drugs. The drugs kill the active form of the parasite but have no effect on the dormant stage. The need for treatment depends on the severity and duration of symptoms, evidence of serious damage to vital organs, any underlying medical problems, and whether or not the patient is pregnant. People taking these drugs must be monitored

Toxoplasmosis

regularly because the side effects can include toxicity due to bone marrow depression. Treatment with a drug called folinic acid is used in adults to reverse these effects.

In Pregnancy

Treatment of toxoplasmosis acquired during pregnancy decreases but does not eliminate the chance of a congenitally infected infant. Unfortunately, little can be done to reverse any damage already done to the fetus. In cases where the patient chooses to begin drug therapy, sulfa drugs alone are the treatment of choice because pyrimethamine can cause birth defects.

In the Newborn

If the mother has been diagnosed as having toxoplasmosis during pregnancy and has received treatment, the baby is usually begun on treatment at birth, whether the infection is symptomatic or not. The drugs are given for as long as a year, and if started early in infancy, can significantly reduce the chance of serious complications later in life. In infants born with severe toxoplasmosis, further damage may be prevented by adding corticosteroids to the pyrimethamine/sulfa drug regimen.

Transmission

Emptying kitty-litter boxes and handling raw meat without washing the hands immediately afterward are two of the most common ways people become infected. Unknowingly, people carry the parasites from their hands to their mouth and ingest them. Eating raw or undercooked meat is also risky. The parasites have been found in pork, mutton, and beef. In addition, infection may be transmitted through blood transfusions, organ transplants, and laboratory accidents.

Role of the Cat

Only cats are known to shed *Toxoplasma* organisms in their feces. This is why the common household cat plays a major role in human *Toxoplasma* infections.

Like other animals that harbor the toxoplasmosis parasite in their tissues and organs, the cat shows no sign of infection. If a cat eats infected birds or rodents, the parasites multiply within the cat's intestine. The cat excretes the parasites for 10 days or longer in the form of microscopic egg-like capsules known as oocysts. Generally, once a cat has been infected and has excreted oocysts, it will not shed oocysts if it becomes infected again. Thus, it can transmit the parasite only around the time of its first infection.

The oocysts mature two to four days after being expelled in cat feces. When mature, each oocyst contains infectious organisms known as sporozoites, which can remain infective for months in moist soil. Similarly, a litter box used by an infected cat is a significant reservoir of oocysts.

How People are Exposed

When a person accidentally ingests mature oocysts, the sporozoites are released in the intestine. The parasites penetrate the intestinal wall, spread throughout the body in the bloodstream, and multiply within the host's cells. Eventually, the body's immune defenses cause the parasite to transform into cysts, which usually remain dormant in the tissues for the rest of the person's life.

Transmission to the Fetus

If a woman is first exposed to the parasite during her pregnancy, the parasite can be transmitted to the fetus. The ingested parasite travels through the woman's intestinal tract, where it enters the bloodstream and reaches the fetus through the placenta.

Prevention

Fortunately, there are several preventive measures one can take to avoid toxoplasmosis. Naturally, many of these center around the cat.

- A cat can be maintained free of infection by feeding it only well-cooked meat or commercial cat food. It should also be kept indoors and not allowed to hunt mice and birds. These strict precautions are especially important if a woman is planning to become or is already pregnant. The pregnant woman should avoid close contact with the animal throughout her pregnancy.

    Testing the cat is not recommended because the results may be misleading. Positive results could mean that the cat has been infected, has shed oocysts, will probably not shed oocysts again, and is therefore not a threat to a pregnant woman. Negative results could mean that the cat was never infected, was so recently infected that antibodies have not yet appeared, or was infected in the past but for some reason did not develop antibodies.

- Someone other than the expectant mother should be responsible for regularly changing the kitty litter. This should be done daily, since excreted organisms are not infectious when passed but become infective within two to four days. The empty litter pan should be filled with boiling water and allowed to stand for a least five minutes. If the pregnant woman must change the litter, disposable gloves should be used and hands washed immediately afterward.

- Similar care should be taken when working in gardens that cats have access to. Hands should be kept away from the face and thoroughly washed when finished. Homegrown foods should also be thoroughly washed or cooked before being eaten.

- Children's sandboxes may be a prime source of contaminated cat feces. When not in use, keep the sandbox covered. If the sandbox does become contaminated with cat feces, discard all sand and replace it.

- Prevent flies and cockroaches from getting into food since these insects are capable of carrying infectious oocysts from cat feces to food.

- All meat should be well cooked—especially pork, mutton, and lamb, which should be cooked at 151°F (66°C) or higher.

- Finally, hands should be washed after touching uncooked meat.

Research

Much of what is known about the link between cats and toxoplasmosis derives from work supported by the National Institute of Allergy and Infectious Diseases (NIAID). NIAID continues to fund a broad spectrum of research on toxoplasmosis.

Improving Diagnostic Tests

The chemical make-up of the parasite is being analyzed, and methods of detecting very small amounts of these chemicals are being developed. The end result may be more sensitive and rapid tests for diagnosis of congenital and acquired toxoplasmosis.

Testing New Drugs

NIAID-supported scientists are developing better methods of treatment and prevention of *Toxoplasma* infections. Studies of the antibiotic spiramycin are being extended to test its effectiveness in congenital toxoplasmosis. Preliminary results suggest that highly specific monoclonal antibodies, made in the laboratory, may have a protective effect. Perhaps with further testing, these antibodies may one day be used to prevent human toxoplasmosis.

Finding Who Gets Toxoplasmosis

Other NIAID-supported research includes studies to ascertain whether certain people are at greater risk for the disease or if there is a genetic tendency to develop it. They are also studying children born with asymptomatic *Toxoplasma* infections, to see how many will develop complications later in life. To assess the need for widespread pre-pregnancy screening, the U.S. Public Health Service is currently doing studies to get a clearer estimate of the number of pregnancies affected by toxoplasmosis.

Investigating What Happens During Pregnancy

Other NIAID-supported scientists are studying various aspects of human toxoplasmosis. Of particular interest is the way the immune system responds to *Toxoplasma* during pregnancy. Scientists are investigating the relationship between the immune response, the transmission of the parasite to the fetus, and spontaneous abortion.

Understanding Immune-Deficiency Responses

NIAID grantees are studying *Toxoplasma* infections in persons whose immune systems are not working properly because of other medical problems. Specifically, the researchers are studying the signs of infection, how the deficient immune system responds, and better ways of diagnosing the infection, which is often fatal in immunosuppressed people.

Past and Present Goals of Biomedical Research

Earlier research solved the mysteries of what caused toxoplasmosis and how the parasite was transmitted. Current research holds the promise of finding more effective ways to diagnose and treat persons with this potentially handicapping, and sometimes fatal, disease.

Chapter 41

Cytomegalovirus Infection

People rarely hear about cytomegalovirus (CMV) because it seldom causes illness, even though it's very common. Most people become infected before they reach three years of age, and by the time they reach adulthood, up to 85% of the U.S. population may be infected. The immune system of a healthy person may not prevent CMV from infecting the body, but it normally does inactivate the virus and confine it to a dormant state throughout a person's life. If CMV is acquired for the first time later in a person's life, it can cause a brief mononucleosis-like illness. CMV's greatest threat is to immune-deficient patients and babies whose mothers are infected during early pregnancy.

Transmission

CMV is present in nearly all human body fluids, particularly urine, saliva, semen, breast milk, and blood. It is commonly transmitted in day-care centers, where the children and staff members come into contact with infected children's saliva or urine-soaked diapers. The virus then can be carried from unwashed hands or shared toys to the mucosal tissue of the mouth or nose. CMV also can be transmitted from one sexual partner to another. A woman can transmit the virus to her baby before it is born or at delivery, through contact with cervical fluids. In addition, it is possible to acquire CMV from transfused blood or transplanted organs.

National Institute of Allergy and Infectious Diseases (NIAID), October 1994.

In Immune-Deficient Patients

People undergoing organ transplantation or cancer chemotherapy must take drugs that suppress the immune system. Many of these patients had acquired CMV earlier in life, and their weakened immune system permits the previously dormant virus to reactivate, resulting in life-threatening illness. If people are exposed to CMV for the first time while they are taking immune-suppressant drugs, the virus can cause severe illness. Similarly, in patients with immune-deficiency diseases such as AIDS, CMV can cause pneumonia, hepatitis, encephalitis (brain inflammation), colitis, and a serious eye infection called retinitis.

Effects on Babies

CMV infection is of concern if a woman is in early pregnancy when she is first infected with the virus. Some of the babies born to these women may eventually develop minor impairments affecting hearing, vision, or mental capacity. A small percent of the babies are born with severe neurologic damage, including mental retardation or profound hearing loss. Prenatal tests of amniotic fluid can offer some evidence that fetal infection may have occurred.

CMV Mononucleosis

While CMV infection occurs uneventfully in most people, it can sometimes cause an acute form of mononucleosis. The symptoms include fever that lasts 2 to 3 weeks, hepatitis, and occasionally a rash. The doctor may do a blood test to see if the number of white blood cells is higher than normal. CMV mono is a self-limiting disease and, for people who do not have a serious immune deficiency, the prognosis is excellent.

Diagnosis

Because antibody levels vary from person to person, and also fluctuate in each individual, testing for CMV is difficult. The present antibody tests show only that a person has been infected at some point in life. Further clues as to how recently a person may have been infected can be obtained through follow-up tests, in which doctors can compare changes in antibody levels. Researchers are working to develop tests that will be more specific. The current tests are probably most useful for immune-deficient patients, for whom testing can provide a way of measuring the effectiveness of therapy.

Treatment

Two antiviral drugs, ganciclovir and foscarnet, now are available for treating CMV infection (such as retinitis) in immune-deficient patients. Such treatment is not recommended for people with healthy immune systems because the risk from disease is small compared with the side-effects of the drugs.

Prevention

Good hygienic practices such as handwashing, especially in day-care settings, can reduce the risk of transmission. However, intensive infection-control measures generally are not practical in dealing with a virus as common as CMV. A preventive vaccine is in early stages of development.

Chapter 42

Syphilis

Syphilis, once a cause of devastating epidemics, now can be effectively controlled with antibiotic therapy. Yet, in many cities of the United States both adult and congenital syphilis are on the rise. In 1990, about 134,000 cases were reported to the U.S. Public Health Service. Although treatment is available, the early symptoms of syphilis can be very mild, and many people do not seek treatment when they first become infected. Of increasing concern is the fact that a person with syphilis sores who has sex with someone infected with HIV (the virus that causes AIDS) is at high risk for developing HIV infection.

Syphilis is a sexually transmitted disease (STD) caused by a bacterium called *Treponema pallidum*. The bacterium can move throughout the body, damaging many organs over time. Medical experts describe the course of the disease by dividing it into four stages—primary, secondary, latent, and tertiary (late). An infected person who does not get treatment may infect others during the first two stages and during the early latent stage, which usually lasts 1 to 2 years. In its late stages, untreated syphilis, although not contagious, can cause serious heart abnormalities, mental disorders, blindness, other neurological problems, and death.

The bacterium spreads from the sores of an infected person to the mucous membranes of the genital area, the mouth, or the anus of a sexual partner. It also can pass through broken skin on other parts

National Institute of Allergy and Infectious Diseases (NIAID), NIH Pub. No. 95-9091, June 1992.

of the body. The syphilis bacterium is very fragile, and the infection is rarely, if ever, spread by contact with objects such as toilet seats or towels. A pregnant woman with syphilis can pass the bacterium to her unborn child, who may be born with serious mental and physical problems as a result of this infection.

The most common way to get syphilis is to have sex with someone who has an active infection. People at increased risk for syphilis, like those at high risk for other STDs, are those who have had multiple sex partners, have sexual relations with an infected partner, have a history of STDs, and do not use condoms (rubbers).

Symptoms

The first symptom of primary syphilis is a sore called a chancre ("shan-ker"). The chancre can appear within 10 days to 3 months after exposure, but it generally appears within 2 to 6 weeks. Because the chancre is ordinarily painless and sometimes occurs inside the body, it may go unnoticed. It is usually found on the part of the body exposed to the bacteria, such as the penis, the vulva, or the vagina. A chancre can also develop on the cervix, tongue, lips, or other parts of the body. The chancre disappears within a few weeks whether or not treatment is obtained. If not treated during the primary stage, the disease may progress through three other stages.

Secondary syphilis is marked by a skin rash that appears anywhere from 3 to 6 weeks after the chancre appears. The rash may cover the whole body or appear only in a few areas, such as the palms of the hands or soles of the feet. Because active bacteria are present in these sores, any physical contact—sexual or nonsexual—with the broken skin of an infected person may spread the infection at this stage. The rash usually heals within several weeks or months. Other symptoms may also occur, such as mild fever, fatigue, headache, sore throat, as well as patchy hair loss, and swollen lymph glands throughout the body. These symptoms may be very mild and, like the chancre of primary syphilis, will disappear without treatment. The signs of secondary syphilis may come and go over the next 1 to 2 years.

If untreated, syphilis then lapses into a latent stage during which the disease is no longer contagious and no symptoms are present. Many people who are not treated will suffer no further consequences of the disease. However, approximately one-third of those infected go on to develop the complications of late, or tertiary, syphilis, in which the bacteria damage the heart, eyes, brain, nervous system, bones, joints, or almost any other part of the body. This stage can last for years, or even for decades. Late syphilis, the final stage, can result in mental illness, blindness, other neurological problems, heart disease, and death.

Neurosyphilis

The syphilis bacterium frequently invades the nervous system during the early stages of infection, and approximately 3-7 percent of persons with untreated syphilis develop neurosyphilis. Some persons with neurosyphilis never develop any symptoms. Others may have headache, stiff neck, and fever that result from an inflammation of the lining of the brain. Some persons develop seizures. In those whose blood vessels are affected, symptoms of stroke can occur with resulting numbness, weakness, or visual complaints. In some instances, the time from infection to the development of neurosyphilis may be up to 20 years. Neurosyphilis may be more difficult to treat, and its course may be different, in people with HIV infection.

Diagnosis

Syphilis has sometimes been called "the great imitator" because its early symptoms are similar to those of many other diseases. People who have more than one sex partner should consult a doctor about any suspicious rash or sore in the genital area. Those who have been treated for another STD such as gonorrhea should be tested to be sure they have not also acquired syphilis.

There are three ways to diagnose syphilis: a doctor's recognition of its signs and symptoms, microscopic identification of syphilis bacteria, and blood tests. These approaches are usually used together to detect syphilis and decide upon the stage of infection.

To diagnose syphilis by identifying the bacteria, the doctor takes a specimen from a chancre and examines it under a special "darkfield" microscope to detect the organism itself. Blood tests also provide evidence of infection, although they may give false negative results (not show signs of infection despite its presence) for up to 3 months after infection. Interpretation of blood tests for syphilis can be difficult, and repeated tests are sometimes necessary to confirm the diagnosis.

The blood-screening tests most often used to detect evidence of syphilis are the VDRL (Venereal Disease Research Laboratory) test and the rapid plasma reagin (RPR) test. These tests can result in false-positive results (show signs of infection when it is not present) in people with autoimmune disorders, certain viral infections, and other conditions.

Confirmatory blood tests are, therefore, used when the initial test is positive. These tests include the fluorescent treponemal antibody-absorption (FTA-ABS) test that can accurately detect 70 to 90 percent of cases. Another specific test is the *T. pallidum* hemagglutination assay (TPHA). These tests detect syphilis antibodies (proteins made by a person's immune system to fight infection). They are not useful for diagnosing a new case of syphilis in patients who have had the disease previously, because once antibodies are formed, they remain in the body for many years. These antibodies do not, however, protect against a new syphilis infection. In some patients with syphilis (especially in the latent or late stages), a lumbar puncture (spinal tap) must be done to check for infection of the nervous system.

Treatment

Syphilis is usually treated with penicillin, administered by injection. Other antibiotics can be used for patients allergic to penicillin. A person usually can no longer transmit syphilis 24 hours after beginning therapy. However, some people do not respond to the usual doses of penicillin. Therefore, it is important that people being treated for syphilis have periodic blood tests to check that the infectious agent has been completely destroyed. Persons with neurosyphilis may need to be retested for up to 2 years after treatment. In all stages of syphilis, proper treatment will cure the disease, but in late syphilis, damage already done to body organs cannot be reversed.

Effects of Syphilis in Pregnant Women

It is likely that a pregnant woman with active syphilis who is not treated will pass the infection to her unborn child. About 25 percent of these pregnancies result in stillbirth or neonatal death. Between 40 and 70 percent of such pregnancies will yield a syphilitic infant.

Some infants with congenital syphilis may have symptoms at birth, but most develop symptoms between 2 weeks and 3 months later. These symptoms may include skin sores, rashes, fever, weakened or hoarse crying sounds, swollen liver and spleen, yellowish skin (jaundice), anemia, and various deformities. Care must be taken in handling an infant with congenital syphilis because the moist sores are infectious.

Syphilis

Often the symptoms of syphilis go undetected in infants. As infected infants become older children and teenagers, they may develop the symptoms of late-stage syphilis including damage to their bones, teeth, eyes, ears, and brain.

Prevention

The open sores of syphilis may be visible and infectious during the active stages of infection. Any contact with these infectious sores and other infected tissues and body fluids must be avoided to prevent spread of the disease. As with many other sexually transmitted diseases, methods of prevention include limiting the number of sex partners and use of condoms during sexual intercourse. Testing and treatment early in pregnancy is the best way to prevent syphilis in infants and should be a routine part of prenatal care.

Research

Developing better ways to diagnose and treat syphilis is an important research goal of scientists supported by the National Institute of Allergy and Infectious Diseases (NIAID). New tests are being developed that may provide better ways to diagnose syphilis and define the stage of infection.

Tissue culture systems are being used as models to determine how the syphilis bacterium infects tissues—whether it moves through or between cells. NIAID-supported scientists have found the syphilis organisms to be very mobile, able to slip through tight junctions between cells. Learning how the bacteria enter tissues may lead to effective ways to block that mechanism and limit the spread of syphilis in the body.

Scientists are also learning about the body's natural defenses against syphilis. Important disease-fighting cells called macrophages have the ability to engulf and destroy syphilis organisms. Scientists are exploring how this mechanism works in hopes of boosting the ability of these immune system cells to combat the bacterium.

In an effort to stem the spread of syphilis, vaccine research is under way. Molecular biologists are learning more about the various surface components of the syphilis bacterium that stimulate the immune system to respond to the invading organism. This knowledge will pave the way for development of an effective vaccine that can ultimately prevent this age-old sexually transmitted disease.

Part Seven

Research Initiatives

Chapter 43

Maternal Heat Exposure and Neural Tube Defects

Over a century ago, heat was found to be a teratogen in chickens.[1] Subsequently, many experimental studies using various mammalian species concluded uniformly that heat was teratogenic[2-8] and that the central nervous system was especially vulnerable. For the past two decades, many reports have emerged suggesting a teratogenic role for heat in humans, including not only fever,[9-15] but hot tub and sauna use.[10,16,17] Notwithstanding these reports, in 1978, *Lancet*[18] and *British Medical Journal*[19] editorialists and, later, Warkany[1] concluded that the evidence concerning hyperthermia as a teratogen in humans was still tenuous. Given these uncertainties, we aimed to assess the relationship between early pregnancy heat exposure and subsequent neural tube defects (NTDs) in a large cohort of pregnant women.

About This Study

Objective. To determine if exposure to hot tub, sauna, fever, or electric blanket during early pregnancy was associated with an increased risk for neural tube defects (NTDs).

Design. Prospective follow-up study.

Setting. Mostly private obstetric practices, primarily in New England.

From *JAMA*, August 19, 1992—Vol. 268, No. 7, pp. 882-85; copyright 1992 American Medical Association; reprinted with permission.

Participants. A cohort of 23,491 women having serum alpha-fetoprotein screening or an amniocentesis were identified. Complete exposure and outcome information was available for 97% of these women.

Outcome Measures. Relative risks (RRs) were used to compare incidence of NTD in those exposed to heat with those who were not exposed to any heat. Crude RRs were calculated directly from the data. Unconfounded RRs were calculated using logistic regression.

Results. Women reporting any heat exposure (sauna, hot tub, fever, or electric blanket) in early pregnancy had a crude risk of their fetuses developing NTD of 1.6 (95% CI [confidence interval], 0.9 to 2.9). Women reporting exposure to sauna, hot tub, or fever in early pregnancy had a crude risk of their fetuses developing NTD 2.2 times that of women without heat exposure (95% CI, 1.2 to 4.1). For hot tub use, the crude RR was 2.9 (95% CI, 1.4 to 6.3); for sauna, 2.6 (95% CI, 0.7 to 10.1); for fever, 1.9 (95% CI, 0.8 to 4.1); and for electric blanket, 1.2 (95% CI, 0.5 to 2.6). Multivariate adjusted RRs for individual heat sources, after controlling for maternal age, folic acid supplements, family history of NTD, and exposure to other heat sources, were for hot tub use, 2.8 (95% CI, 1.2 to 6.5); sauna, 1.8 (95% CI, 0.4 to 7.9); fever, 1.8 (95% CI, 0.8 to 4.1); and electric blanket, 1.2 (95% CI, 0.5 to 2.6). When only hot tub, sauna, and fever were considered and the women's exposure to each tallied, compared with no heat exposure, the RR for NTDs increased from 1.9 (95% CI, 0.9 to 3.7) after one type of heat exposure to 6.2 (95% CI, 2.2 to 17.2) after two types of heat exposure.

Conclusions. Exposure to heat in the form of hot tub, sauna, or fever in the first trimester of pregnancy was associated with an increased risk for NTDs. Hot tub exposure appeared to have the strongest effect of any single heat exposure. Exposure to electric blanket was not materially associated with increased risk for NTDs.

Methods

This study is part of a larger investigation of pregnancy outcomes in a cohort of women receiving prenatal care or an amniocentesis. The details of recruitment are described elsewhere.[20] In brief, pregnant women were identified through 100 participating obstetricians; 96%

of the pregnancies were between 15 and 20 weeks' gestation when identified. Thirty-three percent of the subjects lived in the Boston area, 48% elsewhere in Massachusetts, 5% elsewhere in New England, and 14% in states outside New England.

Trained nurse interviewers (with institutional review board approval) contacted the women by telephone and asked questions regarding family, medical, and genetic history. In addition, information about diet, medication, illness, and environmental exposures (including heat exposures), during the first trimester of pregnancy was obtained. Interviews were conducted with 23,491 individuals.

Heat Exposure Information

As part of the interview, each woman was asked, "During the first 2 months of pregnancy, did you use a sauna? Hot tub? Electric blanket?" In addition, each woman was asked, "During the first 3 months of pregnancy, did you have a fever ≥100°F?" Duration of pregnancy was defined by last menstrual period. Responses were classified as "yes" or "no" or "unknown."

Pregnancy Outcome Information

Overall pregnancy outcome information was obtained from completion of a brief questionnaire mailed to the delivering physician (76.5%) or directly to the women in the study (23.5%) if the physician failed to respond. The information requested included prenatal test results, presence of birth defects or chromosomal abnormalities, complications of pregnancy or delivery, complications in the newborn, and perinatal maternal illness. An NTD was defined as any occurrence of spina bifida, anencephaly, or encephalocele alone or in combination with other defects. Among NTD cases, 86% of the outcome information was obtained from physicians and 14% was obtained from mothers (not specifically verified). All cases of prenatally diagnosed NTDs, stillbirths, and live births were included in this study.

Data Analysis

For crude analyses, risks and relative risks (RRs) were calculated directly from the data; we used test-based approximate confidence limits.[21] To control confounding, we fit a multiple logistic regression model and estimated RR from the odds ratio (OR), which approximates the risk ratio when risks are small, as they are for NTDs. Information about diagnosis of NTDs, exposure to sauna, hot tub, fever, electric blanket, folic acid supplements, and family history of NTDs was dichotomous ("yes" or "no"), and each variable was entered into the model as a single term. We divided maternal age into three categories (less than 25, 25 to 35, and more than 35 years) and represented age in the logistic model with two indicator terms. Information that was "unknown" was treated as missing data and excluded from analyses.

Results

We excluded one subject from the cohort of 23,491 women interviewed because of missing heat exposure information. An additional 736 women were excluded because of missing outcome information.

A total of 5,566 women were exposed to at least one heat source. There were 1,254 women exposed to hot tub (hot tub exposure was unknown for 55 women), 367 exposed to sauna (unknown for 35 women), 1,865 who had a fever (unknown for 128 women), and 2,883 women exposed to electric blanket (unknown for 61 women). There were 17,188 women who were not exposed to any of these heat sources.

A total of 49 pregnancies ended with an NTD. These cases included 23 outcomes of spina bifida alone, one case of spina bifida with cleft lip and palate, three cases of spina bifida with chromosome abnormalities (a triploid partial mole, a trisomy 13, and a balanced translocation in an infant whose parents had normal karyotypes), two cases of spina bifida with multiple defects (one infant had ventricular septal defect, the other had multiple defects and a short umbilical cord), one case of iniencephaly with rachischisis, three cases of encephalocele, 15 cases of anencephaly, and one case of anencephaly with encephalocele and rachischisis. Numbers were too small to stratify data by type of defect.

The RR between any heat exposure (sauna, hot tub, electric blanket, and fever) and NTD was 1.6 (95% CI, 0.9 to 2.9).

When the electric blanket was excluded as a potential heat source, the RR was 2.2 (95% CI, 1.2 to 4.1). We also evaluated the heat sources individually and obtained the following results:

- hot tub use, RR, 2.9 (95% CI, 1.4 to 6.3)
- sauna use, RR, 2.6 (95% CI, 0.7 to 10.1)
- fever of ≥100°F (37°C), RR, 1.9 (95% CI, 0.8 to 4.1)
- electric blanket use, RR, 1.2 (95% CI, 0.5 to 2.6)

Maternal Heat Exposure and Neural Tube Defects

We used logistic regression to control for the age of the mother (less than 25, 25 to 35, and more than 35 years), folic acid supplementation taken within the first 6 weeks of pregnancy, family history of NTD, and exposure to more than one study heat source. The multivariate adjusted RRs for exposure to hot tub, sauna, or fever combined was 2.2 (95% CI, 1.2 to 4.2). The multivariate adjusted RRs for the individual heat sources were as follows:

- hot tub, RR, 2.8 (95% CI, 1.2 to 6.5)
- sauna, RR, 1.8 (95% CI, 0.4 to 7.9)
- fever, RR, 1.8 (95% CI, 0.8 to 4.1)
- electric blanket, RR, 1.2 (95% CI, 0.5 to 2.6)

Duration or frequency of exposure to heat was not available from the interview data. We were, however, able to use the number of different types of heat exposures as a proxy for exposure frequency. We first excluded electric blanket as a heat source at this point in the analysis after observing no increased RR. We grouped sauna, hot tub, and fever and tallied the subjects' exposure to zero of three, one of three, two of three, or all three of these heat sources. Compared with those with no heat exposure, the RR for NTD increased from 1.9 (95% CI, 0.9 to 3.7) when subjects were exposed to one heat source to 6.2 (95% CI, 2.2 to 17.2) when exposed to two of the three heat sources. Only 22 women were exposed to three heat sources, too few for evaluation.

Comment

The data presented are especially noteworthy since they were drawn from a large, prospective, broad-based study of the antecedents to congenital defects and pregnancy complications. At the time of the interview, 66% of the women whose pregnancy ended in NTD knew the results of their amniocentesis. Among the subjects who knew their amniocentesis results, the RR for any heat exposure was 2.3 (95% CI, 0.8 to 5.7). Among subjects who did not know the results, the RR was 2.0 (95% CI, 0.4 to 7.3). Therefore, recall bias is not a likely explanation for the increased risk found in women exposed to heat. However, we considered the possibility of follow-up bias as an explanation for the findings. Since the physicians did not know the mothers' responses to the questionnaire, follow-up bias was only a possibility for the mothers themselves. We therefore analyzed the subset of the data pertaining to those women whose follow-up information came from a physician. All the associations with heat exposure among this subgroup were stronger than those found in the entire cohort, with the exception of the association with hot tubs, for which the RR was 2.5 (95% CI, 0.9 to 6.1). Although this RR was numerically different from the overall RR of 2.9 from physician-derived information, it is not substantively different, and certainly insufficient to influence any conclusion. This difference is much more likely to reflect sampling variability rather than any important bias in follow-up.

We found a stronger relation between hot tub use and NTD than for sauna use. Perhaps immersion in hot water raises the core temperature to higher levels for a longer period of time than the sauna, in which perspiration and cooling through evaporation are less efficient at reaching the same body temperature for as long a period. The smaller association for fever may reflect the nature of the question about fever, which referred to the first 3 months of pregnancy. Clearly, fever during the third month of gestation would have no effect on neural tube closure occurring within 6 weeks (menstrual dates) of conception (4 weeks, fetal age). The resulting misclassification would lead to an underestimate of any fever effect.

Heat has been found to be teratogenic in all mammalian species studied, including chickens,[22] rats,[2] mice,[23] guinea pigs,[5] hamsters,[5] rabbits,[24] sheep,[4] monkeys,[7] and pigs.[3] It is reasonable to infer that heat is also teratogenic in humans, a conclusion reinforced by our data and largely supported by earlier, though frequently uncontrolled, studies.[9-17]

In 1984 in Ontario, Canada, Hunter[25] did a retrospective study of families who had had a child with an NTD from 1969 through 1981, using both records and patient contact. Thirty-two of 264 reported fever during pregnancy. Thirteen of these 32 had fever during the first 4 weeks and nine of these 13 ended with anencephaly. Interestingly, 10% of pregnancies resulting in anencephaly were associated with fever vs. 1.7% for spina bifida.

In 1978, Smith et al.[9] reported 11% (7/63) of pregnancies with anencephalic fetuses had associated maternal fever of ≥102°F (38.9°C to 40°C) at the presumed time of neural tube closure. Two of these exposures also included sauna bathing. Sauna was discounted as a cause of NTDs, given its frequent use in Finland,[25,27] where the frequency of NTD is about the lowest anywhere. Apparently, Finnish women have an average duration of sauna use between 6 to 12 minutes.[28] Moreover, women in Finland shorten their time in the sauna during pregnancy.[27] Prolonged sauna use may, however, be teratogenic.[2]

Maternal Heat Exposure and Neural Tube Defects

In 1981, Fisher and Smith[13] reported maternal fever in four of 17 offspring with occipital encephalocele. Overall, combined retrospective studies[10,12,13] included 170 cases of anencephaly, meningomyelocele, and posterior occipital encephalocele. A history of heat exposure during the week of neural tube closure (21 to 28 days, fetal age), averaged 10% compared with none in a control group of friends and relatives.

In 1980, Layde et al.[11] in another retrospective study, noted fever in the first trimester among 13.5% (19/141) of pregnancies ending with spina bifida. However, Kleinebrecht et al.[29] in Germany noted *no* association of any congenital defects with fever in 7,870 pregnancies, including 38 with NTDs.

The possible mechanism by which heat exposure may interfere with the cells involved in neural tube closure is unknown. Intracellular damage, inhibition of mitosis and hence cell proliferation and migration, or cell death may all occur following heat injury. Heat causing cell death in the early rat embryo may result in anencephaly.[8] Cell damage within minutes and cell death within hours after heating may occur in guinea pig embryos.[30,31] Other mechanisms of cell injury due to heat may involve microvascular lesions (as in the chick embryo),[22] placental necrosis (rats),[32] and placental infarction (monkeys).[7] Heat may also interfere with genetically programmed activation and inactivation of cells.[33]

The intensity, duration, and frequency of heat exposure necessary for teratogenicity is unknown. Edwards[8] found from his own studies and literature review that the lowest temperature with an adverse effect in animals was 1.5°C above the core temperature, which for humans would approximate 38.9°C. Edwards[8] emphasized that for other mammalian species it remains uncertain whether the absolute temperature reached or the speed of temperature elevation is most important to reach a teratogenic threshold. Prolonged hyperthermic episodes or multiple temperature spikes were more teratogenic at lower temperature elevations than a single spike.[8] Possibly, body temperatures reach higher levels and remain higher for a longer time from hot tub use than from sauna use. Electric blanket use is highly unlikely to raise core temperatures as easily or as high as hot tubs, skin discomfort or burning occurring in all likelihood before a rise in the core temperature occurs.

Harvey et al.[28] recorded vaginal temperatures of 20 nonpregnant women while in hot tubs set at 39.0°C or 41.1°C and in the sauna with an average temperature of 81.4°C. Five women remained in the 39°C hot tub and six in the 41.1°C tub until their temperature reached 38.9°C. It took at least 15 minutes in the 39°C tub and 10 minutes in the 41.1°C tub to reach 38.9°C. The rest left the tub because of discomfort, even though their temperatures were lower than 38.9°C. None of the 20 women were able to remain in the sauna long enough for temperatures to reach 38.9°C.

Pleet et al.[14] reviewed the central nervous system defects and facial dysmorphia following heat exposure in 24 individuals. The most frequent neurologic abnormalities were neuronal heterotopias, mental retardation, hypotonia, and microphthalmia. Other claims implicating heat exposure in the first trimester and yet to be substantiated have included Hirschsprung's disease,[34] microphthalmia,[14,35,36] oromandibular and limb defects,[37] hypospadias and cardiac defects,[33] holoprosencephaly,[15] and Möbius syndrome.[38] Our database contains too few of these other outcomes to provide useful conclusions.

It is not possible to control for all confounding variables in this type of study. For example, the role of infection rather than height or duration of temperature could not be assessed. It is also impossible to determine from this study at which temperatures (eg, >100°F [37.8°C] or >102°F [38.9°C]) or with which type of infection an effect on neural tube closure occurred. Clearly, heat exposure or infection after the first 6 menstrual weeks of pregnancy would have no effect on neural tube closure. While extremely unlikely, we could not exclude the possibility that certain women's health behavior (which may include hot tub use) is the marker for some unknown association with an increased RR for NTDs.

Our findings reveal an increased risk for NTDs among offspring of women exposed to heat in the form of hot tub, sauna, or fever during early pregnancy. Exposure to electric blanket was not materially associated with increased risk for NTDs. Hot tub exposure had the strongest effect, while exposure to multiple heat sources led to an even greater risk. More confirmatory studies are needed to evaluate the effects of timing, frequency, intensity, and duration of heat exposure on the risk for NTD to support any clinical recommendations.

This study was supported by U.S. Public Health Service grant NS 19561 from the National Institute of Neurological Disorders and Stroke.

We acknowledge with great appreciation the sterling work of the interviewing team and especially that of Carol Bruell, MS, Marsha Thomas Lanes, MS, Brenda Flomenhaft, MS, Shirley Kasten, Maryanne Megliola, RN, and Nancy Powell, BSN. We are also very indebted to the many obstetricians and their staff members for allowing us to study their patients and for providing outcome data and to the many patients who so graciously participated in this study.

—by Aubrey Milunsky, MBBCh, DSc, FRCP, DCH; Marianne Ulcickas, MPH; Kenneth J. Rothman, DrPH; Walter Willett, MD; Susan S. Jick, MPH; and Hershel Jick, MD

From the Center for Human Genetics and the Department of Pediatrics (Dr. Milunsky), the Boston Collaborative Drug Surveillance Program (Ms. Ulcickas, Ms. Jick, and Dr. Jick), and the Department of Medicine and Epidemiology (Dr. Rothman), Boston (Mass) University School of Medicine; and the Departments of Epidemiology and Nutrition, Harvard School of Public Health, Channing Laboratory, Harvard Medical School, and the Brigham and Women's Hospital, Boston (Dr. Willett).

References

1. Warkany J. Teratogen update: hyperthermia. *Teratology* 1986; 33:365-371.

2. Cockcroft DL. New DAT: abnormalities induced in cultured rat embryos by hyperthermia. *Teratology* 1978;17:277-283.

3. Umpierre CC, Dukelow WR. Environmental heat stress in the hamster. *Teratology* 1978;16:155-158.

4. Hartley WJ, Alexander G, Edwards MJ. Brain cavitation and micrencephaly in lambs exposed to prenatal hyperthermia. *Teratology* 1974;9:299-303.

5. Kilham L, Ferm VH. Exencephaly in fetal hamsters following exposure to hyperthermia. *Teratology* 1976;14:323-326.

6. Edwards MJ. Congenital defects in guinea-pigs following induced hyperthermia during gestation. *Arch Pathol Lab Med* 1967;84:42-48.

7. Hendrickx AG, Stone GW, Hendrickson RV, Matayoshi K. Teratogenic effects of hyperthermia in the bonnet monkey (*Macaca radiata*). *Teratology* 1979,19:177-182.

8. Edwards MJ. Hyperthermia as a teratogen: a review of experimental studies and their clinical significance. *Teratogenesis Carcinog Mutagen* 1986;6:563-582.

9. Smith DW, Clarren SK, Harvey MAS. Hyperthermia as a possible teratogenic agent. *J Pediatrics* 1978;92:878-883.

10. Miller P, Smith DW, Shepard TH. Maternal hyperthermia as a possible cause of anencephaly. *Lancet* 1978;1:519-21.

11. Layde PM, Edmonds LD, Erickson JD. Maternal fever and neural tube defects. *Teratology* 1980;21:105-108.

12. Chance PF, Smith DW. Hyperthermia and meningomyelocele and anencephaly. *Lancet* 1978;1:769-770.

13. Fisher NL, Smith DW. Occipital encephalocele and early gestational hyperthermia. *Pediatrics* 1981;68:480-483.

14. Pleet H, Graham JM, Smith DW. Central nervous system and facial defects associated with maternal hyperthermia, at four to 14 weeks' gestation. *Pediatrics* 1981;67:785-789.

15. Shiota K. Neural tube defects and maternal hyperthermia in early pregnancy: epidemiology in a human embryo population. *Am J Med Genet* 1982;12 281-288.

16. Edwards MJ. Influenza, hyperthermia and congenial malformations. *Lancet* 1972;1:320-321.

17. Saxen L, Holmberg PC, Nurminen M, Kuosma E. Sauna and congenital defects. *Teratology* 1982;26:309-313.

18. Hyperthermia and the neural tube. *Lancet* 1978;2:560-561. Editorial.

19. Is hyperthermia a teratogen? *BMJ* 1978;2:1586-1587. Editorial.

20. Milunsky A, Jick H, Jick SS, et al. Multivitamin/folic acid supplementation in early pregnancy reduces the prevalence of neural tube defects. *JAMA* 1989;262:2847-2852.

21. Miettinen OS. Estimability and estimation in case-referent studies. *Am J Epidemiol* 1976;103:226-235.

22. Nilsen NO. Vascular abnormalities due to hyperthermia in chick embryos. *Teratology* 1984;30:237-251.

23. Webster WS, Edwards MJ. Hyperthermia and the induction of neural tube defects in mice. *Teratology* 1984;29:417-425.

24. Brinsmade AB, Rübsaamen H. Zur teratogenetisehen Wirkung von unspezifischem Fieber auf den sich entwickelnden Kaninchenembryo. *Beitr Pathol Anat* 1957;117:154-164.

25. Hunter AGW. Neural tube defects in eastern Ontario and western Quebec: demography and family data. *Am J Med Genet* 1984;19:45-63.

26. Sohar E, Shoenfeld Y, Shapiro Y, Ohry A, Cabili S. Effects of exposure to Finnish sauna. *Isr J Med Sci* 1976;12:1275-1282.

27. Uhari M, Mustonen A, Kouvalainen K. Sauna habits of Finnish women during pregnancy. *BMJ* 1979;1:1216.

28. Harvey MAS, McRorie MM, Smith DW. Suggested limits to the use of the hot tub and sauna by pregnant women. *Can Med Assoc J* 1981;125:50-53.

29. Kleinebrecht J, Michaelis H, Michaelis J, Koller S. Fever in pregnancy and congenital anomalies. *Lancet* 1979;1:1403.

30. Edwards MJ, Mulley R, Ring S, Wanner RA. Mitotic cell death and delay of mitotic activity in guinea-pig embryos following brief maternal hyperthermia. *J Embryol Exp Morphol* 1974;32:593-602.

31. Wanner RA, Edwards MJ, Wright RG. The effect of hyperthermia on the neuroepithelium of the 21-day guinea-pig foetus: histological and ultrastructural study. *J Pathol* 1976,118:235-244.

32. Arora KL, Cohen BJ, Beaudoin AR. Fetal and placental responses to artificially induced hyperthermia in rats. *Teratology* 1979;19:251-260.

33. German J. Embryonic stress hypothesis of teratogenesis. *Am J Med* 1984;76:293-301.

34. Lipson A. Hirschsprung disease in the offspring of mothers exposed to hyperthermia during pregnancy. *Am J Med Genet* 1988;29:117-124.

35. Fraser FC, Skelton J. Possible teratogenicity of maternal fever. *Lancet* 1978;2:634.

36. Spragget K, Fraser FC. Teratogenicity of maternal fever in women—a retrospective study. *Teratology* 1982;25:78A.

37. Superneau DW, Wertelecki W. Brief clinical report: similarity of effects—experimental hyperthermia as a teratogen and maternal febrile illness associated with oromandibular and limb defects. *Am J Med Genet* 1985;21:575-580.

38. Graham JM, Edwards MJ, Lipson AH, Webster WS. Gestational hyperthermia as a cause for Moebius syndrome. *Teratology* 1988,37:461-462.

Chapter 44

Investigating Prenatal Causes of Mental Retardation and Developmental Disabilities

Fetal Protein Malnutrition

The Mental Retardation and Developmental Disabilities (MRDD) Branch is currently supporting a program project that evaluates the behavioral, neurophysiologic, immunocytochemical, and neuroanatomical consequences of mild to moderate protein malnutrition in a rat model. The animals receive a 6% protein diet during the prenatal period, resulting in adequate physical growth but impaired brain function, and a 25% diet on which maximal physical and brain growth occurs. The animal model has the advantage over the human because of the ability to control potentially confounding variables which often co-exist with the human condition, and also because of the possibility of performing interdisciplinary research on various components of brain function. This research is being undertaken with an emphasis on a major brain model system, the hippocampal formation, which is known to play a role in learning and memory processing.

There is selective vulnerability on behavioral tasks in prenatal malnutrition, in contrast to the overwhelming effects in the neurophysiology, neurochemistry, and neuroanatomy of the hippocampal formation. For example, prenatally malnourished rats have greater difficulty giving up a previously learned response under a new set of

From *The Mental Retardation and Developmental Disabilities Branch Report to Council*, January 1993, National Institute of Child Health and Human Development (NICHD).

conditions. This inflexibility is maladaptive and may well relate to the human condition. When challenged with drugs that are known to block certain brain receptors, striking deficits were observed in prenatally malnourished rats on a standard test of hippocampal function (e.g., water maze) which otherwise revealed no such deficits. Thus, these findings suggest that "compensatory responses" to prenatal malnutrition can be "uncovered" by additional challenge to the CNS.

The main findings in the Neurophysiology Division are that prenatal protein malnutrition:

1. results in pathological inhibition in the hippocampal formation resulting in a faulty gating of information inflow to the hippocampus

2. retards the development of hippocampal theta rhythm

3. affects the ability of the animal to respond to neuroplastic events

This means that information inflow to the hippocampus is perturbed resulting in deficits in information processing in a brain structure associated with learning and memory. The significance of this is that long-term deficits in learning and memory appear to be due to these altered gating mechanisms, i.e., the hippocampus formation cannot take in and process information.

The Immunocytochemistry Division has examined a number of different neurotransmitter systems in the hippocampal formation of prenatally malnourished rats. A 20% decrease was found in the serotonin fiber plexus innervating the hippocampal formation as well as a decrease in the serotonin uptake sites. Similarly, a 25-30% decrease in the cholinergic M2 receptors was observed. In contrast, a 25-30% increase in the tensity of the kainate receptors for excitatory amino acids and a 20% increase in the benzodiazepine receptors were observed. These alterations in neurotransmitter-specific neurons and/or receptors occur early in development and continue throughout the postnatal period despite dietary rehabilitation. These data suggest changes in the basic neurobiological organization of the hippocampal formation that may underlie the alterations in learning, memory and attention that occur in prenatally malnourished rats.

Neuroanatomic studies demonstrate convincingly that the effects of prenatal malnutrition on the individual neurons are almost identical to changes following chronic malnutrition, suggesting that the "critical" period for their postnatal development in the rat is during gestation.

Effect of Prenatal and Postnatal Lead Exposure on Intellectual Development

The MRDD Branch has been supporting a longitudinal study of a regional sample of children with varying degrees of exposure to environmental lead. The children were evaluated with developmental tests and intelligence tests at 6, 12, 18, 24, and 57 months, and again at the time of their 10th birthday. Infants were originally recruited for follow-up if the lead blood level from the umbilical cord fell in one of three groups: below the 10th percentile of all babies born in a university-affiliated hospital in a northeastern city, i.e., <3 micrograms per deciliter (µg/dL); approximately the 50th percentile (6.5 µg/dL); or above the 90th percentile (≥10 µg/dL). Postnatal exposure was assessed by blood levels and, for some children, dentine lead levels in shed deciduous teeth. Overall, the sample consisted of children from white, intact families with college-educated parents and relatively well functioning children with low lifetime exposures to lead (mean— between 6.3 and 7.8 µg/dL blood levels on all postnatal tests between 6 and 57 months). At 10 years the average was 2.9 µg/dL, with a standard deviation of 2.4 (range 0.5-16).

Higher prenatal lead levels were associated with depressed performance on early infant tests, but this effect was attenuated over time; at 57 months there was no significant association between prenatal lead and cognitive development, as tested by the McCarthy Scale. However, higher levels of lead in the blood at age two were related to poorer scores on the McCarthy test at 57 months. At age 10, 88% of the children who were seen at 57 months were assessed with the Wechsler Intelligence Scale (WISC-R) and a standardized achievement test. The 10-year test scores averaged approximately one standard deviation above the population mean. Nevertheless, higher levels of blood lead at age 24 months (but not blood levels at other ages) were significantly associated with lower IQ and achievement test scores, even after adjustment for potential confounding variables. Over the range of about 0 to 25 µg/dL, an increase of 10 µg/dL in blood level at 24 months was associated with a 5.8 point decline (>1/3 standard deviation) in IQ score, and an 8.9 point decline (>1/2 standard deviation) in achievement test score.

Mechanisms of Ischemic/Anoxic Brain Damage

The developing brain is particularly sensitive to ischemic or anoxic insults. Brief insufficiencies can trigger a cascade of biochemical events leading to irreversible brain damage which results in mental retardation and other developmental delays. Although ischemia and anoxia can result from several diverse causes, the resultant pathophysiology seems to center on calcium overload and overstimulation of excitatory amino acid (EAA) pathways, particularly those involving the NMDA (N-methyl-D-aspartate) subtype of glutamate receptors. Research into the prevention of ischemic/anoxic brain damage has focused on calcium homeostasis, early excitatory pathways, and the pharmacology of excitatory receptors.

One project funded by the MRDD Branch provided evidence that in the early brain, the excitatory amino acid, glutamate, is directly responsible for anoxic/ischemic pathophysiology. Two embryonic systems, chicken retina cultures and 10 day old rat pups, were used in order to assess the effects of pharmacological agents in the prevention of ischemic/hypoxic damage. Most of the existing animal models were not adequate, because they do not address the mechanisms that may predominate at these early stages. Initial studies demonstrated that the histopathology resulting from ischemic insult resembles that seen with exogenous administration of glutamate. Pretreatment with the MK-801, an antagonist of the NMDA receptor, prevented most of the pathology. Moreover, this protection was uniform across all the affected brain regions, suggesting that in the developing brain most, if not all, of the histopathology induced by ischemic/hypoxic conditions is mediated through the action of endogenous glutamate at NMDA receptors. This is in contrast to adult brain, which is less sensitive to the toxic action of glutamate.

Another project is aimed at developing clinically safe NMDA antagonists for the treatment of ischemia and hypoxia. Using the rat pup model, two NMDA compounds are being evaluated for their ability to prevent neurotoxicity in ischemic animals. Related studies will be performed in cultures of human CNS neurons. They are also examining the possibility that nitric oxide modifies the function of NMDA receptors.

Other studies have focused on the role of glycosphingolipids in cellular processes that lead to neural damage. In some pathways, glycolipids serve as "second messengers," initiating a cascade of cellular events. In cultured oligodendrocytes (cells that normally produce myelin in the brain), hypoxic conditions depress the synthesis of glycosphingolipids, which then reduces organellar movement, as well as altering the phosphorylation of key myelin proteins. There is also evidence that glycosphingolipids play a role in calcium homeostasis through the regulation of ion channels. Current studies are aimed at determining whether the glycolipids have any role in the regulation of excitatory neurotransmitter receptors.

AIDS

In the next few years, HIV will become the largest infectious cause of mental retardation and developmental disabilities in children. The majority of children with HIV show intellectual impairment manifested in deceleration of development; loss of previous developmental achievements or failure to acquire new ones; deterioration in school performance and on tests of intelligence; language delay, attention deficit hyperactivity disorder; and, social incompetence requiring specialized supportive living. The MRDD Branch is currently supporting research on the neuropathology of HIV infection in brain, and its effect on neuronal development.

One study involves a neuroanatomical investigation of the effect of HIV infection on a developing brain, focusing on CNS atrophy and microcephaly. This is complicated by the dynamic nature of the developing infant brain, and the difficulty of obtaining suitable autopsy material. In a study of AIDS and age-matched control brains, careful measurement of 28 brain structures indicate that the volume and surface area of all major brain regions (except the ventricles) are reduced in pediatric AIDS. Along the fronto-occipital axis, the reduction in volume is more pronounced toward the occipital pole. Current studies are examining the pattern of neuropathological lesions, and attempting to determine which cell populations are most affected in pediatric AIDS. This will provide an anatomical basis for understanding the clinical progression of HIV encephalopathy in pediatric AIDS.

Another study, which is part of a larger program project on neuronal growth and calcium-dependent phenomena, will focus on the mechanism of HIV neurotoxicity in the CNS in order to develop clinical strategies for blocking this damage. Previous studies have shown that picomolar amounts of the HIV coat protein gp120 are toxic to CNS neurons in culture. It appears to involve calcium-mediated mechanisms similar to those acting through NMDA receptors to trigger the neuronal damage associated with stroke, trauma, and other neurodegenerative diseases. This suggests that the administration of NMDA antagonists might delay HIV toxicity. In these studies, various NMDA antagonists will be tested on HIV-exposed neurons in culture, then in HIV-infected rat pups. Indirect mechanisms of neurotoxicity involving monocytes, macrophages, and oligodendrocytes will also be examined using cultured cells.

Chapter 45

Assessment of Outcomes Following Neonatal Asphyxia

Stedman's medical dictionary[16] defines asphyxia as "1) Unconsciousness due to suffocation or interference of any kind with oxygenation of the blood. 2) Absence of the pulse beat. 3) Cyanosis, local or general, through interference with the circulation." Because we are especially interested in perinatal asphyxia, consider the definition of Snyder and Cloherty,[17] "Perinatal asphyxia is an insult to the fetus or the newborn due to lack of oxygen (hypoxia) and/or lack of perfusion (ischemia) to various organs."

Because of the problems posed by multiple different definitions, some investigators have replaced the definition of asphyxia with correlates of asphyxia including:

- Meconium passage *in utero*;
- Fetal heart (tocographic) monitoring abnormalities;
- Low pH values of scalp or umbilical cord blood;
- Low Apgar scores at either 1 or 5 minutes; and
- Low biophysical profile scores.

Problems with these correlates of *fetal distress* have been identified by others.[18,19] For example, in the Collaborative Perinatal Project, expulsion of meconium during labor occurred in 18 percent of babies.[20] Are we to assume that 18 percent of babies are asphyxiated?

From *Report of the Workshop on Acute Perinatal Asphyxia in Term Infants*, National Institute of Child Health and Human Development (NICHD), NIH Pub. No. 96-3823, March 1996.

A committee opinion published by the American College of Obstetricians and Gynecologists included the following: "Intrapartum asphyxia implies fetal hypercarbia and hypoxemia, which, if prolonged, will result in metabolic acidemia. Because the intrapartum disruption of uterine or fetal blood flow is rarely, if ever, absolute, *asphyxia* is an imprecise, general term. Terms such as *hypercarbia, hypoxia, metabolic acidemia,* and *respiratory or lactic acidemia* are more precise."[21] Indeed, recently published articles have addressed the neonatal and later characteristics of babies with neonatal acidemia.[22-27]

Although the level of acidemia required for a definition of asphyxia varies the pH cut off for defining *pathologic fetal acidemia* appears to be closer to 7.0 than to 7.2.[22-25] The value of cardiac dysfunction[28] and biophysical profile[29,30] are also gaining greater acceptance as indicators/predictors of early neonatal well being.

The limitations of arterial blood gas assessments[31] have directed attention away from peripheral blood to measures and correlates of intracranial energy metabolism. This has prompted some to emphasize the brain when seeking early expressions of the presumed adverse developmental effects of asphyxia, including:

- Expressions of damage to brain, especially MRI abnormalities;[6,14]
- Newborn encephalopathy;[19]
- Impaired cerebral blood flow regulation;[32,33] and
- Near infrared spectrographic documentation of energy metabolism disorders.[34,35]

Criteria for Outcomes

The criteria for selecting appropriate outcome measures for a given situation generally require that the outcomes be linked to anatomical/physiologic derangement, or be derived from another theoretical framework. The importance of a well specified theoretical model lies not only in the ability to strengthen understanding of the pathogenesis and potential prevention of adverse outcome, but also to anticipate potential confounders, i.e., factors that may contribute to or even account for the observed outcomes other than the event of interest. The lack of a well articulated model incurs the risk of using available, not necessarily appropriate, outcome measures, and failing to ascertain or control for important correlates of outcome.

The criteria for defining asphyxia have already been noted. Most of these criteria can be characterized as clinical markers of generalized physiologic derangement but not specific anatomic damage or alteration in function. Much of the information in potential anatomic and functional impact of this derangement is derived from animal studies and postmortem examination of humans, neither providing a sound basis for predicting specific later morbidity in surviving children. Thus, the selection of outcome measures has been driven largely by what is available. However, even in applying available measures, investigators have often failed to consider the theoretical context of some outcome measures in their interpretation and selection of covariates.

General Selection Criterion Validity and Reliability

Valid measures are an expression of the concept or construct intended to be measured. An often tacit assumption is that the concept or construct being measured has been adequately specified and the factors influencing the measure are known. For example, not only does the concept of health include indicators of well-being or illness, but also influences on health such as poverty and the consequences of poor health such as death, disability and the need for health services. Establishing validity is complex and may involve examination of the content of measures, comparisons with previously established measures (sensitivity/ specificity is a subset of this type of validity testing), and repeated use under a variety of conditions.

Reliability refers to the ability of a given measure to provide the same response on repeated observations. Intrarater reliability assesses the extent to which repeated observations on the same individual by the same observer yield the same response. Interrater reliability reflects the ability of different observers to obtain similar responses.

We have already argued that the concept or construct of neonatal asphyxia still lacks specification and agreement. That, in and of itself, does not preclude selecting outcome measures of potential relevance. In doing so, however, it is essential that attention be paid to the conceptual basis of the outcome measure.

Specific Outcome Measures and Concerns

Mortality. Mortality tends to be validly and reliably measured. Attribution of mortality to asphyxia, however, requires elimination of other causes of death. Obvious major malformations of known natural history represent a straightforward case. Less clear are some cases of immaturity or sepsis.

Specific Diagnoses. The most frequently reported diagnoses associated with asphyxia are cerebral palsy (CP) and seizure disorders. Shaywitz[37] has identified many of the issues involved in the diagnosis of CP. The general consensus is that CP is a "nonprogressive disorder of movement and posture due to a defect or lesion of the immature brain" (Bax as quoted by Shaywitz).[37] Eliminated are progressive or transient disorders, and CP associated with well defined congenital malformations. However, as Shaywitz notes, little agreement surrounds the age of assessment, classification of types of CP, or severity. Thus, the outcomes being measured may differ substantially across studies.

Shaywitz[37] also reports on the interrater reliability of the diagnosis. Among six experienced clinicians the percent agreement was 50 percent with Kappa in the range of 28 percent. Thus, even with agreement in definitions, detection would also vary substantially across observers.

Similar concerns can be raised concerning the diagnosis of seizure disorders. Seizures in the neonatal period are sometimes difficult to diagnose because of their variable appearance and occasional lack of correlation between clinically apparent seizures and electroencephalographic findings.[38]

Abnormalities on Physical/Neurologic Examination. Other studies have avoided the pitfalls of diagnostic validity by reporting observed abnormalities. In their review, Bryce et al.[1] note outcomes such as *neurologically abnormal*, *abnormal tone* and *abnormal grasp*. Such measures incur two difficulties. While not well documented in the literature, they are likely to incur the low interrater reliability associated with most maneuvers on the physical examination.[39] In addition, the prognostic significance of isolated abnormal signs or single neurologic examinations is often unclear. Standardized approaches[40,41] depend on assessing a number of neurologic functions over time to assess the presence of a neurologic abnormality.

Mental Retardation/Cognitive and Social-Emotional Developmental Delay. In contrast, reliance on cognitive assessments as outcome measures is attractive because of the availability of well standardized assessment instruments with established prognostic significance. Difficulty arises in the specificity of the linkage between the

Assessment of Outcomes Following Neonatal Asphyxia

signs of neonatal asphyxia and alterations of development. Several factors may influence causal inferences between perinatal events and later developmental outcomes.

- Developmental abnormalities observed early in infancy may be transient or of limited prognostic significance. Thus, permanent, significant residua are best assessed later in infancy or early childhood.

- The etiology and natural history of variations in developmental patterns are not well established. While overall scores, some major subscales and individual items may have population norms, the significance of more subtle groups of relative strengths and abnormalities is not well established. For example, the most frequently used infant test, the Bayley, has two major components: mental and motor scales. Further refinement into more subscales remains unconventional, and the significance of differential development across these subscales is still unknown.

- Higher order development and its failure, which may result in school difficulties or learning disabilities, should not be assessed until substantially later in childhood. Assessments at later ages, however, may well be highly confounded by intervening events. For example, extensive evidence supports the adverse effects of poverty on cognitive development and maternal mental health on social-emotional development—effects that may far outweigh the influence of all but the most severe perinatal events.[42,43]

Disability/Handicap. (In reviewing past studies, we have used the terminology that was specified in each report realizing that, in many cases, disability would be a more appropriate term than handicap.) Because of the infrequency and variability of abnormalities potentially encountered, investigators have categorized outcomes in terms of functional impact, described as disability or handicap. As has been pointed out in other contexts,[44,45] the definitions of disability/handicap, and its severity, tend to be idiosyncratic to the individual report. Moreover, such categorizations tend to be composites of performance on standardized tests and/or diagnoses and neurologic abnormalities, thus incurring previously mentioned concerns about reliability and validity.

Moreover, much of the literature on disability/handicap antecedes or lacks modern and standardized approaches. Over the past 10 years, several investigators have modified/extended the types of measures of limitations of activities of daily living (ADLs) suitable for adults to be appropriate for children.[46-48] Such approaches are derived from extensive experience[46] or comprehensive theoretical models of health status.[47,48] More recently, the Institute of Medicine examined the issue of disability, laying out both a conceptual approach and specific definitions.[49] At least one group has operationalized this approach in their examination of outcomes of one neonatal problem, very low birth weight.[50]

Assessment Criteria

For purposes of this report, the outcomes in the studies reviewed were assessed for the presence of the following criteria.

- Clear and specific definition of the population studied;

- Clear and specific definition of the outcome measure(s);

- Specification of assessment techniques (e.g., type of assessor, training and experience, reliability checks if appropriate, timing);

- Comparability of outcomes with a) nature of neonatal insult (i.e., causal influence) and b) later outcomes if appropriate (i.e., predictive value);

- Appropriate attention to the underlying theoretical model of the outcome measure with identification and ascertainment of confounders; and

- Explicit recognition of the statistical properties of the outcome measures and their effect on statistical power.

Despite the fact that we prefer using the term *neonatal encephalopathy* or *neonatal depression* rather than hypoxic-ischemic encephalopathy or asphyxia, we have used the original terminology used by the authors in each of the reports reviewed.

Outcome Studies (Table 45.1). The most extensive studies that have been published recently are by Robertson and Finer.[12,51-53] They include follow-up of a group of 167 term infants born between 1974 and 1979 with evaluations performed at 6, 12 and 27 months, 3.5, 5.5 and 8 years. The criteria used for entry into the study were a diagnosis of hypoxic-ischemic encephalopathy (HIE) defined as an abnormal neurological examination after 1 hour of age and at least one of the following: intrapartum fetal distress, based on abnormal heart-rate patterns; immediate neonatal distress indicated by a low 1- or 5-minute Apgar score (<5); and/or immediate neonatal resuscitation, including bag and mask ventilation or intubation with ventilation. The neurological exam was abnormal if an alteration in consciousness, muscle tone or abnormal primitive reflexes were noted. The HIE was classified into one of Sarnat's three stages: *stage 1 or mild*—hyperalertness, hyperexcitability; *stage 2 or moderate*—lethargy, hypotonia, suppressed primitive reflexes; and *stage 3 or severe*—stupor, flaccidity, absent primitive reflexes.

Outcome measures evaluated included the following handicaps: cerebral palsy, cognitive delay, visual impairment, epilepsy, and neurosensory hearing loss > 70 dB. IQ was measured by the Stanford-Binet Intelligence Scale. Visual motor integration, speech and language development, fine and gross motor skills were also assessed as were school readiness and language development at age 5.5 years. At 8 years, a full battery of school performance measures were tested.

IQ tests were administered by a psychologist, speech and language by a speech pathologist, hearing by an audiologist, motor assessments by a physical therapist and developmental pediatrician, and educational testing by a reliability-tested educator; testers were unaware of the patients' neonatal courses. Comparable groups of children with normal healthy neonatal courses were also studied at 5.5 and 8 years. Potential confounding factors such as socioeconomic status, mother's language and intervening illnesses were evaluated.

Eleven percent of the 226 children died and of the 200 survivors, 19 percent had handicap: 11 percent with severe cognitive delay, 10 percent with cerebral palsy, 6.5 percent with convulsive disorders, 5.5 percent with visual loss and 2 percent with deafness. Outcome was significantly related to severity of encephalopathy with *all* of the severe encephalopathy group developing severe disability, none of the mild encephalopathy children developing disability and 21 percent of the moderate encephalopathy infants developing later disability. In those with moderate encephalopathy, an abnormal neurological exam at the time of discharge and the occurrence of seizures in the neonatal period appeared to be related to worsened outcome. At the 5.5 and 8 year assessments, children who had mild encephalopathy performed as well as their control peers. This led the authors to question whether these infants should be classified to have had encephalopathy at all. Children with moderate and severe encephalopathy however, did less well than their peers on assessments of school readiness and later school performance.[51-53]

Adsett et al.[3] used criteria for perinatal asphyxia including: fetal distress (not further defined), Apgar score <6 at 5 minutes, necessity

AUTHOR	NUMBER OF PATIENTS	ENCEPHALOPATHY CLASSIFICATION	RESULTS	OTHER PREDICTORS OF OUTCOME
Robertson (1985, 1988, 1989)	226	Yes	11% Mortality 19% Handicap 10% CP 11% Cognitive delay 5.5% Visual impairment 6.5% Convulsive disorder	Abnormal neurological exam at discharge
Adsett (1985)	56	No	14% Mortality 23% Normal 8% Mild handicaps 42% Major handicaps 27% Indefinite	CT scan
Levene (1986)	122	No	11% Mortality 8% Severe neurologic abnormality	Apgar scores
Ishikawa (1987)	86	No	15% Mortality 76% Normal 9% Mild abnormalities 15% Major abnormalities	Abnormal neurological exam at discharge Persistent abnormal neurological findings Neonatal seizures
Low (1988)	37	Yes	50% Normal 27% Minor abnormalities 13% Major abnormalities	Degree metabolic acidosis
Perlman (1988)	36	No	6% Mortality 17% Abnormal outcome	Renal injury
Shankaran (1991)	28	Yes	14% Mortality 42% Spastic quadriplegia or hemiplegia 50% Microcephaly & seizure disorder 25% Vision impairment 17% Hearing 54% Language delay 50% Normal cognitive development 38% Severe cognitive delay	Cardiac injury Renal injury Pulmonary injury Hematologic injury Seizures, EEG, CT
Lam (1992)	40	Yes	10% Mortality 7.5% Normal outcome 10% Mild handicap 2.5% Moderate handicap 2.5% Severe handicap	Renal injury

Table 45.1. Summary of outcome studies of infants with diagnosis of perinatal asphyxia

Assessment of Outcomes Following Neonatal Asphyxia

for positive pressure ventilation for ≥2 minutes, and metabolic acidosis with pH <7.2 in the first 2 hours of life. Fifty-six full-term infants met these criteria, 48 of whom survived and were evaluated by a neurologist or pediatrician at ages 4-23 months with outcomes reported as: *Normal*—normal neurological examination and development at one year or older; *Mild handicap*—mild delay in development without definite neurological deficits, or equivocal neurological abnormalities resulting in minor impairment of function; and *Major handicap*—definite permanent neurological deficits. Only 23 percent were reported as normal, 8 percent as mild handicap, 42 percent as major handicap, and 27 percent as indefinite. CT scans performed on all patients were found to add to prediction of outcome with normal and patchy (areas of hypodensity) abnormalities correlating with better outcomes and diffuse and global (extensive areas of deceased density) abnormalities correlating with poor outcomes. Assessment techniques used were not reported nor was the evaluation of potential confounding factors such as socioeconomic status or intervening illness.

Levene's group[54] evaluated 122 patients with perinatal asphyxia (definition not provided) born between 1980-1984 and assessed between 1-5 years (median 2.5 years). As in Robertson's studies, patients were categorized as having *mild* (minor disturbance of tone, hyperalertness, and slight feeding difficulties, recovering by 48 hours after birth); *moderate* (lethargy, more pronounced abnormalities of tone, poor feeding, and convulsions, with signs of recovery by 7 days); and *severe* (coma, failure to maintain adequate ventilation, profound hypotonia, and seizures). Children were evaluated by a neurologist and a psychologist (Bayley Scales of Infant Development) if abnormalities were suspected. Outcome was defined as presence or absence of severe neurological abnormality (cerebral palsy sufficient to impair independent locomotion, developmental delay severe enough to warrant special education, sensorineural hearing loss, visual impairment, or epileptic seizures requiring medication) or death. Fourteen patients died. Of the 108 survivors, 8 percent developed severe neurological abnormalities; all with severe handicap had moderate or severe perinatal encephalopathy. Apgar scores were not found to be good predictors of outcome. The evaluation of potential confounders was not described.

Ishikawa et al.[55] evaluated 86 full-term infants in whom asphyxia was defined by the following criteria: 1-minute Apgar score of ≤6; neurological complications including: (a) findings of stupor or lethargy, hypotonia, weakness of proximal limbs, abnormal breathing patterns, and jitteriness or seizures, and (b) one or more abnormal findings on laboratory test such as cerebrospinal fluid, cranial ultrasound, cerebral angiography, electroencephalogram, or brain CT scan. Children were evaluated from ages 3-13 years (mean 8 yrs, 5 mos) using outcome measures including neurological exam, hearing assessment, and intelligence quotient (IQ) as measured by a clinical psychologist (Wechsler or Tanaka-Binet intelligence tests).

Of the 55 patients followed (75 percent), 15 percent developed *major developmental abnormalities* (cerebral palsy, mental retardation or epilepsy); and 9 percent developed *mild abnormalities* (normal function in daily life). Neonatal factors that were found to be of predictive value included: an abnormal neurological exam on discharge; an absent Moro reflex for >6 days; disturbance of consciousness over 6 days; and the occurrence of neonatal seizures and poor sucking over 28 days. No evaluation of potential confounders was noted.

In a report of 37 term infants with neonatal asphyxia, Low et al.[11] used criteria for neonatal asphyxia that included evidence of a metabolic acidosis at delivery (umbilical artery buffer base <34 mmol/L). As Robertson and Levene did, infants were divided into three groups by severity: *mild* (hyperalertness, irritability, jitteriness, transient hypertonia or hypotonia); *moderate* (lethargy, severe hypotonia, occasional seizures); and *severe* (coma, multiple seizures, and recurrent apnea). Patients were evaluated at 6 and 12 months of age with a neurological examination, the Bayley Scales of Infant Development, and the Uzgiris and Hunt scale.

A control group of 76 healthy infants with no history of neonatal complications was also assessed. Twenty-seven percent of the infants with asphyxia developed minor deficits and 13 percent major deficits; 60 percent were reported as normal compared to 92 percent normal in the control group. Assessments of potential confounders such as maternal education or socioeconomic status were not reported.

Perlman and Tack[7] assessed renal injury in another follow-up evaluation of infants with neonatal asphyxia. Asphyxia criteria included one or more of the following: 1) 5-minute Apgar score ≤5 with or without need for intubation; 2) 5-minute Apgar 6 if required intubation; and/or 3) umbilical cord arterial pH <7.20 or umbilical cord arterial PCO_2 > 50mm Hg. Thirty-six full-term infants born between 1985-1986 were assessed at age 12-18 months with methods that were not reported. Of the six patients with persistent oliguria, only one had a normal outcome; the rest had cerebral palsy and seizures. Transient

Assessment of Outcomes Following Neonatal Asphyxia

oliguria and normal urine output were associated with a much better outcome. Overall 17 percent of patients had abnormal outcomes and 5 percent died. Little further information about these infants including potential confounders was provided.

Shankaran et al.[4] thoroughly evaluated a small group of 24 survivors with perinatal asphyxia as defined by satisfying at least three of the following four criteria: fetal distress documented on fetal heart monitor (late or variable decelerations); presence of meconium stained amniotic fluid with the neonate in a vertex position; the need for endotracheal intubation at delivery; and the occurrence of abnormal muscle tone and seizures within 24 hours of age. Infants were all full-term and delivered between 1980-1982. Sarnat stages of encephalopathy were assigned to each patient. Patients were evaluated at 3, 6, and 12 months, and then yearly up to 5 years of age with neurological exams and age appropriate standardized developmental assessments (Bayley Scales of Infant Development and McCarthy Scales of Children's Abilities), language and hearing assessments. Information regarding socioeconomic status was routinely collected. During the neonatal time period, information regarding multisystem function including cardiac, renal, pulmonary, hematologic and neurological systems was also evaluated. At 5 years of age, 58 percent of infants had normal motor exams; and the remaining 42 percent had spastic quadriplegia or hemiplegia. Fifty percent had microcephaly and seizure disorders; 25 percent vision impairment; 17 percent hearing and 54 percent language delay; 38 percent had normal cognitive development while 50 percent had very abnormal cognitive development. Factors that were found in multiple regression analysis to be predictive of lower cognitive scores were: lower socioeconomic status, neonatal seizures, renal problems, cardiac problems, need for cardiopulmonary resuscitation, and poor head growth at 3 months of age. Potential confounders including socioeconomic status and intervening illness (meningitis, postnatal brain injury) were also evaluated.

The last report to be reviewed is that of Lam et al.[10] describing the outcome of 40 full-term newborns delivered in 1985-1987 who met the single criterion for asphyxia of having an Apgar score of ≤3 at 1 minute. These infants were classified using Amiel-Tison's staging: (Stage Ia) hyperexcitability and mild abnormalities of tone for ≤7 days, (Ib) for >7 days; (Stage IIa) CNS depression such as lethargy or light coma without seizures, (IIb) with seizures; (Stage III) Deep coma and repetitive seizures without brainstem signs and the presence of spontaneous respiratory efforts, (IIIb) with brainstem signs and the absence of spontaneous respiration efforts. Outcome assessment measures included a full neuro-developmental exam performed by a neurologist at 2 years of age. Outcome was reported as: *Normal*—within the average age development and no evidence of handicap; *Mild handicap*—variations from normal on neurologic or developmental examination without a specific diagnosis; *Moderate handicap*—trainable retardation, severe behavioral disorders and/or convulsive disorders, mild or moderate neurosensory deafness, spastic diplegia, hemiplegia, visual impairment; *Severe handicap*—spastic quadriplegia, severe psychomotor retardation, severe neurosensory deafness or blindness; and *Death*. Fully 75 percent had a normal outcome, 10 percent had mild handicap, 5 percent had moderate or severe handicap and 10 percent died. In this study, again outcome was related to the severity of the initial neonatal classification. All children who had stage III encephalopathy developed moderate to severe handicap or death and none of the patients with stage I or II developed later significant sequelae. Severe renal impairment was also again a predictor of poor outcome. Potential confounders were not evaluated.

Conclusions

In summary, studies of the outcome of infants with perinatal asphyxia remain cumbersome to compare because of differences in the basic definitions of *asphyxia* essential to defining the population of infants being studied, differences in measuring outcomes and in evaluating potential confounding factors that also contribute to those outcomes. Trends in the past 8 years, however, appear to clarify that using only simple criteria such as low Apgar scores or blood pH to define the population at risk for adverse outcome is not sufficient. Classifying the severity of neonatal encephalopathy, as five of the eight studies reviewed in this paper did, appears to augment the ability to predict outcome. The diagnosis of mild encephalopathy, on the other hand, appears to be unnecessary as the outcome of these patients appears to be universally good. The majority of these studies also attempted to use evidence of actual end-organ insult as demonstrated by persistent abnormal neonatal neurological state, seizures or evidence of injury to other organ systems such as the kidneys or heart and found this to provide better prediction of risk for an adverse outcome. Perhaps with new, more precise methods of assessing CNS injury and clear definitions of neonatal encephalopathy with criteria that are universally applied, the group at greatest risk of poor outcome will also be better identified so that interventions can be offered as early as possible to optimize potential development. Likewise, in the continuing follow-up of these infants, standard methods of assessment, use of comparison groups and evaluation of factors such as socioeconomic status and parental education should routinely be utilized in the analysis of outcome results. Until these definitions and methods of assessment are standardized, studies can not be compared and results can not be generalized to the general population of infants.

References

1. Bryce RL, Halperin ME, Sinclair JC. Association between indicators of perinatal asphyxia and adverse outcome in the term infant: A methodological review. *Neuroepidemiol* 4:24-38, 1985.

2. Goldberg RN, Moscoso P, Bauer CR et al. Use of barbiturate therapy in severe perinatal asphyxia: A randomized controlled trial. *J Pediatr* 109:851-856, 1986.

3. Adsett DB, Ritz CR, Hill A. Hypoxic-ischaemic cerebral injury in the term newborn: Correlation of CT findings with neurological outcome. *Dev Med Child Neurol* 27:155-160, 1985.

4. Shankaran S, Woldt E, Koepke T et al. Acute neonatal morbidity and long-term central nervous system sequelae of perinatal asphyxia in term infants. *Early Hum Dev* 25:135-148, 1991.

5. Roland EH, Jan JE, Hill A, Wong PK. Cortical visual impairment following birth asphyxia. *Pediatr Neurol* 2:133-137, 1986.

6. Lupton BA, Hill A, Roland EH et al. Brain swelling in the asphyxiated term newborn: Pathogenesis and outcome. *Pediatrics* 82:139-146, 1988.

7. Perlman JM, Tack ED. Renal injury in the asphyxiated newborn infant: Relationship to neurologic outcome. *J Pediatr* 113:875-879, 1988.

8. Blair E, Stanley FJ. Intrapartum asphyxia: A rare cause of cerebral palsy. *J Pediatr* 112:515-519, 1988.

9. Riikonen RS, Kero PO, Simell OG. Excitatory amino acids in cerebrospinal fluid in neonatal asphyxia. *Pediatr Neurol* 8:37-40, 1992.

10. Lam BCC, Yeung CY. Perinatal features of birth asphyxia and neurologic outcome. *Acta Pædiatr JPN* 34:17-22, 1992.

11. Low JA, Galbraith RS, Muir DW et al. Motor and cognitive deficits after intrapartum asphyxia in the mature fetus. *Am J Obstet Gynecol* 158:356-361, 1988.

12. Robertson C, Finer N. Term infants with hypoxic-ischemic encephalopathy: Outcome at 3.5 years. *Dev Med Child Neurol* 27:473-484, 1985.

13. Naeye RL, Peters EC, Bartholomew M, Landis JR. Origins of cerebral palsy. *Am J Dis Child* 143:1154-1161, 1989.

14. Barkovich AJ, Truwit CL. Brain damage from perinatal asphyxia: Correlation of MR findings with gestational age. *AJNR* 11:1087-1096, 1990.

15. Foley J. Dyskinetic and dystonic cerebral palsy and birth. *Acta Paediatr* 81:57-60, 1992.

16. Taylor NB (ed). *Stedman's Medical Dictionary*. Baltimore: The Williams and Wilkins Company, 19th Revised Edition, pp 137, 1957.

17. Snyder EY, Cloherty JP. Perinatal asphyxia. In: Cloherty JP, Stark AR (eds). *Manual of Neonatal Care*. Boston: Little Brown and Company, pp 393-419, 1991.

18. Hollander DI, Wright L, Nagey DA et al. Indicators of perinatal asphyxia. *Am J Obstet Gynecol* 157:839-43, 1987.

19. Nelson KB, Leviton A. How much of neonatal encephalopathy is due to birth asphyxia? *AJDC* 145:1325-1331, 1991.

20. Nelson KB, Ellenberg JH. Obstetric complications as risk factors for cerebral or seizure disorders. *JAMA* 251:1843-1848, 1984.

21. Committee on Obstetrics: Maternal and Fetal Medicine. Utility of umbilical cord blood acid-base assessment. American College of Obstetricians a Gynecologists Committee Opinion Number 91, 1991.

22. Fee SC, Malee K, Deddish R et al. Severe acidosis and subsequent neurologic status. *Am J Obstet Gynecol* 162:802-806, 1990.

23. Low JA, Muir DW, Pater EA, Karchmar EJ. The association of intrapartum asphyxia in the mature fetus with newborn behavior. *Am J Obstet Gynecol* 163:1131-1135, 1990.

24. Goldaber KG, Gilstrap LC 3rd, Leveno KJ et al. Pathologic fetal acidemia. *Obstet Gynecol* 78:1103-1107, 1991.

25. Mires GJ, Agustsson P, Forsyth JS, Patel NB. Cerebral pathology in the very low birthweight infant: Predictive value of peripartum metabolic acidosis. *Eur J Obstet Gynecol Reprod Biol* 42:181-185, 1991.

26. Winkler CL, Hauth JC, Tucker JM et al. Neonatal complications at term as related to the degree of umbilical artery acidemia. *Am J Obstet Gynecol* 164:637-641, 1991.

27. Goodwin TM, Belai I, Hernandez P et al. Asphyxial complications in the term newborn with severe umbilical acidemia. *Am J Obstet Gynecol* 167:1506-1512, 1992.

28. Gill AB, Weindling AM. Echocardiographic assessment of cardiac function in shocked very low birthweight infants. *Arch Dis Child* 68:17-21, 1993.

29. Vintzileos AM, Campbell WA, Rodis JF et al. The relationship between fetal biophysical assessment, umbilical artery velocimetry, and fetal acidosis. *Obstet Gynecol* 77:622-626, 1991.

30. Walkinshaw S, Cameron H, MacPhail S, Robson S. The prediction of fetal compromise and acidosis by biophysical profile scoring in the small for gestational age fetus. *J Perinat Med* 20:227-232, 1992.

31. Dudell G, Cornish JD, Bartlett RH. What constitutes adequate oxygenation? *Pediatrics* 85:39-41, 1990.

32. Pryds O. Control of cerebral circulation in the high-risk neonate. *Ann Neurol* 30:321-329, 1991.

33. Wyatt JS, Edwards AD, Cope M et al. Response of cerebral blood volume to changes in arterial carbon dioxide tension in preterm and term infants. *Pediatr Res* 29:553-557, 1991.

34. Bucher H-U, Edwards AD, Lipp AE, Duc G. Comparison between near infrared spectroscopy and ^{133}xenon clearance for estimation of cerebral blood flow in critically ill preterm infants. *Pediatr Res* 33:56-60, 1993.

35. Hirtz DG. Report of the National Institute of Neurological Disorders and Stroke workshop on near infrared spectroscopy. *Pediatrics* 91:414-417, 1993.

36. Carmines EG, Zeller RH. *Reliability and validity assessment.* Quantitative Applications in the Social Sciences Series, #17, Beverly Hills: Sage Publications, 1979.

37. Shaywitz BA. The sequelae of hypoxic-ischemic encephalopathy. *Sem Perinatol* 11:180-190, 1987.

38. Mizrahi EM. Neonatal seizures: Problems in diagnosis and classification. *Epilepsia* 28:546-555, 1987.

39. Feinstein AR. A bibliography of publications on observer variability. *J Chron Dis* 38:619-32, 1985.

40. Amiel-Tison C, Grenier A (eds). *Neurological Assessment During the First Year of Life.* New York: Oxford University Press, 1986.

41. Swanson MW, Bennett FC, Shy KK, Whitfield MF. Identification of neuro-developmental abnormality at four and eight months by the movement assessment of infants. *Dev Med Child Neurol* 34:321-337, 1992.

42. McCormick MC, Brooks-Gunn J, Workman-Daniels K et al. The health and developmental status of very low birth weight children at school age. *J Am Med Assoc* 267:2204-2208, 1992.

43. McCormick MC, Workman-Daniels K. Brooks-Gunn J. The behavioral and emotional well-being of school-age children with different birthweights. *Pediatrics* (in press).

44. Kitchen WH, Ryan MM, Rickards A et al. Changing outcome over 13 years in very low birth weight infants. *Seminars in Perinatol* 6:373-389, 1982.

45. Escobar GJ, Littenberg B, Petitti DB. Outcome among surviving very low birthweight infants: A meta-analysis. *Arch Dis Child* 66:204-211, 1991.

46. Stein REK, Jessop DJ. Functional Status II(R). A measure of child health status. *Med Care* 28:1041-1055, 1990.

47. Eisen M, Donald CA, Ware JE et al. *Conceptualization and Measurement of Health of Children in the Health Insurance Study*. R-2313-HEW. Santa Monica: The Rand Corporation, 1980.

48. Kaplan RM, Anderson JP. A general health policy model: Update and applications. *Health Serv Res* 23:203-235, 1988.

49. Institute of Medicine. *Disability in America*. Washington, DC: National Academy Press, 1991.

50. Schreuder AM, Veen S, Ens-Dokkum MH et al. Standardised method of follow-up assessment of preterm infants at the age of 5 years: Use of the WHO classification of impairments, disabilities and handicaps report from the collaborative project on preterm and small for gestational age infants (POPS) in The Netherlands, 1983. *Pædiatr and Perinatal Epidemiol* 6:363-380, 1992.

51. Robertson CMT, Finer NN. Educational readiness of survivors of neonatal encephalopathy associated with birth asphyxia at term. *J Dev Behav Pediatr* 9:298-306, 1988.

52. Robertson CMT, Finer NN, Grace MGA. School performance of survivors of neonatal encephalopathy associated with birth asphyxia at term. *J Pediatr* 114:753-60, 1989.

53. Robertson CMT, Finer NN. Long-term follow-up of term neonates with perinatal asphyxia. *Clin Perinatol* 20:483-499, 1993.

54. Levene MI, Sands C, Grindulis H, Moore JR. Comparison of two methods of predicting outcome in perinatal asphyxia. *Lancet*: 67-69, 1986 (Jan).

55. Ishikawa T, Ogawa Y, Kanayama M, Wada Y. Long-term prognosis of asphyxiated full-term neonates with CNS complications. *Brain Dev* 9:48-53, 1987.

Chapter 46

Long-Term Outcome in Birth Asphyxia—The Role of Encephalopathy in Prediction

Introduction

The long-term outcome of birth asphyxia that is of central interest to a neurologist, and probably to most others including parents, is neurologic status. In asking the long-term neurologic outcome of birth asphyxia, we encounter a number of problems. First, there is no generally available means for the objective measurement of birth asphyxia, allowing surety as to whether nonspecific clinical signs in the neonate are appropriately attributable to asphyxia. Second, we have far too few good studies of the natural history of birth asphyxia, studies in defined populations that were not selected for factors that might have an impact on outcome, that included clear and reasonable criteria for asphyxia, that followed the studied children to a time when some reasonably homogeneous outcome condition could be reasonably reliably ascertained, and that were large enough to permit conclusions about relationships between uncommon events and uncommon outcomes.

In addition to these difficulties and a number of others, we have probably been compounding our problems by using the same words, *birth asphyxia*, to mean a number of different things. Birth asphyxia occurs in a wide range of degrees, from the normal low oxygen tension of the intrauterine environment and of birth, to acute total and

---

From *Report of the Workshop on Acute Perinatal Asphyxia in Term Infants*, National Institute of Child Health and Human Development (NICHD), NIH Pub. No. 96-3823, March 1996.

prolonged absence of gas exchange. The same words have in general been employed for all of these. Crudely diagrammed (Figure 46.1), the outer boundary of birth asphyxia, BA-I, represents *some* degree and duration of asphyxia differing from whatever norms are employed. BA-I may be useful to obstetricians and to neonatologists as a signal of need for increased vigilance lest problems progress. The second circle, BA-II, represents the degree and duration of asphyxia that is associated with a substantial risk of irreversible brain injury in the term fetus who survives it. BA-II is a subset, and a fairly small subset, of BA-1, as indicated by repeated observations that in term infants, whatever definitions the various studies have employed, the majority of survivors of even severe and lengthy asphyxia are later clinically normal.[1-3] One reason interventions designed to prevent damage from birth asphyxia have apparently not been associated with lower rates of perinatal mortality or of later neurologic morbidity may be that the monitoring methods have identified BA-I and not BA-II, resulting in interventions directed largely at mother-baby pairs in whom there would not have been an excess of long-term morbidity

Degrees of Birth Asphyxia and Their Relationship to Outcome

BA-I = some birth asphyxia

BA-II = irreversibly injurious birth asphyxia

BA-III = injurious & obstetrically preventable

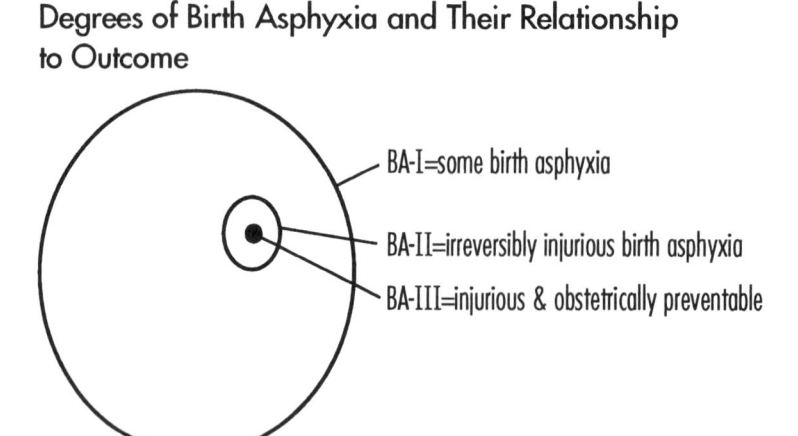

Figure 46.1. The outer circle, BA-I, represents the presence of some degree of birth asphyxia. BA-II, a subset, represents the degree and duration of birth asphyxia required to produce irreversible brain injury in a term fetus/neonate. BA-III, the size of which relative to the others is not known, represents the degree and duration of birth asphyxia required for irreversible brain injury, and obstetrically preventable.

even without the intervention. (Other possibilities have been discussed by Grant.)[4] A third circle, BA-III, its relative size entirely unknown, is a subset of BA-II, and represents the degree and duration of birth asphyxia that is injurious to brain *and is obstetrically preventable*.

Another range of differences encompassed by our use of the words *birth asphyxia* has to do with *when* in the course of illness a defect of gas exchange occurs. Some infants thought to be asphyxiated, perhaps with demonstrated poor cerebral perfusion, are born following such obstetric catastrophes as placental abruption, cord prolapse with lengthy occlusion, or maternal shock. More often no such clearcut obstetrical antecedent is identified. We have no convincing answers as to why these infants are affected. It is probably not reasonable to assume without investigation of other possible risk factors that the initiating pathology must have been acutely asphyxial in all or most such cases, since many pathogenetic mechanisms trigger changes in the biology of cells that, once they are underway, can result in ischemia as a late result. For example, Leviton[5] has recently noted that tumor necrosis factor, associated with infection and inflammation, can produce hypotension which can in turn lead to ischemia; he has raised the possibility that agents such as tumor necrosis factor and other cytokines known to play a role in triggering preterm birth, might themselves contribute to brain pathology in prematurely born infants, or in those born at term. Leviton's focus was on factors that might contribute to injury to white matter, but experimental evidence also suggests that certain cytokines can affect neurons in developing brain in exceedingly low concentrations the effects differing by developmental stage.[6] Whether or not these interesting hypotheses prove correct, the point for this discussion is that ischemia is a late common path for many kinds of illnesses. Ultimately most of us die of asphyxia, in a sense; is it a medically interesting sense?

Ignoring the chain of events that precedes hypoxia or ischemia may prevent focus on real and important differences, and may discourage needed clinical research such as, for example, investigating whether certain maternal or pregnancy conditions, including infectious or inflammatory illnesses, predispose to hypotension or cerebral hypoperfusion in the term or preterm neonate.

Once hypoxemia or poor cerebral blood flow is identified in the infant, consideration of trials of therapy may be warranted in an attempt to interrupt the chain of damage whatever the cause. However, therapy at that point is damage control; if we are to develop better strategies for primary prevention, it is necessary that we learn to identify the instigating pathology. The implications are quite different if ischemia is the end stage of a process that began with chorionitis or immune disturbance, for example, than if the defect in gas exchange arose by way of placental abruption or maternal shock. Using the words birth asphyxia an ischemia for these quite different situations may also have unwarranted implications concerning responsibility and blame.

The difficulties we face in approaching questions of the relationship of birth asphyxia to outcome are real and formidable. Using the same words to mean a range of different things is one part of the problem that we can and should avoid.

What Prenatal or Neonatal Factors that Might Be Related to Birth Asphyxia Predict Long-Term Neurologic Outcome?

Consideration is limited to term singleton infants (free of major malformations), because for low birthweight infants or those multiply born other issues may arise, and also because evidence is even more sparse, selected, and heterogeneous than for term singletons.

What long-term neurologic outcomes have we have reason to think might be related to birth asphyxia? Sameroff wrote, "The intellectual outcomes for children (mental retardation and learning disorders) were far better explained by the small set of *family* factors than on any combination of the multitude of *biomedical* variables."[7] Paneth recently noted,[8] "A very consistent finding in the literature is that when adverse perinatal events are implicated in the causation of a neurodevelopmental disorder, cerebral palsy is invariably present." Current evidence indicates that the outcome to track in studying the long-term outcome of birth asphyxia is cerebral palsy (CP), which may be accompanied by mental retardation, seizure disorder, or other associated neurologic or sensory disability.

Obstetric Factors

Three obstetric conditions especially linked with asphyxial birth are placenta previa, abruptio placentae, and prolapsed umbilical cord. All these conditions are uncommon, the most common of them, abruption, occurring in 1.7 percent of births.[9] All these conditions are

Long-Term Outcome in Birth Asphyxia

associated with increased risk of preterm delivery, so they are even less common in term births. In a cohort of more than 50,000 live births, only one of these conditions—placenta previa—was associated in infants over 2,500 g with a risk of CP that significantly exceeded the risk in children whose births were uncomplicated, and the absolute magnitude of risk in term survivors was less than 2 percent.[9] These asphyxial obstetric conditions were not strikingly powerful as predictors of long-term neurologic deficit.

Furthermore, even these seemingly acute obstetric catastrophes have histories that may go far back into pregnancy. Placenta previa is obviously determined at the time of implantation. If there are disadvantages to the fetus who has his or her placenta implanted in the isthmic area of the uterus rather than in the fundus, then those disadvantages have been present in pregnancies with placenta previa for a long time before labor begins. Placenta previa is associated with higher rates of spontaneous abortion, with male fetuses, advanced maternal age, parity, impaired fertility, smoking, and developmental defects of the fetus.[10,11] Placenta previa may be recurrent in the same gravidae.[10] Whether the increase in risk of cerebral palsy associated with placenta previa is fully preventable by obstetric interventions at the time of birth is not known.

Abruption too may have early precursors including maternal age, smoking history, cocaine exposure or frequent use of marijuana, preeclampsia, chorionitis, and fetal malformation.[12,13] Cord prolapse is often associated with breech birth, which is disproportionately often associated with conditions characterized by weakness or hypotonia in the fetus.

So even previa, abruption and cord prolapse were not strikingly good as predictors of CP, and these conditions are not necessarily bolt-from-the-blue acute hypoxic or ischemic events that begin during labor or delivery. These factors have their own histories, some of which have implications for development. Although all of these can be associated with fetal hypoxemia, the relationship of each with fetal neurologic condition may be considerably more complicated than the words *birth asphyxia* imply.

Neurologic Signs

Among signs apparent in the newborn immediately after birth that might be evaluated as predictive of long-term outcome are those recorded in the Apgar score. Low Apgar scores are indeed predictors of marked increase in risk of CP in term survivors, but only at the rare extreme: it is very low scores (3 or less) very late (after 10 minutes) that are strongly predictive.[2] These very low late scores are very uncommon and when they do occur are often not survived.[2] Nevertheless, extremely deviant Apgar scores have high positive predictive value for later CP in survivors.

Do low Apgar scores identify asphyxial birth? Very low late scores, those that are associated with adverse outcome, might have antecedents different from factors that predispose to transient mild depressions of Apgar score; I know of no examination of this possibility.

Hypotonia, respiratory delay, difficulty in maintaining respiration, and poor reflex responsivity all are or can be evidence of neurologic dysfunction. When such signs of neurologic depression are recognized in the delivery room they are called low Apgar scores. The same signs identified in the neonatal nursery, with or without the addition of seizures and with some variously defined exclusions, are often referred to as *hypoxic-ischemic encephalopathy*. Low Apgar scores are not specific to any etiology, and neither is a constellation of similar signs observed over the next days of life. Defining birth asphyxia by Apgar scores alone is no longer acceptable.

Neurologic signs that appear or persist after the first minutes or hours of life are also predictors of neurologic outcome. Indeed, obstetrical complications were predictive only if other neurologic signs were present in the neonatal period.[14] Subdivided to give special attention to neonatal seizures, these factors show a striking relationship with rate of later CP.[15] Obstetrical complications or low Apgar scores were related to CP risk only if followed by neonatal encephalopathy, and then there was dramatic increase in risk. Children with that combination of ominous predictive factors were 0.06 percent of term infants.[15] They contributed 16 percent of the CP in that population.

Levene et al.[16] found low Apgar scores to predict CP, but reported that "No handicapped children were found who had had low Apgar scores alone without encephalopathy." Hadders-Algra et al.[17] made a similar observation: "The Apgar score was the sole obstetrical variable which contributed significantly to an increased risk of neurological handicap, but only in the presence of neonatal (neurologic) deviancy."

Klipstein and McBride[18] noted that number of days on respirator, days to full oral feeds, and days to normal level of activity were predictive of CP in term newborns they considered asphyxiated at birth. Clearly, all these are measures of presence and severity of neurologic disturbance.

Long-Term Outcome in Birth Asphyxia

A substantial body of evidence indicates that in the term baby, if a complicated birth is not followed by neurologic symptomatology, and usually by symptomatology also in other organ systems, then there is no increase in risk of CP. Asphyxial birth is not associated with heightened risk of unfavorable neurologic outcome unless there is neonatal encephalopathy (Figure 46.2). The pathway from asphyxial birth to long-term bad outcome is via neonatal encephalopathy.

Asphyxia Associated with Long-term Adverse Outcome Only When Neonatal Encephalopathy is Present

Asphyxial birth → Neonatal encephalophy → Bad outcome

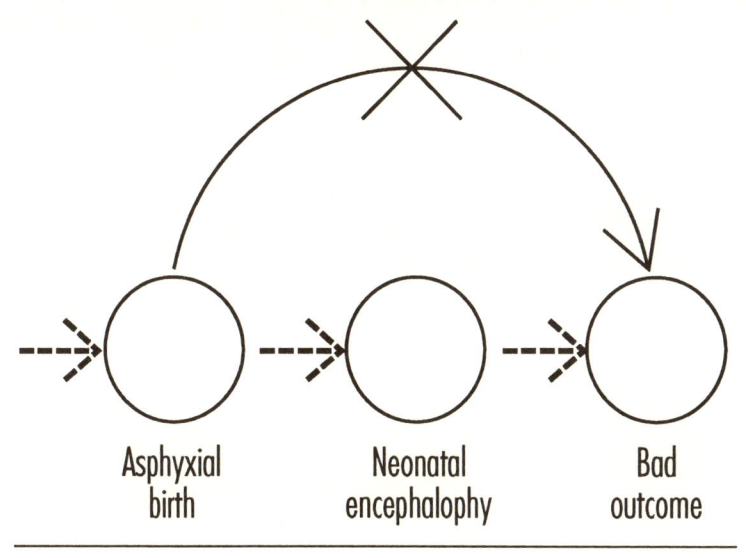

Figure 46.2.

A major predictor of long-term neurologic disability, then, is short-term neurologic abnormality, neonatal encephalopathy. Evidence from the National Collaborative Perinatal Project suggests that neonatal depression present from birth and with continuing manifestations that culminate in neonatal seizures is a particularly dire predictor.[15] This cluster of factors needs evaluation in a current dataset.

Low Apgar scores and low pH account for only a small minority of encephalopathy in term babies.[19] There are obviously causes of neonatal encephalopathy other than asphyxial birth and some or many of these may evade our short list of exclusions. For CP we have some ideas about other possible causes,[20,21] but we have only scattered and nonconvergent ideas of what these factors are. Can infection and the associated lactic acidosis predispose to encephalopathy in the neonate? If the mother or placenta are infected, can factors associated with infection such as cytokines reach the fetus and affect it even if the fetus is not itself infected? There is great need for clinical examination of hypotheses derived from the experimental neurosciences.

The only study I know of to examine a whole range of clinical factors as possible antecedents of neonatal encephalopathy in term infants is an investigation now underway in the Western Australia Research Institute for Child Health. Evidence from the pilot phase of that study suggests some surprises: births in neonates with encephalopathy were not strikingly different in most regards from births of controls, but administration of thyroid hormone to mothers and maternal fevers in labor were observed in significant excess in infants who manifested encephalopathy as neonates as compared with controls.

Most CP, and virtually all of mental retardation, learning disorders, and so on, in children who do not also have CP, has causes other than birth asphyxia. So, it appears likely, does neonatal encephalopathy. The contribution of these other predictors of neonatal encephalopathy to later neurologic disability remains to be determined in studies that *investigate* rather than *assume* etiology.

Acid-Base Measures

Low pH at or soon after birth, especially with a metabolic component, is a factor associated with multiorgan problems including signs of neonatal encephalopathy.[23] Selection factors in most existing studies make judging frequency difficult, but this is an uncommon combination: the 98 term children Portman et al.[23] considered to be asphyxiated came from 2 years of births in a population base of 60,000 to 75,000 births per year which, assuming a middle-range of 135,000 births, suggests a rate of moderate or severe asphyxia by their criteria of about 0.07 percent in term infants.

Studies starting with a defined denominator have found that pH, with or without Apgar scores, accounts for very little of neonatal encephalopathy: most infants with encephalopathy are not acidotic, and most acidotic—even severely acidotic—infants are not encephalopathic.[19] Only weakly predictive of encephalopathy in the newborn period, measures of acid-base balance including umbilical artery pH have not been shown to be good predictors of long-term outcome.[24-26] It would seem reasonable to guess, and recent studies suggest,[26,27] that pH may operate as a predictor in a manner similar to that of Apgar scores, predictive chiefly at the rare extremes. If that is so, then there is likely to be a very high rate of false positive identification, and very large studies will be required to demonstrate relationships. An important additional consideration is that other prenatal factors may influence or determine outcome: in two recent studies of infants with pH below 7.00, a majority of those with adverse outcome had prenatal abnormalities.[27,28]

Studies of pH have seldom been performed in large and unselected populations in which outcome is systematically evaluated in a manner permitting estimations of magnitudes of risk. Information on the natural history of children with low pH values with or without base deficit and combining that information with Apgar score would be very desirable if we hope to use pH and base deficit, or combinations of acid-base measures and Apgar scores, as important factors in selecting babies for trials of new therapies for birth asphyxia.

Conclusions

- A major predictor of long-term neurologic outcome is short-term neurologic outcome, neonatal encephalopathy. We need substantially more information on the differential diagnosis of this nonspecific clinical syndrome, and more information also on the natural history of its specific subsyndromes.

- Defining birth asphyxia by Apgar scores alone is no longer acceptable. Many definitions of birth asphyxia now proposed include acidosis. This is probably an advance, but acidosis is also not etiologically specific. We need more information on differential diagnosis and natural history of specific combinations of factors proposed for the definition of birth asphyxia, as well as of factors that modify risk. This is especially critical if we are to use these criteria as a basis for selecting babies to receive experimental treatments soon after birth.

- When defective oxygenation is identified or suspected, it may be important to clarify at what point in the clinical course inadequate oxygenation is thought to have arisen.

- The incorporation into perinatology and neonatology of new findings in cell biology and in particular of developmental neurobiology is likely to contribute greatly to our understanding of developmental neurologic abnormalities. Oxygen is not the only molecule important to the developing nervous system. Developmental neurobiology may also help us to anticipate and avoid some unintended harms in trials of experimental therapies.

- Current evidence is that irreversible brain damage from asphyxia during birth in term infants is very uncommon, and that the signs available at the times when decisions must be made as to whether to intervene are low in specificity: the fetus/infant who is truly in trouble may share similar early signs with a very much larger number of other fetuses/infants, the great majority of whom would fare well if they survive without new interventions. In seeking to prevent irreversible brain injury from birth in a small proportion of term infants, we are faced with the possibility that interventions that may save a small number of babies might increase risk for a much larger number. To establish a basis for comparing risks and benefits, as well as costs, we must make wise use of randomized clinical trials.

—by Karin Nelson, M.D.

Dr. Nelson is affiliated with the Neuroepidemiology Branch (NEB), National Institute of Neurological Disorders and Stroke (NINDS), National Institutes of Health, Bethesda, Maryland.

References

1. Scott H. Outcome of very severe birth asphyxia. *Arch Dis Child* 51:712-716, 1976.

2. Nelson KB, Ellenberg JH. Apgar scores as predictors of chronic neurologic disability. *Pediatrics* 68:36-44, 1981.

3. Seidman D, Paz I, Laor A et al. Apgar scores and cognitive performance at seven years of age. *Obstet Gynecol* 77:875-878, 1991.

4. Grant A. Epidemiological principles for the evaluation of monitoring programs—the Dublin experience. *Clin Invest Med* 16:149-158, 1993.

5. Leviton A. Preterm birth and cerebral palsy: Is tumor necrosis factor the missing link? *Develop Med Child Neurol* 35:549-558, 1993.

6. Brenneman DE, Schultzberg M, Bartfai T, Gozes I. Cytokine regulation of neuronal survival. *J Neurochem* 58:454-460, 1992.

7. Sameroff A. Forward. In: Broman S, Bien E, Shaughnessy. *Low Achieving Children: The First Seven Years*. Hillsdale, NJ: Erlbaum Associates, pp. vii-xi, 1985.

8. Paneth N. The causes of cerebral palsy, recent evidence. *Clin Invest Med* 16:95-102, 1993.

9. Nelson KB, Ellenberg JH. Obstetric complications as risk factors for cerebral palsy or seizure disorders. *J Am Medical Assoc* 251:1843-1848, 1984.

10. Kelly JV, Iffy L. Chapter 63. Placenta previa. In: Iffy L, Kaminetzky HA (eds). *Principles and Practice of Obstetrics and Perinatology*. New York: Wiley & Sons, Vol 2, pp. 1105-1117, 1981.

11. Iyasu S, Saaftlas AK, Rowley DL et al. The epidemiology of placenta previa in the United States, 1979 through 1987. *Am J Obstet Gynecol* 168:1424-1429, 1993.

12. Naeye RL. *Disorders of the placenta, fetus, and neonate: Diagnosis and clinical significance*. St. Louis: Mosby, 1992.

13. Williams MA, Lieberman E, Mittendorf R et al. Risk factors for abruptio placentae. *Am J Epidemiol* 134:965-972, 1991.

14. Nelson KB, Ellenberg JH. The asymptomatic newborn and risk of cerebral palsy. *Am J Dis Child* 141:1333-1335, 1987.

15. Ellenberg JH, Nelson KB. Cluster of perinatal events identifying infants at high risk for death or disability. *J Pediatr* 113:546-552, 1988.

16. Levene MI, Grindulis M, Sands C, Moore JR. Comparison of two methods of predicting outcome in perinatal asphyxia. *Lancet* 1:67-68, 1986.

17. Hadders-Algra M, Huisjes HJ, Touwen BCL. Perinatal correlates of major and minor neurological dysfunction at school age: A multivariate analysis. *Develop Med Child Neurol* 30:472-481, 1988.

18. Klipstein CA, McBride MC. Predictors of cerebral palsy in perinatal hypoxic-ischemic encephalopathy (abstract). *Ann Neurol* 32:478, 1992.

19. Nelson KB, Leviton A. How much of neonatal encephalopathy is due to birth asphyxia? *Am J Dis Child* 145:1325-1331, 1991.

20. Nelson KB, Ellenberg JH. Antecedents of cerebral palsy. I. Univariate analysis of risks. *Am J Dis Child* 139:1031-1038, 1985.

21. Torfs CP, van den Berg BJ, Oechsli FW, Cummins S. Prenatal and perinatal factors in the etiology of cerebral palsy. *J Pediatr* 116:615-622, 1990.

22. Adamson SJ, Alessandri LM, Badawi N, et al. Predictors of neonatal encephalopathy in full-term infants. *Brit Med J* 311:598-602, 1995.

23. Portman RJ, Carter BS, Murphy MG et al. Predicting neonatal morbidity after perinatal asphyxia: A scoring system. *Am J Obstet Gynecol* 162:174-182, 1990.

24. Fee SC, Malee K, Deddish R et al. Severe acidosis and subsequent neurologic status. *Am J Obstet Gynecol* 162:802-806, 1990.

25. Dennis J, Johnson MA, Mutch LM et al. Acid-base status at birth in term infants and outcome at 4.5 years. *Am J Obstet Gynecol* 161:213-220, 1989.

26. Goldaber KG, Gilstrap LE III, Leveno KJ et al. Pathologic fetal acidemia. *Obstet Gynecol* 78:1103-1107, 1991.

27. Goodwin TM, Belai I, Hernandez P et al. Asphyxial complications in the term newborn with severe umbilical acidemia. *Am J Obstet Gynecol* 162:1506-1512, 1992.

28. Winkler CL, Hauth JC, Tucker M et al. Neonatal complications at term as related to the degree of umbilical artery acidemia. *Am J Obstet Gynecol* 164:637-41, 1991.

Chapter 47

Research Update: Pre-Term and Low Birthweight Infants

Summary

Preterm birth is the single greatest cause of newborn and infant mortality, and those who survive may develop lifelong sequelae. Furthermore, the high prematurity rate explains the United States relatively high infant mortality compared to that of other countries. Studies continue to clarify the normal onset of labor, the etiology of premature labor, and how it might be stopped without detrimental effects.

A significant number of deaths are caused by disorders of the newborn and many survivors suffer long-term disabilities. For the newborn, the continuous process of growth and maturation extends from the intrauterine milieu to the external environment where the infant must adapt to new conditions. Remarkable advances in the care of the small infant have taken place, but many problems remain. An overlapping goal of this area of research and that of preterm labor and birth is to reduce the risk of being born with a low birthweight, and not mature enough to adapt successfully.

Research Project Grants

Maternal psychosocial and physical stressors have been implicated in the birth of low birthweight infants. An investigator is attempting

From *Pregnancy and Perinatology Branch, National Institute on Child Health and Human Development (NICHD), Report to the National Advisory Child Health and Human Development (NACHHD) Council,* September 1995.

to identify previously unaccounted-for stressors in the workplace and home environment. A cohort of 600 women are being studied prospectively throughout pregnancy, with redesigned instruments to increase their sensitivity to the actual social, economic, cultural, and regional conditions of the individual woman.

An ongoing study is examining fetal cerebrovascular regulatory mechanisms and adaptations under normoxic conditions and in response to relatively prolonged hypoxemia. The investigator measured α_1 adrenergic receptors and/or inositol 1,4,5-triphosphate (in-P)$_3$ responses. It was determined that in near-term fetal and newborn sheep there is a marked variation in potencies of norepinephrine (NE) in contracting common carotid and middle cerebral arteries. Density of α_1-adrenergic receptors was high in the carotid and modestly high in combined anterior middle and posterior cerebral arteries and in cerebral micro vessels with the density decreasing as a function of developmental age. Marked regional differences were determined in cerebral vascular (in-P)$_3$ response to NE. Alpha, receptor density and (in-P)$_3$ responses in premature fetal cerebral vessels were less than in the near-term fetus. Of interest is that the magnitude of (in-P)$_3$ responses did not necessarily correlate with α_1-receptor density. The researcher speculates that decreased α_1-receptor-inositol coupling in the pre-term fetus may be an important factor in dysregulation of cerebrovascular blood flow in the premature infant.

Cerebral palsy (CP) is a leading cause of permanent neurologic impairment. Premature birth has emerged as a major risk factor for CP and, because of an increase in the number of surviving premature infants the prevalence of CP is rising. Two epidemiologic studies have demonstrated an inverse association between maternal magnesium sulfate (MgSO$_4$) administration and subsequent CP in the offspring. Whether MgSO$_4$ was used for seizure prophylaxis in preeclampsia or for tocolysis of preterm labor, the result was a lowered rate of CP. Based on findings in adult experimental animals, where Mg caused cerebrovasodilation, an investigator studied its potential effect on the newborn brain. In newborn piglets it was shown to cause cerebral vasodilation in a dose-dependent fashion.

Preeclampsia remains a major cause of maternal and fetal morbidity. In both preeclampsia and intrauterine growth retardation (IUGR), there may be marked alterations in the physiological dilatation of the spiral arteries characteristic of normal pregnancy. Consequently, maternal blood flow to the placenta may not be sufficient to provide oxygen and nutrients required for normal fetal growth and development. Investigators using the macaque model are determining the cellular mechanisms involved in the intravascular migration of trophoblast cells into the maternal spiral arteries and their role in modeling the arterial wall. They have identified a type IV collagenase enzyme (gelatinase A or MMP-2) which appears to be active in the invasive process and in the subsequent remodeling. It seems that this collagenase, and probably other proteinases, are active throughout gestation to accommodate the developing fetus.

The problem of preterm birth in the U.S. has failed recently to respond to major clinical intervention programs. A significant insight into the nature of the problem may be provided by an awardee who examined fetal growth. It had been suggested by several previous studies that preterm birth is associated with suboptimal fetal growth. In an observational cohort study, the awardee found for the first time that the type of fetal growth restriction is related to the cause of preterm birth. Specifically, infants delivered after spontaneous preterm labor or preterm premature rupture of membranes were symmetrically (or proportionally) smaller, whereas those delivered preterm for obstetric or medical indications had asymmetric growth patterns. These findings suggest that fetal growth retardation in the former spontaneous delivery group may start early in pregnancy and reflect a more chronic deprivation or stress. Thus, factors such as inadequate placentation and periconceptional nutrition may be possible factors in spontaneous preterm birth and probably deserve enhanced research attention. Also, clinical interventions in later pregnancy may not be effective in cases in which an earlier insult has already occurred.

Animal models have suggested that the combination of antenatal steroid and increased thyrotropin may enhance fetal lung maturity. A multi-center randomized controlled trial is assessing the effects of combined prenatal administration of corticosteroids and thyrotropin-releasing hormone to mothers in preterm labor on the incidence of chronic lung disease. Surfactant therapy is administered as required to the premature neonates. This study, which will be completed in 1996, will complement the findings of the Neonatal Research Network and the Consensus Development Conference on Antenatal Steroids.

Development of exogenous surfactant replacement therapy represented a major breakthrough in reducing the morbidity and mortality associated with preterm birth. An investigator has made a major contribution to the understanding of the pathophysiology of respiratory distress syndrome and the metabolism of surfactant proteins in replacement preparations. Studies of surfactant function and metabolism are complex because of its multicomponent lipid and protein nature, and the multiple form transitions, inactivation, and recycling events that occur in the alveolus. This laboratory has recently quantitated and integrated measurements of surfactant component metabolism and function in order to provide information to optimize surfactant therapy for respiratory distress syndrome. They have characterized surfactant activation, the effect of gestational age on endogenous surfactant effectiveness and activation of exogenous surfactant. They determined that activity of replacement surfactant containing SP-B is dependent on ventilation using positive end-expiratory pressure, and have obtained information regarding the amount of SP-B required to supplement the *in vivo* function of bovine surfactant. They are currently testing the hypothesis that ventilation style alters surfactant function and metabolism. This information combined with measurement of surfactant function from samples collected from SP-B and SP-C metabolism studies provides a uniquely integrated evaluation of surfactant within the preterm lung with respiratory distress syndrome.

Normal newborn pulmonary function involves control of pulmonary vascular tone. Endothelium-derived nitric oxide (NO), produced by the enzyme NO synthase (NOS), is a critical mediator of vasomotor tone in the developing lung. It plays a key role in the normal transition to extrauterine life and the pathophysiology of persistent pulmonary hypertension of the newborn (PPHN). One investigator is studying the mechanisms by which pulmonary endothelial NO production is modified by changes in oxygen and maturation. It was shown that prolonged *in vivo* hypoxia in the rat attenuates pulmonary endothelial NO production and that this process is unique to the pulmonary circulation. This suggests that decreased NO production may contribute to the pathogenesis of hypoxic pulmonary hypertension, which complicates many primary respiratory and cardiac disease states in the newborn, older children and adults. The studies of NOS protein and mRNA expression in this model indicate that diminution in pulmonary endothelial NO production may be related to impaired NOS function or altered availability of cofactors necessary for NOS activity. Experiments delineating the ontogeny of pulmonary endothelial NO production and NOS gene expression indicate that NO production is developmentally regulated, and that NOS gene expression is maximal late in gestation. These findings increase our understanding of the fundamental processes prerequisite for successful transition from fetal to postnatal existence. Finally, this investigator has established a pulmonary artery endothelial cell tissue culture system with which the processes regulating the activity of NOS can be investigated. Studies of 24-hour exposure to exogenous NO reveal upregulation of NOS expression and suggest that brief treatment with inhaled NO may not adversely affect the abundance of NOS *in vivo*.

Cooperative Agreements

In 1986, the National Institute of Child Health and Human Development (NICHD) established an administrative framework to conduct multicentric randomized clinical trials and other prospective clinical studies in both obstetrics and neonatology (MFMU and NICU Networks).

Why were the Networks established? A critical factor was the negligible decline in the rate of low birth weight during the last 40 years. Currently, more than 270,000 low birth weight infants (less than 2500 grams) are born annually in the U.S., with 48,000 of them considered "very low birth weight" (less than 1500 grams). These infants account for a disproportionately large share of infant morbidity and mortality, and subsequent developmental problems, such as cerebral palsy. The improvement in infant survival rates in the U.S. in recent years is largely attributed to increasingly effective neonatal intensive care of low birth weight infants.

However, in the neonatal intensive care nurseries, principles of management and innovative methodologies in this highly technical environment were changing within months, before rigorously controlled studies of their safety and efficacy could be initiated, much less completed. Further progress in perinatal health will depend not only in designing appropriate therapeutic regimens, but also on prevention of low birth weight. The primary purpose of the MFMU Network is to promote research emphasizing such prevention.

What are the advantages of clinical trials done within the Networks? First, the Networks provide a large enough population (approximately 60,000 births/year in the MFMU; and, 108,000 inborn infants/year of which more than 3,500 are ≤1500 grams birth weight in the NICU) to conduct studies with adequate statistical "power" to resolve many research questions. Inadequate sample size is a common limitation of many published clinical trials. Second, the study population is diverse, so that if a test management is shown to be effective across an array of ethnic and socio-economic backgrounds and health care settings, such a management is more likely to prove effective in "realworld" clinical practice. Third, the Biostatistics Coordinating Center attached to the Networks has sufficient resources to assure excellent data quality. Fourth, the collaborative Network approach is efficient and cost-effective because the administrative systems are developed and functioning. Thus, new trials can be brought "on-line" relatively rapidly.

The Networks provide one solution to the need for clinical trials in neonatology and obstetrics, especially those relating to the prevention of low birth weight infants and their management. They build upon previous contributions to the clinical trials field, but are somewhat unusual in that they rely to a greater extent on shared responsibility and commitment.

Investigators in both Networks agreed to collaborate using common protocols, definitions, and data forms and are linked by a common Biostatistics Center and distributed data entry computer system. Protocols are developed by the investigators with the aid of the NICHD staff and the BCC, and externally reviewed by both an Advisory Board and external reviewers.

For each Network a Data Safety and Monitoring Board has been established to ensure that the trials are safe and on target. The two Networks are achieving their purposes in a cost-effective manner, each center is awarded a minimal base budget, and is provided capitated funds for enrollment in specific protocols.

Maternal-Fetal Medicine Units (MFMU) Network

An important factor leading to the establishment of the Network was the growing recognition that modern obstetrical management—especially of high-risk pregnancies—has sometimes utilized treatments that have not been adequately tested for efficacy. Like most other medical specialties, maternal-fetal medicine has enthusiastically adopted certain managements, only to have to modify or replace them after extensive clinical experience has failed to confirm their promise. Thus, a purpose of the Network was to foster research that would provide better scientific evidence on which to base obstetric practice, particularly before widespread application of new approaches.

The Network originally included seven MFMU divisions at leading U.S. research universities, and was expanded in 1991 to encompass 11 centers. NICHD is closely involved in the selection of research topics, in the study designs, in analysis of data, and also provides funding for the Network.

Research Update: Pre-Term and Low Birthweight Infants

To illustrate the productivity of the Network, three examples of completed Network studies are presented:

Preeclampsia prevention in low-risk patients. Preeclampsia is a leading cause of fetal and maternal morbidity and death. Low-dose aspirin administration reportedly reduces the incidence of preeclampsia among pregnant women with certain medical and obstetrical risk factors for this condition. Our Network investigators wished to evaluate the possible benefit and safety of aspirin in healthy nulliparous women. Accordingly, 3,135 normotensive nulliparous women were entered into a randomized, double-blind clinical trail, one-half receiving matching placebo, starting during the second trimester of pregnancy. We observed a 26% reduction in the incidence of preeclampsia in the aspirin group, but this missed being statistically significant. Furthermore, patients taking aspirin did not experience any advantage in perinatal morbidity, but did show a higher risk for abruptio placenta. It was concluded, on the basis of these and other results, that low-dose aspirin should not be recommended to healthy nulliparous women. This conclusion may or may not apply to women with specific risk factors for preeclampsia, such as diabetes mellitus.

Antibiotic treatment of preterm labor with intact membranes. Preterm birth is the leading cause of perinatal morbidity and mortality. Adjunctive antibiotics to prolong pregnancy in patients with preterm labor with intact membranes have reportedly been effective in some randomized clinical trials. However, these studies have not demonstrated an improvement in perinatal morbidity and mortality as a result of antibiotic treatment. Our Network designed a randomized, double-blind, placebo controlled trial to assess the effect of intravenous and oral ampicillin and erythromycin or matching placebos, added to standard therapies of preterm labor, including tocolytics and steroids. Primary outcome variables were a composite of perinatal morbidity and mortality and pregnancy prolongation and frequency of preterm birth. Surprisingly, no significant difference in outcomes could be detected in the 277 patients studied. The power of the study was high in terms of assessing effects on pregnancy prolongation and preterm birth, but lower than expected for the effect on perinatal morbidity and mortality. This was so because of a lower than estimated prevalence of adverse perinatal outcome (14% actual versus 40% estimated). Thus, the investigators concluded that adjunctive antibiotics do not appear to be beneficial in the overall patient group having preterm labor with intact membranes. From a research standpoint, it may be reasonable to re-assess this intervention at a point in the future when, and if, subclinical infection can be identified rapidly in patients presenting in preterm labor.

Predictive factors for spontaneous preterm birth. This protocol addressed the difficult problem of identifying women at risk for spontaneous preterm birth so that preventive efforts can be focused on them. Several tests currently advocated to predict preterm birth were evaluated individually, and in combination, to determine their predictiveness. Tests included demographic, behavioral, psychosocial, anthropometric and historical profiles, cervical examination both digital and by ultrasound, genital tract vaginoses, genital tract fetal fibronectin, and various serum protein markers. Nearly 3,000 asymptomatic patients from the general obstetric population were evaluated. Three major findings have emerged so far: (1) The occurrence of bacterial vaginosis at 28 weeks gestation was associated with increased risk of spontaneous preterm birth, odds ratio (OR) 1.84, (95% C.I. 1.15-2.95 p<0.01); (2) Risk of preterm birth increases as cervical length (measured by ultrasound) decreases, with cervical length below the 10th percentile being the most predictive of preterm birth less than 35 weeks and (3) A positive cervical or vaginal fetal fibronection at 24 weeks predicted more than half of the spontaneous preterm births less than 28 weeks, making it one of the most promising biomarkers for preterm delivery ever identified.

Neonatal Intensive Care Units (NICU) Network

The original NICU Network was composed of seven participating university units, and later restructured to include 12 centers. They have expanded their original mission by planning studies including Full Term (FT) infants and updated its designation to NRN.

The first protocol initiated by the original Network was a 2,400 subject randomized trial of intravenous gamma globulin (IVIG) to prevent sepsis in infants ≤1500 grams. The trial demonstrated that IVIG is not effective in decreasing the incidence of nosocomial infection in very low birth weight (VLBW) infants. Subsequent to the publication of the trial, use of this expensive therapy has decreased dramatically. A second controlled randomized trial tested two major forms of exogenous surfactant replacement therapy for the treatment of respiratory distress syndrome (n=600). The trial demonstrated that the two surfactants were equally effective in preventing death and chronic lung disease in VLBW infants.

The Network has recently completed randomized controlled trials of "early" vs "late" steroids to decrease the time to successful extubation (n=370) in VLBW infants at risk for chronic lung disease and antenatal phenobarbital to prevent intracranial hemorrhage and early death in infants ≤33 weeks gestation (n=668 infants). The results of these studies are not yet available.

Currently the Network is collaborating with 10 Canadian centers in a randomized trial (n=250) testing the efficacy of inhaled nitric oxide to decrease the risk of death or extracorporeal membrane oxygenation (50% to 30%) in term and near-term infants with hypoxemic respiratory failure. Half the sample size has already been recruited. The Network is also participating in a randomized trial jointly cosponsored by the National Eye Institute (n=880) to test the efficacy of supplementary oxygen to prevent the progression of prethreshold retinopathy of prematurity. This 23-center trial requires computerized bedside adjustment of the infants' oxygen saturation and verified serial ophthalmologic examinations. A trial of supplementary vitamin A (n=780) to prevent chronic lung disease and nosocomial infection in VLBW infants is ready to begin enrollment. Because high vitamin A levels are teratogenic to the developing fetus, a pilot study (n=90) was completed to establish the appropriate dosing regimen for the intramuscular injections. Finally, three centers are comparing two state-of-the-art methods, DNA diagnosis and continuous blood culture reading, for the early diagnosis of neonatal infection. This pilot will provide information for a larger interventional trial.

An early activity of the Network was the creation of a detailed generic data base (GDB) on all infants born at ≤1500 grams. Designed to provide data on the consequences of neonatal disease and therapy, and to generate hypotheses for future studies, the GDB now has detailed data on more than 18,000 infants ≤1500 gms. Several summary papers on the status of newborn care have been published including a recent publication which documents improved survival without an increase in morbidity or length of hospital stay among 1804 inborn VLBW infants cared for between November 1989 and October 1990. The latest GDB paper on infants admitted in 1991-1992 (n=4279) reports a continued decline in mortality and morbidity in all VLBW birth weight classes over a five-year period. Although the overall survival for infants 501-1500 grams at birth is 81%, it is ≥ 92% in infants over 1000 grams at birth.

The Network has done a number of observational studies in the last five years, in addition to the randomized controlled trials. A bedside method to predict jaundice in healthy term infants was tested by measuring end tidal carbon monoxide in the exhaled breath. The study concluded that end tidal carbon monoxide levels may be helpful in understanding the mechanisms of jaundice in these infants in a variety of conditions.

A number of observational studies done document the impact of therapy on outcome. The introduction of artificial surfactant treatment of 2,780 infants 601-1300 grams at birth was associated with a sharp reduction in mortality from 27.8% before to 19.9%, suggesting that adoption of surfactant as part of routine clinical care would be widely effective. This conclusion was subsequently verified with a one-year decrease in the infant mortality rate of 6.2%. A Network study on the effectiveness of antenatal steroid (ANS) treatment of pregnant women to enhance fetal maturity in 9,949 VLBW infants revealed that ANS use was associated with a decreased risk for mortality, intracranial hemorrhage (ICH), respiratory distress syndrome, and chronic lung disease among 28-day survivors, even after artificial surfactants were introduced. Despite their demonstrated efficacy, ANS use ranged widely among centers (1 to 33%) in 1992; current Network use in VLBW infants is 81%. Among protective factors against severe ICH in VLBW infants, ANS was the only effective therapeutic intervention; protective factors included ANS treatment, black race, female infant gender, maternal hypertension, increasing gestational age, and increasing birth weight. Network studies indicate that the incidence and severity of severe ICH in VLBW infants is decreasing; comparable data on ICH term infants will soon be available.

The Network has undertaken several studies to predict outcome of care, resource utilization, and quality of care in VLBW infants. Among an entire birth weight cohort of 501-1500 gm inborn infants (n=3603), black race was associated with a decreased risk of mortality; however, among the tiniest infants 501-800 grams (n=1087), race had no discernable effect on survival but female gender had a survival advantage equivalent to a 112 g increase in birth weight. Observed survival ranged from 10 to 82% and total hospital days from 95 to 202 per survivor in these infants at the threshold of viability. These studies have concluded that until more accurate predictive models are developed and validated and the relationships between outcomes and care practices are better understood, the models should

Research Update: Pre-Term and Low Birthweight Infants

not be relied on for evaluating the quality of care provided in different NICUs.

Adequate nutrition and growth represents a critical issue in the outcome of VLBW infants. Studies to generate new growth curves for VLBW infants (n=1614) and to validate gestational age dating by early physical examination (n=1758) have recently been completed, but the data is not yet available. Finally, a standardized followup protocol for evaluating outcome of infants ≤1000 grams at 18-22 month corrected age has been defined and implemented. The followup protocol will provide the largest standardized followup assessment to date of infants <1000 grams at birth, which will be enhanced by detailed information from the GDB. The standardized followup protocol will also provide the ability to evaluate the outcome of the randomized trials.

Four Research Network sites are participating in a longitudinal observational study of the sequelae of intrauterine drug exposure cosponsored by NICHD, Agency for Children, Youth, and Families, National Institute on Drug Abuse, and Center for Substance Abuse Treatment. This study, dubbed the Maternal Lifestyle Study (MLS), includes mothers of infants of all gestational ages and compares the outcome of infants exposed to opiates or cocaine versus "background" exposure to alcohol, nicotine, and marijuana. Families are evaluated at nine visits during a 3-year period with pediatric developmental followup as well as a state-of-the art neurodevelopmental assessment battery. The battery includes a broad set of measures to look at infant physiologic state, attention and temperament, maternal-child interaction and attachment, maternal stress and depression, the neighborhood, ongoing exposure to drugs and violence, etc.

During the first two-years, MLS recruited over 19,000 mothers who were approached in the hospital after delivery. A history of their pregnancy and drug exposure was taken on all consenting mothers, their infants were examined, and meconium sent for drug testing. Approximately 1375 infants have been enrolled in the 3-year longitudinal followup study (a potential total of 12,375 followup visits). At each visit, ongoing drug abuse, the stability of the household, parenting skills, the services to which they have been referred, the type of interventions in which they and the baby are participating, exposure to violence, etc. will be assessed. A formal home visit is conducted at 10 months. Case managers and social workers are available at each clinic visit and by phone to refer the mother and baby to required services.

Networks Bibliography

Neonatal Research Network Publications

Fanaroff A, et al. Intravenous immunoglobulin: Prevention and treatment of disease. NIH Consensus Development Conference, May 21-23, 1990. Bethesda, MD pp.61-67.

Hack M, Horbar JD, Malloy MH, Tyson JE, Wright E, Wright L: Very low birth weight outcomes of the National Institute of Child Health and Human Development Neonatal Network. *Pediatrics* 1991; 87:587-597.

Malloy MH, Onstad L, Wright E and the NICHD Neonatal Research Network. The effect of cesarean delivery on birth outcome in very low birth weight infants. *Obstet Gynecol* 1991; 77:498-503.

Uauy RD, Fanaroff AA, Korones SB, Phillips EA, Phillips JB, and Wright LL for members of NICHD Neonatal Research Network. Necrotizing enterocolitis in very low birth weight infants: Biodemographic and clinical correlates. *J Pediatr* 1991; 119:630-8.

Horbar JD, Wright EC, Onstad L and the members of the NICHD Neonatal Research Network. Decreasing mortality associated with the introduction of surfactant therapy: An observational study of neonates weighing 601-1300 grams at birth. *Pediatrics* 1993; 92:191-196.

Horbar JD, Onstad L, Wright E, NICHD Neonatal Research Network. Predicting mortality risk for infants weighing 501 to 1500 grams at birth: A National Institute of Health Neonatal Research Network report. *Crit Care Med* 1993; 21:12-18.

Horbar JD, Wright LL, Soll RF, Wright EC, Fanaroff AA, Korones SB, Shankaran S, Oh W, Fletcher BD, Bauer CR, Tyson JE, Lemons JA, Donovan EF, Stoll BJ, Stevenson DK, Papile LA, Philips JB for the NICHD Neonatal Research Network. A multicenter randomized trial comparing two surfactants for the treatment of neonatal respiratory distress syndrome. *J Pediatr* 1993; 123:757-766.

Fanaroff AA, Korones SB, Wright LL, Wright EC, Poland RL, Bauer CR, Tyson JE, Philips JB, Edwards W, Lucey JF, Catz CS, Shankaran S, Oh W. A controlled trial of intravenous gamma globulin infusions to reduce nosocomial infections in very-low-birth-weight infants. *N Engl J Med* 1994; 330:1107-1113.

Stevenson DK, Vreman HJ, Oh W, Fanaroff AA, Wright LL, Lemons JA, Verter J, Shankaran S, Tyson JE, Korones SB, Bauer CR, Stoll BJ, Papile LA, Okah F, Ehrenkranz RA. Bilirubin production in healthy term infants as measured carbon monoxide in breath. *Clin Chem* 1994; 40:1934-1939.

Vreman HJ, Stevenson DK, Oh W, Fanaroff AA, Wright LL, Lemons JA, Wright E, Shankaran S, Tyson JE, Korones SB, Bauer CR, Stoll BJ, Papile LA, Donovan EF, Ehrenkranz RA. Semiportable electrochemical instrument for determining carbon monoxide in breath. *Clin Chem* 1994; 40:1927-1933.

Etches PC, Ehrenkranz RA, Wright LL. Clinical monitoring of inhaled nitric oxide. *Pediatr* 1995; 95:620-621.

Hack M, Wright LL, Shankaran S, Tyson JE, Horbar JD, Bauer CR, Younes N. Very-low-birthweight outcomes of the National Institute of Child Health and Human Development Neonatal Network, November 1989-October 1990. *Am J Obstet Gynecol* 1995; 172:457-464.

Shankaran S, Bauer CR, Bain R, Wright LL, Zachary J for the NICHD Neonatal Research Network. Antenatal steroid administration reduces grade III-IV intracranial hemorrhage in low birth weight infants. *Am J Obstet Gynecol* 1995; 173:305-12.

Stoll BJ, Fanaroff AA and the NICHD Neonatal Research Network. Early-onset coagulase negative staphylococcal sepsis in preterm neonate. *Lancet* 1995; 345:1236-7.

Wright LL, Horbar JD, Gunkel H, Verter J, Younes N, Andrews E, Long W. Evidence from multicenter networks on the current use and effectiveness of antenatal corticosteroids in low birthweight infants. *Am J Obstet Gynecol* 1995; 173:263-69.

Wright LL, Verter J, Younes N, Stevenson DK, Fanaroff AA, Shankaran S, Ehrenkranz RA, Donovan EF. Antenatal corticosteroid administration and neonatal outcome in very low birthweight infants: the NICHD Neonatal Research Network. *Am J Obstet Gynecol* 1995; 173:269-74.

Maternal Fetal Medicine Units Network Publications

Sibai BM, Caritis SN, Thom E, Klebanoff M, McNellis D, Rocco L, Paul RH, Romero R, Witter F, Rosen M, Depp R, and The National Institute of Child Health and Human Development Network of Maternal-Fetal Medicine Units. Prevention of preeclampsia with low-dose aspirin in healthy, nulliparous pregnant women. *N Engl J Med* 1993; 329:1213-1218.

Sibai BM, Reply to: Prevention of preeclampsia with low dose aspirin in healthy, nulliparous pregnant women. *N Engl J Med* 1994; 330:795.

Romero R, Sibai B, Caritis S, Paul R, Depp R, Rosen M, Klebanoff M, Sabo V, Evans J, Thom E, Cefalo R and McNellis D. Antibiotic treatment of preterm labor with intact membranes: A multicenter, randomized, double-blinded placebo-controlled trial. *Am J Obstet Gynecol* 1994; 169:764-774.

Romero R and Thom E. Reply to: Randomized controlled trials of antibiotics in preterm labor. *Am J Obstet Gynecol* 1994; 171:865-866.

NICHD Network of Maternal-Fetal Medicine Units. A clinical trial of induction versus expectant management in postterm pregnancy. *Am J Obstet Gynecol* 1994; 170:716-723.

Caritis S, Thom E, and McNellis D. Reply to: Comment on the effectiveness of induction of labor for postterm pregnancy. *Am J Obstet Gynecol* 1995; 172:241.

McNellis D and Caritis S. Reply to: On prolonged pregnancy. *Am J Obstet Gynecol* 1995; 172:1321-1322.

Landon M, Harger J. McNellis D, Mercer B, Thom E, for the MFMU Network of the NICHD. Prevention of neonatal group B streptococcal (Gbs) infection. *Obstet and Gynecol* 1994; 84:460-462.

Landon M, McNellis D, Thom E. Reply to: Prevention of neonatal group B streptococcal infection. *Obstet and Gynecol* 1995; 85:160-161.

Sibai B, Gordon T, Caritis S, McNellis D, Paul R, Thom E, Klebanoff M, Romero R, Depp R and Witter F. Risk Factors for preeclampsia in

Research Update: Pre-Term and Low Birthweight Infants

healthy nulliparous women: A prospective multicenter study. *Am J Obstet Gynecol* 1995; 172:642-648.

Sibai B, Caritis S, Thom E, Shaw K, McNellis D and the NICHD MFM Network, Bethesda, MD. Low-dose aspirin in nulliparous women: Safety of epidural and correlation between bleeding time and maternal-neonatal bleeding complications. *Am J Obstet Gynecol* 1995; 172:1553-1557.

Guinn D, Goldenberg R, Hauth J, Andrews W, Thom E, Romero R, The Department of Obstetrics and Gynecology at The University of Alabama at Birmingham, Birmingham, AL and The Biostatistics Center, The George Washington University, Rockville, MD and NICHD MFMU Units Network, Bethesda, MD. Risk factors for the development of preterm premature rupture of the membranes following arrest of preterm labor. *Am J Obstet Gynecol* (Accepted)

Iams J, Goldenberg R, Meis P, Mercer B, Moawad A, Das A, Thom E, McNellis D. Copper R, Johnson F, Roberts J, Miodovnik M, Van Dorsten J, Caritis S, Thurnau G, Bottoms S and the NICHD Maternal Fetal Medicine Unit Network, Bethesda, MD. The preterm prediction study: cervical sonography and risk of spontaneous prematurity. *N Engl J Med* (Accepted)

Meis P, Goldenberg R, Iams J, Mercer B, Moawad A, McNellis D, Roberts J, Das A, Copper R, Thom E, Johnson F, Andrews W, Miodovnik M, Van Dorsten J, Caritis S, Thurnau G, Bottoms S and the NICHD Maternal Fetal Medicine Unit Network, Bethesda, MD. The preterm prediction study: Significance of vaginal infections. *Am J Obstet Gynecol* (Accepted)

Goldenberg R, Iams J, Mercer B, Meis P, Moawad A, Copper R, Das A, Thom E, Johnson F, Roberts J, McNellis D, Miodovnik M, Van Dorsten J, Caritis S, Thurneau G, Bottoms S and the NICHD MFMU Network, Bethesda, MD. The preterm prediction study: Early fetal fibronectin testing predicts early spontaneous preterm birth. (Submitted *N Engl J Med*)

Chapter 48

Perinatal Emphases Research Centers

This program started in 1977 under the name of Major Research Programs (MRP) and the designation was changed to PERC (Perinatal Emphases Research Centers) in 1984 to highlight its importance to perinatology. The program is undergoing a further change in order to incorporate the eight active centers with other multidisciplinary projects in the same overall area. The final designation of the program is not yet decided but a working name being considered is Perinatal Research Program (PRP). The purpose of the program has not changed since its inception, the intent is to promote and support multidisciplinary research where knowledge gaps are not being sufficiently addressed by ongoing investigations or there are needs to stimulate and intensify efforts in promising research areas. Two PERCs are in the area of "Diabetes in Pregnancy," two centers support studies on "Intrauterine Growth Retardation (IUGR)," one is in "Fetal Hypoxia during Development," one addresses the issue of "Prematurity and the Initiation of Labor," one is examining "Fetal Maturation," and the latest center studies "Development of Infant Sleep." A multidisciplinary program has been reviewed recently centering on rural health with a major emphasis on infections, it will be incorporated in the PERCs. PERC investigators and NICHD staff meet every year to discuss goals, scientific achievements, and directions for future research. Summaries follow some of the accomplishments achieved since last report.

From *Pregnancy and Perinatology Branch, National Institute on Child Health and Human Development (NICHD), Report to the National Advisory Child Health and Human Development (NACHHD) Council*, September 1995.

Investigators interested in diabetes during pregnancy are studying the consequences of disorders of fetal metabolism on the mother and the newborn infant while obtaining normative data in humans describing the adaptive response of the mother during pregnancy. Studies involve women with gestational diabetes. One subproject is quantifying changes in gluconeogenesis and in the metabolism of a non-essential amino acid, serine, in normal pregnant women with advancing gestation. For that purpose, the group has developed a novel micromethod to quantify gluconeogenesis *in vivo*, using deuterium bound to carbon 6 of glucose at safe and acceptable doses. Another subproject is investigating the impact of the dietary mix of carbohydrate and exercise on maternal glucose and insulin responses to feeding and exercise, and on the rate and quality of placental and fetal growth and development. To date, in a relatively small number of subjects randomized to either a low glycemic diet and exercise or to a high glycemic diet, the results show striking differences. The first group has minimal glycemic and insulin responses to food intake, they gain less weight, have relatively slow mid-trimester placenta growth, and smaller placentas and infants at term.

Animal experiments (rats) were carried out to investigate the mechanisms responsible for metabolic alterations caused when fed a milk-formula high in carbohydrate (HC) derived calories during the suckling period. Rats fed the HC diet show early evidence of increased pancreatic insulin content and ß-cell hypertrophy which persists to adulthood, whereas those fed a high fat diet during the suckling period show no changes in pancreatic islets, glucose tolerance, or body weight. The HC fed group became obese in adult life. Female rats, artificially reared on the HC formula had hyperinsulinemia but were normoglycemic before and during pregnancy. Their offsprings, nursed by their own mothers and weaned onto a laboratory stock diet, also became obese. Therefore, the metabolic changes, which occurred in the first generation, were passed to the second generation, although these animals were fed a regular diet.

Since 1977, a center in the area of Diabetes in Pregnancy, continues with the overall objective of exploring the pathogenesis and pathophysiologies of the perinatal complications in the infants of diabetic mothers. One interesting aim was to clarify the mechanisms of early phase insulin release in pregnant women as a function of exercise training. A study encompassing 3 groups of women (non-pregnant, normal pregnant, and with gestational diabetes [GD]) concluded that glucose intolerance characterizing GD is not mediated by resistance to insulin suppression of glucose production but results from peripheral insulin resistance. Exercise training elicited similar physiologic changes in pregnant and non-pregnant states. In response to maternal exercise duration fetal heart rate increases and the amplitude of this effect augments with advancing gestational age.

A longitudinal study is accumulating anthropometric data on infants of GD mothers and is assessing the development of adiposity. The data on newborns shows a strong relationship between maternal weight, weight gain in pregnancy, and third trimester glucose values with infant birth weight. Control during pregnancy with insulin and diet versus diet alone correlated with a lower birth weight. At 4 years of age, children of GD mothers were observed resting more often during a free session and in general were rated as less active. The 4 year-old girls of GD mothers had the longest long sleep segment, spent more minutes motionless and more time asleep. Short-term behavioral interventions aimed at mothers during the perinatal period showed beneficial effects in early infant growth and parental adjustment in both the preterm and full-term samples.

A subproject is examining the effect on the brain of glucose homeostasis during the perinatal period. The animal model used simulates the human fetus in women with poorly controlled diabetes. It was observed that hyperglycemia reduces arterial oxygen content, increases brain blood flow and cerebral metabolic rate of oxygen. In addition it was shown that in the ovine fetus the blood-brain-barrier is relatively mature even at 60% gestation.

The long-term aim of a center addressing the issue of IUGR is to define and understand the basic physiology of fetal growth and pathophysiology of growth retardation. A major effort is centered on understanding the role of specific growth factors. Transforming growth factor $ß_1$ (TGF-$ß_1$) TGF-α and epidermal growth factor (EGF) do have a function in the growth and differentiation of distal respiratory epithelial cells during branching morphogenesis of embryonic mouse lung. Developmentally expressed TGF-$ß_1$ is an effector of the developing lung, and TGF-α and EGF treated murine fetal lungs in culture show reduced branching and tubule elongation. Studies with transgenic mice demonstrate pulmonary fibrosis and alveolar-hypoplasia and the mechanisms of TGF-α induction of fibrosis involves a paracrine epithelial to interstitial cell interaction, and occurs in the postnatal period of alveolarization.

A rat model of IUGR was developed, in which newborn rats are injected with EGF on days 0-3 of life, and as they grow they express enhanced differentiation at the expense of cell proliferation. The animals exhibit an asymmetric pattern of retardation, as seen in SGA humans, liver and kidney growth are impaired, whereas brain is relatively unaffected. The effect of EGF may be partially reversed by insulin growth factor I (IGF-I).

Interesting research has focused on the metabolic/thermoregulatory effects of EGF during the postnatal period of physiological adaptation as well as on structure-function relations associated with the terminal differentiation of the epidermis. Researchers were able to determine a quantitative estimate of the rate of stratum corneum formation in the rat fetus, which is approximately 1 layer every 5 hours. This stratum constitutes the rate limiting barrier to heat and water loss in the rat and also man. Its absence in preterm infants is associated with difficulties in water homeostasis and body temperature control. EGF is a potent regulator of epidermal cell growth and of the terminal differentiation of the epidermis. Studies demonstrated that a single dose of maternal glucocorticoid accelerates the appearance of skin surface hydrophobicity, an important adaptational property as shedding of surface water results in decreased latent heat of evaporation and better body temperature control.

Another center addresses the issues of IUGR and metabolism. The aim is to understand how the fetus adapts for survival to reduced energy (glucose) and anabolic hormone (insulin) supply; how these deficiencies lead to fetal growth retardation; and, what the fetal metabolic consequences are. For that purpose they have developed models in large animals that consistently, controllably, and reproducibly produce fetal growth retardation. Using transabdominal ultrasound, investigators examined fetal growth prospectively and developed growth curves from day 50 through 130 in control and heat-stressed ewes. Measurements of fetal abdominal circumference and biparietal diameter confirm asymmetry of fetal growth in this model. The investigators have documented that chronic hypoglycemia of 2-3 weeks duration in pregnant sheep in late gestation resulted in fetal growth retardation; however, growth did not cease, it only slowed down. It was noted that during sustained hypoglycemia fetal glucose utilization decreases, but not to the same extent that umbilical glucose uptake does. These experiments, in combination with leucine tracer studies, demonstrate that the response to chronic glucose deficiency is normal metabolism of this amino acid (aa), which is essential for fetal utilization and growth. Therefore, a slower rate of growth is an adaptation that permits less tissue to be produced, but relatively normal metabolism of that tissue. During marked fetal hypoglycemia, cerebral studies showed little capacity for alternate fuel (lactate) uptake. Fetal effects to glucose and insulin deprivation can begin as early as midgestation, showing acute adaptation with fetal proteolysis and (aa) oxidation and conversion to glucose via gluconeogenesis; while chronically, the adaptation is towards the substitution of a slower rate of growth, substrate utilization, and oxygen consumption in order to preserve a smaller amount of still normally functioning fetal tissue.

Human studies demonstrate in IUGR pregnancies a lower maternal/fetal gradient for (aa) and virtually no demonstrable uptake of (aa) into the umbilical circulation at Cesarean section. These findings suggest that intervention strategies to treat IUGR pregnancies should include attempts to increase (aa) transport across the placenta.

A center interested in fetal hypoxia during development has based their studies on the tenet that understanding the extent of and mechanisms underlying the adaptive responses to limitations in oxygen and nutrient availability of various fetal systems can provide new diagnostic approaches to identify abnormalities induced by growth restrictions, or perinatal drug abuse, and possibly a neurodevelopmental basis for SIDS. Initial studies demonstrated that the neuropeptide corticotropin releasing hormone (CRH) is synthesized and released by the placenta, that placental CRH directly stimulates secretion of glucocorticoid and adrenal androgens from the fetal adrenal, and CRH synthesis is stimulated under conditions of chronic stress such as hypoxia. Clinical evidence suggests that placental CRH may modulate maternal and fetal pituitary-adrenal function in human pregnancy.

These investigators have developed a model for mild chronic fetal hypoxemia and IUGR in the sheep. This model has provided evidence for a broad range of adaptive capacities of the fetus. Despite the presence of elevated catecholamines and significant chronic hypoxemia and hypoglycemia, the renal and cardiovascular functions of these fetuses with IUGR were similar to their controls.

Techniques were developed to permit chronic studies of the fetus of nonhuman primate. A unique tether system suitable for chronic studies in the pregnant baboon was established and studies showed distinctive aspects of the activation of the fetal hypothalamo-hypophyseal axis in response to hypoxia. Normative studies have been done to define the maturational course of fetal breathing activity, cardiorespiratory interactions, diurnal processes, patterns of EEG activity, and behavioral state. It was shown that periodic breathing is present in both quiet and active sleep with a circadian periodicity. Studies are underway to clarify the effect of hypoxia on these parameters.

Studies in preterm infants are exploring their activity and responses to nutrient and oxygen supply. The investigator is examining the effect of variations in nutrient intake on the ratio of the plasma concentration of tryptophan to the sum of other large neutral (aa), and see if increases in this ratio are associated with alterations of physiological and behavioral variables consistent with increased central serotonergic activity.

One of the long standing centers focuses on mechanisms involved in the initiation of human parturition with the aim of clarifying the problem of preterm birth. The clinical component addresses several issues, one of which is the relationship between parturition and the accumulation of mediators of the inflammatory response in amniotic fluid. It was shown that the accumulation is the consequence and not the cause of labor either at term or preterm. Another goal is to define the sequence of appearance of markers of bimolecular adaptations of the myometrium prior to the onset of labor. One of the studies examined the cross-linked interstitial collagens that are the principal source of tensile strength of the fetal membranes. It was demonstrated that they are produced exclusively in the mesenchymal cells of the amnion. The activity of interstitial collagenase which effects the degradation of this collagen is inhibited by tissue inhibitor of metalloproteins-1 (TIMP-1) which is also localized in the mesenchymal cells.

Another component is attempting to define the bimolecular processes that regulate the expression of proteins involved in the transition from uterine quiescence to preparation for labor. These studies use human uterine (decidual and myometrial) cells in culture. They are examining systematically the actions of the components of the endothelin/ enkephalinase-parathyroid hormone-related protein system in the uterus and the amnion-chorion vessels. It was shown that the production of this protein is increased by several transforming growth factors (TGF-ß1, ß2, ß3) in endometrial stromal cells and by TGF- ß1 and ß3 in myometrial smooth muscle cells. These findings suggest that these paracrine-acting factors may be important in modulating smooth muscle activity.

A third component has as a long range goal to characterize pregnancy-induced biochemical changes of myometrial cells, which may play a role in uterine quiescence. One finding showed that the plasma membrane $Ca^{2}+$ and the sarcoplasmic reticulum $Ca^{2}+$ pumps activities were similar in myometrium of pregnant and non-pregnant women leading to the conclusion that adaptations may include progesterone-induced modifications of receptor-mediated increases in $Ca^{2}+$ concentrations.

Also under study is the effect of uterine distention on biochemical and mechanical properties of myometrial tissues. They highlight that during pregnancy cellular adaptations are brought about by mechanical forces that result in marked increases in stress-generating capacity and these are independent of estrogen-induced increases in myosin content. It was also determined that although stretch alone (in the absence of estrogen) induces protein synthesis and increased amounts of myosin, stretch-induced adaptations of uterine smooth muscle during pregnancy are independent of myosin content or the extent of light chain of myosin. The role of nitric oxide (NO) in maintaining myometrial relaxation during pregnancy was examined and findings were not supportive of a direct effect of NO on myometrial smooth muscle during pregnancy.

Research on Sudden Infant Death Syndrome (SIDS) is carried out at one of the centers. The objectives are to characterize the development of circadian and homeostatic sleep mechanisms, sleep architecture, respiration and thermal components in an animal model for SIDS, and a clinical study examining the potential role of environmental and body temperatures in SIDS.

Studies in rat pups have shown that the development of the biological clock affects sleep-wakefulness. The ontogeny of augmented sleep drive clearly precedes the emergence of biological clock-dependent alerting, creating a developmental window of unopposed and augmented sleep drive. An interesting finding points to a brief developmental window during which temperature can have an increased influence on arousal state distribution. Investigators are concentrating efforts to clarify the normal physiology and molecular function of the suprachiasmatic nuclei of the hypothalamus where a circadian pacemaker synchronizes a number of physiologic systems including sleep and temperature control.

Studies examining the development of circadian systems in humans have looked at the effect of the NICU environment on preterm infants. Their biological rhythmicity just before discharge is dominated by ultradian components that correlate highly with feeding highlighting the effect of episodic interventions. Epidemiological data links temperature and SIDS and it is hypothesized that it plays an integral role through its influence on sleep distribution, arousal, and control of breathing. In adults thermal and respiratory control is severely inhibited in active sleep (REM). In newborns (who spend a high percentage of time in REM sleep) it was found that an important thermoregulatory effector mechanism, evaporative water loss, seems to continue to function in some infants during REM sleep. Studies continue to elucidate the relationship between ambient and body temperature with breathing patterns, incidence of obstructive apneas, and arousal responses to changes in the infant's environment.

Investigators at one of the newest centers are directing their efforts to the area of prematurity with the goal of developing new approaches to achieve fetal maturation when preterm birth is likely to occur. The aim is to assess "global" fetal maturation anticipating that it will improve outcomes by minimizing many postnatal complications of prematurity. Researchers are targeting four critical organ systems: kidney, neuroendocrine, vascular, and the lung. Initial studies in 138 day preterm newborn lambs determined the glucocorticoid dose and treatment duration capable of evoking altered cardiovascular and renal adaptations in the immediate postnatal period. The administration of a single 0.5 mg/Kg betamethasone dose 48 hours prior to delivery produced an increased newborn glomerular filtration rate (GFR) and sodium reabsorption in response to acute volume expansion. The increase in GFR results primarily from an increased filtration fraction, due to changes in renal vascular resistance. It also improved the animals ability to maintain blood pressure as it reduced the circulating levels of angiotensin II and arginine vasopressin, two potent vasoactive agents important for the regulation of peripheral vascular tone and renal function. It was also determined that in very immature animals (121 days gestation) there was a modest but significant response to antenatal hormone therapy, manifested by improvement in mean arterial blood pressure, and left ventricular contractility.

Studies regarding Endothelium-Derived Nitric Oxide (EDNO) showed that its role in modulating tone differs between pulmonary arteries and veins in fetal lambs. Antenatal betamethasone potentiates EDNO-mediated relaxation in pulmonary veins of preterm lambs, probably by increasing soluble guanylate cyclase activity in vascular smooth muscle cells. A similar effect was observed in coronary arteries which may contribute to improved myocardial function in the preterm newborn. In addition, steroid treated premature lambs had a higher concentration of DNA in systemic vessels, suggesting cell proliferation. Studies in humans are just beginning, using vascular rings from umbilical cords, to assess their response to vasoconstricting and vasodilating agents. The positive effects of betamethasone treatment is enhanced with the addition of T_4 but only in the lung, no additional increases were observed in the cardiovascular and renal systems.

Part Eight

Resources for Further Help and Information

Chapter 49

National Directory of Hydrocephalus Support Groups

Introduction

The Hydrocephalus Association has produced this National Directory for the purpose of identifying active Hydrocephalus Support Groups. It is the mission of the Association to insure that families and individuals dealing with the complexities of hydrocephalus receive personal support, comprehensive educational materials and access to on-going quality care.

We identified active groups and sent them a questionnaire. The groups listed in the Directory responded and we have described each organization verbatim from the questionnaires. Please notify the Hydrocephalus Association of errors or omissions. (*Denotes non-profit status of groups listed in the Directory.)

Although this Directory was produced by the Hydrocephalus Association of San Francisco, California, it is a wonderful example of the power of networking. We thank all our colleagues for participating in this project.

As Hydrocephalus Support Groups we share a common mission:

- To better the lives of individuals with hydrocephalus and to create a community of patients, families and healthcare professionals

---

Produced by Hydrocephalus Association, 870 Market Street, Suite 955, San Francisco, California 94102, (415) 732-7040, FAX (415) 732-7044, November 1996; reprinted with permission.

addressing the complexities of life-long care for those with hydrocephalus.

Arizona

Phoenix

Children's Hydrocephalus Connection*
909 Brill Street
Phoenix, Arizona 85006
Telephone: (602) 237-4156; Fax: (602) 254-7202
Contact Melani Jaskowiak, BSN, RN, CNRN, Neuroscience Nurse Clinician

Founded in 1993, the Children's Hydrocephalus Connection is sponsored by Phoenix Children's Hospital and promotes family directed care through education and support of children and families with hydrocephalus.

Resources/Programs

- Spring and Fall Meeting/support, education and social
- Annual Fall Conference
- Quarterly Newsletter
- Living with Hydrocephalus, notebook of information from the Hydrocephalus Association as well as community resources
- Parent to Parent support through telephone network.

California

Lakewood

Spirits of Survival (S.O.S.)
12413 Centralia Rd.
Lakewood, California 90715
Telephone: (310) 402-3523; Fax: (310) 924-6666
E Mail: DAFSPLACE.aol.com.
Contact: Debbie Fields

Founded in 1995, Spirits of Survival assists and educates the family, friends, and those affected by hydrocephalus. They are dedicated to

National Directory of Hydrocephalus Support Groups

those people in the Greater L.A. area and have members throughout the state and country.

Resources/Programs

- Bi-monthly meetings/support, education and social
- A booklet for adults written by Debbie Fields
- Distribution of National Hydrocephalus Foundation information materials
- On-going networkings by phone, letter, cassettes and the Internet.

San Francisco

Hydrocephalus Association*
870 Market Street, Suite #955
San Francisco, California 94102
Telephone (415) 732-7040; Fax (415) 732-7044
Office Hours: Mon & Thurs 10-2: Tues & Fri, 9-4: Wed, 10-12 Pacific Time
Emily S. Fudge, Executive Director;
Jennifer Henerlau, Assistant Director

Founded in 1983, the Hydrocephalus Association is a national organization whose goal is to insure that families and individuals, living with the often complex issues of hydrocephalus, receive personal support, comprehensive educational and resource materials, and are empowered by the knowledge of proper medical care.

Resources/Programs

- About Hydrocephalus—A Book for Parents 36 pages in English or Spanish

- The Resource Guide: listing of 319 articles on topics pertaining to hydrocephalus that may be ordered from the Association

- Directory of Pediatric Neurosurgeons: alphabetical/geographical listing of more than 180 pediatric neurosurgeons nationwide

- Fact and Information Sheets: Hydrocephalus, Adult Onset Hydrocephalus, Primary Care of the Child with Hydrocephalus,

Learning Disabilities in Children with Hydrocephalus, Eye Problems Associated with Hydrocephalus, Social Skills Development in Children with Hydrocephalus, Survival Skills for the Family Unit, IEP-Communication Skills for Parents, How to be an Assertive Parent on the Treatment Team, Preparing Your Child for Surgery, Tax Considerations for Parents of Disabled Children

- LINK Program: nationwide network of more than 400 individuals and families listed in Directory format giving members direct access to others

- Quarterly Newsletter

- Regional educational meetings and social gatherings

- Bi-Annual National Conference—4th Conference, January 12-14th, 1996, Monterey, California; 5th Conference, Spring 1998, east coast site.

- Annual Scholarship to a young adult with hydrocephalus to further his/her education

- Annual Research Prize to a Resident in Neurosurgery.

Georgia

Lawrenceville

National Hydrocephalus Foundation*
1670 Green Oak Circle
Lawrenceville, Georgia 30243
(770) 995-9570; FAX (770) 995-8982
Ann Marie Liakos, Executive Director

Founded in 1979, The National Hydrocephalus Foundation is a national organization dedicated to the education, advocacy and support of individuals affected by hydrocephalus, their families, and the professionals who specialize in their education, therapeutic intervention and medical care.

Resources/Programs

- Hydrocephalus Survey
- Educational Video
- Symposiums
- Reference Reading Lists
- Resource Support Library
- Quarterly 20 page newsletter
- Informational Brochures.

Massachusetts

Worcester

Hydrocephalus Support Group*
55 Lake Ave. N.
Worcester, Massachusetts 01655
(508) 856-3403; FAX (508) 856-5074
Kathleen M. Davidson, RN, NP

Founded in 1992, the Hydrocephalus Support Group provides support and education to patients and families.

Resources/Programs

- Monthly support group meeting, some with speakers
- Shunt information available upon request
- Parent to Parent referrals.

Michigan

Detroit

Hydrocephalus Support Group
Children's Hospital of Michigan
3901 Beaubien
Detroit, Michigan 48201
(313) 833-4490; FAX (313) 993-8744
Contact: Mary Smellie-Decker, RN, MSN, Clinical Nurse Specialist, Neurosurgery

Founded in 1992, the Hydrocephalus Support Group provides information and support to families.

Resources/Programs

- Monthly meetings, October-May, to provide support and education

- Quarterly Newsletter—*Channels*

- Brainstormers—Support group for children and adolescents with hydrocephalus

- STARS—Seeking Techniques Advancing Research in Shunts—Fundraising portion of the support group. The group's focus is raising funds for research.

Missouri

Chesterfield

Hydrocephalus Support Group, Inc.*
P.O. Box 4236
Chesterfield, Missouri 63005
(314) 532-8228
Debby Buffa, Founder and Chairman

Founded in 1986, the Hydrocephalus Support Group, Inc. provides information, education and support to anyone dealing with hydrocephalus.

Resources /Programs

- Booklets on hydrocephalus
- Listing of other groups
- Parent information
- List of over 200 research articles dealing with hydrocephalus
- Newsletter
- Yearly day-long conference on hydrocephalus

National Directory of Hydrocephalus Support Groups

New York

Brooklyn

Guardians of Hydrocephalus Research Foundation*
2618 Avenue Z
Brooklyn, New York 11235
(718) 743-GHRF; 1 (800) 458-8655; FAX: (718) 743-1171
Michael Fischetti, Founder, Chairman of the Board; Katherine Soriano, National Vice-President

Founded in 1977, The Guardians of Hydrocephalus Research Foundation offers an information and referral service to the afflicted hydrocephalic, nationwide.

Resources/Programs

- Hydrocephalus information packet
- An Introduction to Hydrocephalus, an information booklet in English and Spanish for parents and lay people
- Video: Hydrocephalus, A Neglected Disease
- Satellite Information Centers and Parent Networking
- Newsletter.

New York City

New York University Medical Center
Auxiliary of Tisch Hospital
560 1st Avenue
New York, New York 10016
(212) 263-5040
Contact: Doris Farrelly or Pat Noel

The Auxiliary of Tisch Hospital and the Division of Pediatric Neurosurgery co-sponsors a yearly symposium on hydrocephalus for families and professionals. The program is held in early June.

Resources/Programs

- HYDRONET (Hydrocephalus Network of Greater New York): A social/support group to assist and support parents of children with hydrocephalus. This group sponsors an annual holiday party and annual summertime picnic for all family members. For more information, please contact: Jackie Pamlanye (516) 588-9402; Maggie O'Brien (516) 797-1027; Cathleen Whelan (516) 294-6219.

Rhode Island

North Kingston

AHEAD (Association of Hydrocephalus Education, Advocacy and Discussion)
29 Water Wheel Lane
North Kingston, Rhode Island 02852
(401) 295-9738
Elizabeth Welker

AHEAD was organized by young adults with hydrocephalus for the purpose of providing telephone support nationwide.

Texas

Dallas

Hydrocephalus Association of North Texas (HANT)*
P.O. Box 670552
Dallas, Texas 75637
(214) 523-1505; FAX (214) 528 8097
Contact: Jana Dransfield

Founded in 1987, the Mission of the Hydrocephalus Association of North Texas is to provide information and support to parents of children with hydrocephalus. They serve the state of Texas and neighboring states. Their primary goal is to meet the needs of the family immediately following the birth of their child with hydrocephalus and to provide support, information and advocacy information to families as their child grows.

Resources/Programs

- Quarterly educational meetings

National Directory of Hydrocephalus Support Groups

- Quarterly Newsletter
- Area Resource List and Referral
- About Hydrocephalus—A Book for Parents
- Periodical and Tape Library
- Information on other local groups as well as access to state advocacy groups and information
- Pilot Parents available for telephone and hospital support
- Annual Conference on Hydrocephalus at Children's Medical Center of Dallas.

Chapter 50

Hydrocephalus Association on the Internet and the World Wide Web

The internet is a growing source of information on all sorts of topics. The Hydrocephalus Association is working on ways to use this resource to help further our mission of support, education and advocacy. One way is to post information about hydrocephalus and our organization where it can be easily found; other ways include having an e-mail address for correspondence and supporting efforts like the HYCEPH-L mail list server at the University of Toronto.

The Hydrocephalus Association has been posting information to the Internet World Wide Web (WWW). Our home page can currently be found at:

http://neurosurgery.mgh.harvard.edu/ha/

What Is the World Wide Web?

Basically this is a vast set of documents stored on thousands of computers around the world; each document is "electronically" linked to other documents on the same computer, as well as to documents on other computers. These documents can contain text as well as pictures, sounds, movies, etc. Most people with a moderately powered personal computer, modem (at least 9600 bps speed) and an account with a "service provider" such as America Online, Compuserve, etc., can access the "web" of documents using a computer application called a "web browser."

From Hydrocephalus Association *Newsletter*, Winter 1996; reprinted with permission.

How can I find information on the WWW?

Web documents have addresses (called URLs) that typically look like the Hydrocephalus Association home page address above. You'll see these in advertisements and articles of most newspapers today. Your web browser application will have a way to open a document where you simply type in this address exactly as it has been specified (with all the colons, forward slash characters, periods, lower-case vs. upper-case, etc.). Some web documents provide ways to search for information when you don't have the address. For example, the document at the address http://www.yahoo.com provides access to a powerful search engine and database of many of the millions of documents available on the World Wide Web.

HYCEPH-L: An Information and Support Forum for Hydrocephalus

HYCEPH-L is an e-mail list for people with hydrocephalus, their friends and family members, health care professionals and anyone else with an interest in the condition. The purpose of the e-mail list is to share information and support in dealing with hydrocephalus. The computer support for this list is donated by the University of Toronto. The list is run by Jayne Butler, currently a doctoral student in Adult Education at the university.

What Is an E-Mail List?

This is a common method on the Internet for a group of people with a common interest to communicate with one another. A list server computer keeps a list of the e-mail addresses of all the people in the group. When a member of that group wants to send an e-mail to all the other members, they send the e-mail to a special address that the computer listens to (in this case "hyceph-l@vm:utcc.utoronto.ca"). Their E-mail is copied by that computer and re-sent to everyone currently on the group list.

When you subscribe to the list you will probably receive anywhere from zero to a dozen e-mail messages from other people on this list every day, asking questions, giving information and discussing various issues related to hydrocephalus.

Hydrocephalus Association on the Internet and the WWW

How Do I Subscribe?

To subscribe to HYCEPH-L, address an e-mail message to the list server computer at:

listserv@vm.utcc.utoronto.ca

In the body of the message put:

subscribe HYCEPH-L Your first name Your last name

The list server computer ignores other fields like the subject of the message. When you send this "subscribe" message, the list server will immediately send you an introductory note containing more information. This information will tell you how to send an e-mail so that it is copied and sent to all other group members, how to send the list server computer other useful commands, and how to correspond with the list owner (a real person).

Go For It!

It may be a bit confusing at first, since you will be using different e-mail addresses: one to send mail to all group members, one to communicate to the list server computer itself, one for questions to the list owner (Jayne Butler), and specific group members addresses for private e-mail to only one or two people. Be patient, give it some time, and you'll soon be an expert!

—by Larry Kenyon, the past President of the Board of Directors and our resident computer expert.

Chapter 51

United Cerebral Palsy Associations on the Internet

Join Us on the Internet

For the last three years, first United Cerebral Palsy Associations' Program Services Department—and now the Technology Projects Group—has been providing leadership in the active pursuit of "electronic avenues" on the ever-changing Internet.

Since August, 1995, multiple UCPA program and technology initiatives have been highlighted in various World Wide Web sites. An initial "gateway" to each site allows users to select from "graphics plus text" or "text only" formats, enabling site visitors to choose the option that meets their sensory, hardware, and time preferences. Point your browser to the listed addresses (URLs), or use the handy links at each of our sites, to check out our Internet locations:

UCPA WWW Site

http://www.ucpa.org/

Our newest site serves as a gateway to our other Internet locations, it features:

- Easy links to other UCPA WWW and Internet locations;
- Easy links to affiliate WWW sites;

From *UCP Across America*, Summer 1996, copyright United Cerebral Palsy Associations; reprinted with permission.

- Downloadable text versions of the United Cerebral Palsy Research & Educational Foundation fact sheets;
- Opportunities to nominate other sites that have great content and access features; and
- A "Donation Station" that invites global talent and equipment donation.

TECH TOTS WWW Site

http://www.ucpa.org/TECHTOTS.html

Visit the TECH TOTS WWW site, for these features:

- Basic information about the TECH TOTS technology lending library network;
- A changing contest for kids;
- A schedule of TECH TOTS training events;
- A growing studio of kids' computer artwork—to which you can contribute;
- A "Donation Station" that invites global talent and equipment donation;
- Links to WWW sites of other TECH TOTS sites;
- A kid-to-kid pen pal service; and
- A challenge to users to nominate "best Internet sites" for kids and families.

Assistive Technology Funding and Systems Change Project WWW Site

http://www.assisttech.com/atfsc.html

UCPA's Assistive Technology Funding and Systems Change Project provides technical assistance and training, and also disseminates information to parents, family members, attorneys, advocates, and others, to assist them in promoting systems change and advocacy activities which remove assistive technology funding barriers. Site features include:

- Text files of documents produced by the project, including reviews of current funding streams, Q&As about funding options, funding decision case reports, and more;
- Key project contact points, featuring direct e-mail access;

United Cerebral Palsy Associations on the Internet

- A changing cartoon feature;

- Links to key Internet locations on complementary topics; and

- An interactive Guest Book featuring a changing mini-poll, to secure input on funding-related questions.

ADA WWW Site

http://www.assisttech.com/SEDBTAC.html

Two of UCPA's ADA grant initiatives, in conjunction with the UCPA Technology Projects Group, host this site. Visit this site for:

- National contact points on the ADA;

- A variety of downloadable text files, including approved press releases, regulations, guidance, small business supports, enforcement updates, and more;

- Information on ADA publications;

- Key contact points, featuring direct e-mail access;

- Links to key Internet ADA resource sites;

- A variety of training supports, including an events calendar, a directory of Southeast ADA trainers, online courses, and reviews of frequent ADA concerns;

- Southeast Regional ADA news updates; and

- A challenge and invitation to users to nominate "great ADA Internet sites," as well as sites that offer exemplary access options.

On the Edge (of Employment) WWW Site

http://www.assisttech.com/edge.html

Two of UCPA's employment-focused projects, in conjunction with UCPA's Technology Projects Group, host this site. Visit this site for these features:

- Text files highlighting UCPA employment projects and services;
- Real-life employment success stories;
- Information on UCPA's employment-focused products;
- Updates on national employment initiatives;
- Key contact points, featuring direct e-mail access; and
- Links to key Internet locations.

For More Information

Do you have questions about any of UCP's national Internet resources? Reach Gretchen Olson at the following contact points, or e-mail staff directly from each Internet site: Phone: (800) USA-5-UCP or (202) 776-0406; Fax: (202) 776-0414; E-mail: golson@ucpa.org

Chapter 52

Resources for People with Facial Differences

The resources listed in this chapter were selected by Betsy Wilson, Director of Let's Face It in the USA and editor of *Resources for People with Facial Difference*, a comprehensive 40-page resource guide that describes organizations, books, videotapes, and much more. The guide is published annually by:

Let's Face It, A Network for People with Facial Difference
Box 29972
Bellingham, WA 98228-1972
(360) 676-7325
e-mail: letsfaceit@faceit.org

The guide contains separate sections for parents, teenagers, and cancer survivors. For a free copy of the complete guide, send a 9x12 self-addressed stamped envelope, with $3.00 postage and a note about yourself to Let's Face It. You can also visit their web site at http://www.faceit.org/~letsfaceit/

Organizations

AboutFace

AboutFace is an international organization providing support and information to families or individuals with facial difference. Networking

Resources listed in this chapter are excerpted from *Resources for People with Facial Difference*, © 1996 Let's Face It; reprinted with permission.

database maintained at each of the national offices and with local chapters and contact people. Resources include newsletters, videos, publications, lending libraries, and more. Publications for families include: "My Newborn has a Facial Difference," "You, Your Child and the Craniofacial Team," "Appert, Crouzon and other Craniosynostosis Syndromes," and a school program package for teachers or parents entitled "We all have different faces. " Another resource, "Making the Difference," is an orientation package for health care providers in community hospitals experiencing the birth of a child with a facial difference. Membership: $20 per year. (Anna Pileggi, AboutFace, 99 Crowns Lane, Toronto, Canada M5R 3P4; 416/944-3223, 800/665-3223; FAX 416/944-2488; U.S. Office, Pam Onyx, Box 93 Limekiln, PA 19535; 800-225-FACE; FAX 610/689-4479; e-mail: abtFace@AOL.com)

The American Cleft Palate; Craniofacial Association (ACPA)

Dedicated to all aspects of facial birth defects, this 53 year old international network of professionals includes over 30 disciplines. With all aspects of patient and family care being represented, they are working to establish standard guidelines for care and for fair insurance coverage. They are encouraging the team approach to the care of all patients. Membership, $125 per year, benefits include the bimonthly "Cleft Palate-Craniofacial Journal," the quarterly newsletter, informational mailings, and discount registration fees to scientific meetings. These meetings are dynamic professional total care meetings. If you are interested in a particular area of care do call the ACPA office to connect with those who have presented on that subject. (Nancy Smythe, 1218 Grandview Avenue, Pittsburgh, PA 15211; 412/481-1376; FAX 412/481-0847)

Craniofacial Foundation of America

Serves as a national resource for patients and families with craniofacial anomalies. It produces educational materials and networks patients and families. The foundation offers financial support for non-medical expenses to patients traveling for evaluation and treatment to the Tennessee Craniofacial Center. Their latest free publication is "Craniosynostosis: Diagnosis and Current Surgical Treatment." (Terri Farmer Tennessee Craniofacial Center, T.C. Thompson Children's Hospital, Erlanger Medical Center, 975 East Third Street, Chattanooga, TN 37403; 423/778-9192, 800/418-3223)

Resources for People with Facial Differences

FACES

The National Association for the Craniofacially Handicapped. People with craniofacial deformities resulting from birth defects, injuries or disease may apply to this nonprofit organization for financial assistance for nonmedical costs. Support is offered on the basis of financial and medical need for such expenses as travel, lodging, and food when traveling to a craniofacial center for reconstructive surgery. Contact FACES for quarterly newsletter, information about craniofacial disorders, support networks and applications for financial assistance. (Lynne Mayfield, Director, Box 11082, Chattanooga, TN 37401; 423/266-1632, 800/332-2373; FAX 423/267-3124)

Foundation for Nager and Miller Syndromes

The foundation's stated goals are to establish awareness among professionals and agencies about the syndrome, to produce information and support to those affected, to obtain information on recent advancements and research, and to seek and finance research. The foundation has a library for families and professionals and also publishes a newsletter. (Margaret Ieronimo and Pam LeBaron, 333 Country Lane, Glenview, IL 60025; 800/507-FNMS)

Mobius Syndrome Foundation

A new foundation dedicated to education and research of this rare disorder. Newsletters, support /meetings and networking. (Box 993, Larchmont, NY 10538; 914/834-6008. Newsletter Mobius Syndrome News in California, 818/908-9288. Support Group in California 805/267-2570)

Mobius Syndrome Network

This growing network has a newsletter and address list for linking up people all over the United States. (Contact Vicki McCarrell, 6449 Gerald Avenue, Van Nuys, CA 91406; Vicki 310/470-2000, or Lori Thomas 805/267-2570)

Moya-Moya Foundation

Two resources for people with this syndrome. Dawn Gruethner, Cedar Rapids, Iowa 800/627-6692 or Peg Garvin, 7652 South Niagra Way, Englewood, CO 80112; 303/721-7563.

National Foundation for Facial Reconstruction

The programs of the NFFR focus on providing support for the care and treatment of individuals, primarily children, with a facial deformity. The foundation provides support to the Institute of Reconstructive Plastic Surgery located at the NYU Medical Center. The NFFR also supports education programs and research in the field. For your copy of an informative book with the proceedings of the November 1992 NFFR National Conference *Special Faces: Understanding Facial Disfigurement* send a $10 check payable to the NFFR to the address below. (Calliope Ligelis, Executive Director, 317 East 34th Street, Room 901, New York, NY 10016; 212/263-6656; FAX 212/262-7534)

National Oral Health Information Clearinghouse (NOHIC)

This information service for special care in oral health is a service of the National Institute of Dental Research. Patients, health professionals and the public can access the oral health database and the many information materials published by the clearinghouse. Many copies of single booklets are free. Do get on their mailing list. (1 NOHIC Way, Bethesda, MD 20892-3500; 301/402-7364; Internet: nidr@aerie.com)

National Organization for Rare Disorders (NORD)

NORD is an educational link for organizations and individuals concerned with a rare disorder. It tracks legislation, researches diseases, advocates for funding, awards grant money and networks individuals. The "Orphan Disease Update," included with the $25 membership fee, is a vehicle for communication about rare disorders and is mailed throughout the world. Annual meeting. Contact NORD about starting a chapter. (NORD, Box 8923, New Fairfield, CT 06812-1783; 203/746-6518; 800/999-6673; Internet—http://www.NORD-RDB.com/-orphan)

National Vascular Malformation Foundation

Bringing together professionals and consumers this important nonprofit organization is dedicated to addressing the complex issues surrounding these malformations. As one doctor said at their first national conference "every single one of these is different." Medical

Resources for People with Facial Differences

referral, printed information, newsletters, national research data and annual conference are some of their services. For an up to date presentation on the issues we found Dr. Wayne F. J. Yakes chapter in *Interventional Radiology* to be very helpful. The title of the chapter is "Diagnosis and Management of Vascular Anomalies." Also, any one who has a hemangioma should sign on to the database of information that is being gathered by Linda Shannon, 518/782-9637. Linda is an educator and mother of a child with a hemangioma. (Mary Burris, 8320 Nightingale Street, Dearborn Heights, MI 48127; 313/274-1243)

Sjogren's Syndrome Foundation

This support and information network has over 170 area coordinators in the U.S. and many in other countries. Their newsletter "The Moisture Seekers," is published 9 times a year. The *Sjogren's Syndrome Handbook* is $24.95 for nonmembers and $19.95 for members. Annual dues: $25 U.S. or $30 Canada. (Rita M. May, Executive Director, 333 N. Broadway, Jerico, NY 11753; 516/933-6365; 800/4-SJOGREN)

Stickler Involved People

This international group began in England in 1989 and the United States branch is now being established. Networking is available for youngsters as well as adults. Membership is free and includes an initial information packet, quarterly newsletter and an information file on the syndrome. An annual conference is held in England. (Contact to International Group Coordinator, KT12 2AZ England; 011-441-932-229421 or contact the U.S. Coordinator, Pat Houchin, 53 Angellina, Augusta, KS 67010: 316/775-2993)

Sturge-Weber Foundation

A clearinghouse of information on all aspects of Sturge-Weber Syndrome. The objectives are to act as a support group; to serve the general public, medical, professional and governmental agencies through the dissemination of information; and to facilitate and fund research. Newsletter, a wonderful new 45 page Resource Guide, annual meetings. Conference videos available. They offer three packets: Parent-Self Pack for $5, School Pack for $5, and a Physicians Pack for $10.

These educational tools are models for us all. Simple, well written, patient, parent and grandparent information, complete educational kit for schools and detailed up-to-date professional packet. (Karen Ball, Box 418, Mt. Freedom, NJ 07970; 800/627-5482)

Von Hippel Lindau Family Alliance

This educational organization is staffed 100 percent by volunteers. They publish a newsletter titled "Family Forum." Their booklet titles include: VHL, Not So Rare After All, What You Need to Know About VHL, The VHL Handbook—A Multifaceted illness that is often not diagnosed. Membership is $25. (171 Clinton Road, Brookline, MA 02146)

Special Organizations for Parents and Families

Apert Support and Information Network

Christine Clark, a mother of a six year-old with Apert Syndrome, was so frustrated with the lack of information about Apert that she has begun this information and support network. Christine's favorite resource about Apert is from the *Medical Journal* "Clinics in Plastic Surgery," April 1991 published by W. B. Saunders Co., Duluth, MN; 800/654-2452. Ask your public library or medical library to get you a copy. Back issues of "Apert News" can be ordered by sending a 9x12" self addressed envelope, stamped with a $2.00 stamp to the address below. (Christine Clark, Director, Apert Support and Information Network, P.O. Box 1184, Fair Oaks, CA 95628; 916/961-1092)

Association of Birth Defect Children

A resource organization for parents of children with environmentally caused birth defects. Focus on parents who served in Vietnam and the Gulf War. Newsletter *The ABDC News*, which includes a special section "Environmental Birth Defect Digest." We urge people to register with their Birth Defect Registry. Your participation is what makes this network able to search for answers. They will provide free information about any birth defect or environmental exposure. Parent Matching and a video titled "Why My Child?" are available. Membership $25. (Betty Mekdeci, ABDC, 827 Irma Ave., Orlando, FL 32803; 407/245-7035; 800/313-2232) The Association has an invaluable

Resources for People with Facial Differences

resource titled "Everything You Want To Know About Your Child's Birth Defect" a comprehensive, personalized report can be up to 150 pages in length. $140 members, $175 nonmembers. (Available from The Health Resource, 564 Locust Street, Conway, AR 72032; 501/329-5272)

Association for the Care of Children's Health

ACCH is a 31 year old international organization for health care professionals and families. Booklets include: Preparing Your Child for Repeated Hospitalizations, Organizing and Maintaining Support Groups for Parents of Children with Chronic Illness and Handicapping Conditions. A free resource catalog lists films and videos, books and bibliographies. A quarterly professional journal publishes research studies. Annual parent and professional meetings. With ACCH membership comes a top notch biannual magazine *The ACCH Advocate*. It is dedicated to Family Centered Care and includes case studies by professionals, and includes information about the cost saving, life saving effects of Family Centered Care. (7910 Woodmont Avenue, Suite 300, Bethesda, MD 20814; 301/654-6549, 800/808-2224)

Carpenter Syndrome Network

Cathy Sponsler has started this support and information network trying to link parents of children with Carpenter Syndrome. If you or any one you know is dealing with this syndrome, contact Cathy. She is on the Internet, her e-mail address is Carpenter.syndrome@php.com. She is going to have a newsletter. (Cathy Sponsler, Box 4215-48, 26661 Bear Valley Road, Tehachapi, CA 93561; 805/821-1313)

Children's Craniofacial Association

Dedicated to supporting the needs of craniofacial patients and their families CCA offers doctor referral and nonmedical patient assistance. They design and manage yearly family retreats and educational programs. Their publications include a newsletter and well written brief guides to understanding the following: Apert Syndrome, Craniosynostosis, Hemangiomas (new), Hemifacial Microsomia, Microtia, and Treacher Collins Syndrome. (Charlene Smith, Director, 9441 LBJ Freeway, Suite 115-LB 46, Dallas, TX 75243; 800/535-3643; Regional Office—Box 306, West Chicago, IL, 60186-0306; 708/876-9664; FAX 708/293-9328)

The Cleft Palate Foundation (CPF)

This public service and education foundation provides services to patients and families. CPF operates a 24-hour toll free **CLEFTLINE service (800-24-CLEFT)** for affected individuals and their families, and offers brochures and fact sheets on various aspects of clefting and other craniofacial anomalies. Some are available in Spanish. A selected bibliography for parents is also available. Provides information about Cleft Craniofacial teams and family support groups. CPF co-sponsors the annual AboutFace Parent-Patient Conference. (Nancy Smythe, 1218 Grandview Avenue, Pittsburgh, PA 15211; 412/481-1376; FAX 412/481-0847)

Ear Anomalies Reconstructed or EAR—The Atresia-Microtia Support Group

Networking and medical information for families whose members have Microtia, Atresia or Craniofacial Microsomia. Meetings, phone support. (Jack Gross 212/947-0770, or Betsy Olds 201/761-5438; 72 Durand Road, Maplewood, NJ 07040)

Forward Face: The Charity for Children with Craniofacial Conditions

The Charity is dedicated to giving practical and financial support to people with Craniofacial conditions. Among its many activities are an active group for teenagers called Inner Faces, a newsletter and regular information and support meetings in New York City. They have workshops on career development, communication, listening skills and self-esteem. Each year Inner Faces produces an off-Broadway show called *Let's Face the Music, A Story of Our Lives*. We are excited about this important production. Video copies of the show are available. Parent networks and Child Life Departments take note! Call the Forward Face office for details. (317 East 34th Street, Suite 901, New York, NY 10016; 212/684-5860 or 800/393-FACE; FAX 212/684-5864)

Foundation for the Faces of Children

An all New England parent network based at the Craniofacial Center at Children's Hospital Medical Center in Boston, Massachusetts.

Resources for People with Facial Differences

Funds raised go for awareness education, research and parent support. Newsletter and lending library. (Cindy Chrisman, Family Liaison Coordinator, Box 1361, Brookline, MA 02146; 617/734-7576)

Freeman-Sheldon Syndrome Parent Support Group

We are delighted to add this network to our resource list. Their resources include a well written brochure describing the syndrome, a newsletter published twice a year, and a bibliography of medical literature. They are a nonprofit volunteer organization which provides emotional support to adults and families affected with the syndrome worldwide. They promote research. (Joyce Dolcourt, 509 East Northmont Way, Salt Lake City, UT 84103; 801/364-7060; e-mail: fspsg@aol.com)

Golden Har Parent Support Network

Hemiofacial Microtia and Ocular Aucicular Vetrebrah Dysplasia are related syndromes that Cathy Rush provides an information packet on. She links parents and keeps the organization informal. (Cathy Rush, 3619 Chicago, Minneapolis, MN 55407-2603; 612/823-3529)

National Information Clearinghouse for Infants with Disabilities and Life-Threatening Conditions

The NIC provides information and referral to appropriate providers of services for families having infants and young children with disabilities. Information Specialists respond to individual requests and assist families in accessing services such as parent support and training, advocacy, health care, financial resources, assistive technology, early intervention, and other information resources. The NIC produces and disseminates materials including bibliographies, fact sheets, and articles on topics related to the care of, and services available to, infants with disabilities and their families. Information materials are available in English, Spanish and alternative formats. The NIC is a collaborative project of the Center for Developmental Disabilities in Columbia, South Carolina and the Association for the Care of Children's Health (ACCH) in Bethesda, Maryland. (Center for Developmental Disabilities, School of Medicine, Department of Pediatrics, University of South Carolina, Columbia, SC 29208; 800/922-9234 ext. 201)

Partners in Intensive Care: A Hand to Hold for Babies and Their Families

This new parent support network is dedicated to extending a helping hand to parents in the D.C./Baltimore area whose babies require intensive care before and/or after birth as well as those who suffer the loss of a baby. Begun by parents who are articulate about what was not there for them, this network is going to be a model for other communities. For their very touching stories and their plans for carrying out their goals, write or call Melanie Morrison Sweeney. (Box 41043, Bethesda. MD 20824-1043; 301/681-2708; FAX 301/681-2707)

Prescription Parents, Inc.

This is an active support network in New England for people with cleft lip and cleft palate. Outreach to parents of newborns with cleft lip or palate, legislative advocacy, a newsletter and social activities are some of the ways in which their energy is focused. (Amy Kapino, 22 Ingersoll Road. Wellesley, MA 02181; 617/431-1398)

STOMP

Specialized Training of Military Parents is a parent-directed network established to help families in the military service who have children with disabilities or specialized educational and health needs. Parents serving in the military in the U.S. or overseas are invited to call STOMP at 800/298-3543; V/TDD 206/588-1741. (12208 Pacific Highway S.W., Tacoma, WA 98499)

Treacher Collins Foundation

This network links families and is directed by Hope Charkins-Drazin and David Drazin, a social worker and a psychologist who have a child with Treacher Collins Syndrome. Hope has written a new book *Children with Facial Difference — A Parents Guide*. Woodbine Press, $16.95 plus $4.00 shipping and handling. An exciting update for the Foundation is that a research team has discovered the location of the gene for Treacher Collins syndrome. Newsletter, new video *"Rare" Should Not Mean "Alone,"* meetings. (Hope Charkins and David Drazin, Box 683, Norwich, VT 05055; 802/649-3050, 800/823-2055)

Resources for People with Facial Differences

Reading for Parents and Families

The Boy David. We are delighted to report that copies of this wonderful book are available. The true account of a facially disfigured Peruvian child adopted by the family of a plastic surgeon. The book documents the story of David Jackson's life and surgeries through text and photographs. Written by Marjorie Jackson. David and his family were featured in a segment of "60 Minutes" on February 14, 1993. Parent Libraries take note—this book can give hope to all who have face, head and neck surgery. ($10 contribution to the Providence Hospital Foundation, 800/423-5801, ask for Eva Forman. Or send a check to the Foundation, Eva Forman, 16001 West 9 mile Road, Fisher Center, 3rd Floor, Southfield, MI 48075).

Building the Healing Partnership, Parents, Professionals and Children with Chronic Illness and Disabilities. This is one of our all time favorite books. Authors Patricia Tanner Leff, a child psychiatrist, and Elaine Walizer, an educator, listened to patient's families and caretakers personal experiences. The book weaves brief vignettes to help the reader experience the essence of caring for a chronically ill child. The authors are explicit and thorough, telling the patient, family and caretakers what to expect and giving permission to experience and adapt to the range of feelings possible when caring for children with chronic illness. The Library Journal said of this book..."The authors spare no punches, the talk is frank, alternately depressing and uplifting. Dozens of entries from parents and healthcare workers seek to educate, invite change, and stimulate personal growth." ($34.95, cloth; $24.95 paperback; discounts available, Brookline Books, Box 1046, Cambridge, MA 02238; 617/868-0360 or 800/666-2665; order via e-mail: brooklinebks@delphi.com).

Cleft Palate Reflections—A Newsletter. A quarterly newsletter free to patients of Shadyside Medical Center, $10 per year to all others. Edited by Dr. Robert E. McKinstry, a maxillofacial prosthodontist who was born with a right sided unilateral cleft lip and palate. The Winter 1995 issue had an article on camouflage make-up. (Shadyside Maxillofacial & Cleft Palate Prosthetics Center, Shadyside Medical Center, 5230 Centre Avenue, Suite 207, Pittsburgh, PA 15232).

The Cleft Palate Story. A comprehensive 218-page parent guide, edited and created by Dr. Samuel Berkowitz, DDS, MS, FCID, is a "primer for parents of children with cleft lip and palate." The book is a clear and accessible resource that is bound to be referred to again and again over a childs lifetime. Dr. Berkowitz and his coauthors have organized the answers to all the questions parents have. This would make a wonderful gift. Ask your public library and hospital gift shop to carry this book. Thank you Dr. Berkowitz. ISBN 0-86715-259-1. ($24.00, plus shipping; Quintessence Publishing Co. Inc., 551 North Kimberly Drive, Carol Stream, IL 60188-1881; 800/621-0387, 708/682-3288).

The Exceptional Parent Annual Directory of National Organizations. A yearly publication of *Exceptional Parent* magazine, it lists the federal parent-to-parent training centers in each state and the varied support available for all pediatric disabilities. Edited by Maxwell Schleifer. ($9.95; Richardson Specialty Books, 1905 Swathmore Avenue, Lakewood, NJ 08701; 800/535-1910).

Genetic Counseling. This 11 page booklet can help families understand and benefit from genetic counseling. Used in clinics across the country. This is one of our favorite "new" resources. (50 Booklets, $12.00; March of Dimes, 1276 Mamaroneck Avenue, White Plains, NY 18703; 800/367-6630).

Genetic Counseling Briefs. Genetic counselors are a vital part of patient services. This article, published in *The Genetic Resource* Vol 6, No. 1, 1991) introduces us to the training and importance of the genetic counselor. For a copy send a self addressed, stamped business envelope to Let's Face It, Box 29972, Bellingham, WA 98228.

Handbook for the Care of Infants and Toddlers with Disabilities and Chronic Conditions. More and more infants and toddlers with special needs are being cared for in centers in their home communities: daycare centers, private homes, early intervention programs or schools. This handbook contains information to help child-care personnel, paraprofessionals, parents and others provide care that will enable children with special needs to reach their maximum potential. Contact Learner Managed Designs, Inc., 2201 K West 25th Street, Lawrence, KS 66047 for a catalog of other professional training resources for health, education and related fields.

Making the Difference: An orientation Package for Health Care Providers. This packet for nurses and other health care providers is an overview of the needs of families whose infants are born with craniofacial anomalies. ($3.00; Contact AboutFace, Box 93 Limekiln, PA 19535; or 99 Crown's Lane, Toronto, Canada M5R 3P4).

A Parent's Guide to Cleft Lip and Palate. "Should be required reading for every new parent of a child with a cleft," says one parent. Chapters range from a basic explanation of the current theory of the cause of clefts to surgical repair and social and psychological development. By Muller, Starr and Johnson. (University of Minnesota Press, 2037 University Avenue SE, Minneapolis, MN 55414).

Physicians' Guide to Rare Disorders. National Organization for Rare Disorders (NORD), in cooperation with Dowden Publishing Company, has provided a resource that will be of great value to physicians as well as patients diagnosed with rare or "orphans" diseases. This 1,224-page reference book includes a key chapter to help physicians communicate more effectively, "Rare Diseases: What Patients Need." Libraries take note. ($69.50; Order from Dowden Publishing Company, 110 Summit Ave, Montvale, NJ 07645-9895).

Someone Like Me — A Booklet for Children Born with Cleft Lip and Palate. Detailed, comforting water colors portray this 30-page story of a child born with Cleft Lip and Palate. The glossary and presentation of the facts would make this a good gift for parents or grandparents of a newborn with a cleft and palate. Written by Michael Fishbaough. ($5.00, Riley Hospital, Diane Wachendorf, 506 Maxine Manor, Brownsburgh, IN 46112).

Other Reading

Complex Craniofacial Problems: A Guide to Analysis and Treatment. Written and edited by Doctors Craig R. Dufresne, Benjamin S. Carson and S. James Zinreich, this 560-page text book charts the history and medical treatment of Craniofacial patients. Many photos and x-ray images help to educate about various syndromes. We think the chapter titled "Patient Family Counseling and Education" should be required reading for all Craniofacial teams. Available through interlibrary loan or medical libraries. ($179.00. Churchill Livingstone, NY, 1992).

Dinner Through a Straw. Another one of our favorite books. Over 130 delicious recipes, on-the-go meals, meals following jaw surgery and calorie counts in this "A Handbook for Oral Fixation" by Patti Rann. She also describes creation of a feeding device. (1 to 5 copies—$6.00 per copy; call for bulk prices; Dethero Enterprises, Box 5742, Cleveland, TN 37320-5742; 423/478-3043).

Let's Do Lunch (and Other Meals), by Beckey Dethero. With their success of selling over 60 thousand copies of *Dinner Through a Straw*, Dethero Enterprises announces the publication of this 58-page handbook for people recovering from mouth and throat trauma. This book has the most up-to-date instructions from doctors and nurses. *Let's Do Lunch* tells how our bodies heal and much more. It's five chapters include: "Keep the Sparkle in Your Smile (Care of Mouth, Teeth, Gums and Body)," "I'm Taking No Chances (Precautions and Limitations)," "Here I Come, World! (Communication, Well-Being, Leaving the Hospital)," "If There's A Way to Eat It, I Can Find It (Dieting and Nutrition)," "We Send Our Best (80 New Recipes to Enjoy)." Both *Dinner Through a Straw* and *Let's Do Lunch* are $6.00 each. Postage is included. Generous discounts for multiple orders. Doctors, nurses and hospital gift shops take note! Order from Dethero Enterprises, Box 5742, Cleveland, Tennessee 37320-5742. Phone or FAX 423/478-3043.

Facial Disfigurement: Problems and Management of Social Interaction and Implications for Mental Health. This article by Frances Cooke Macgregor addresses the impact of facial disfigurement on social interaction during brief encounters, the ramifications of which have the potential for psychological and social destruction. It documents coping mechanisms. Many Let's Face It members have found this article valid and meaningful. From the Fall 1990 issue of the *International Society of Plastic Surgery Journal* (Vol. 14, p. 249). (Send a 9x12 self-addressed envelope with $3.00 postage to Let's Face It, Box 29972, Bellingham, WA 98228-1972).

Genetic Information Via the Internet: Risks and Benefits. The Alliance of Genetic Support Groups asked Dr. Leslie Becker to spell out the advantages and disadvantages of uses of the Internet for medical information. This article is a gift to all of us as we begin to get "with it" and use the Internet. For a copy of this article send a self addressed, stamped, business size envelope to Let's Face It, Box 29972, Bellingham, WA 98228-1972.

After Plastic Surgery: Adaptions and Adjustment. Greenwood Press Publishing Group, Box 5007, 88 Post Road West, Westport, CT 06881; 800/225-5800, ext. 700. ISBN 0275903834.

Resources for People with Facial Differences

Facial Deformities and Plastic Surgery. Written by Macgregor and others, Thomas, Springfield Illinois; 1953.

Transformation and Identity: The Face and Plastic Surgery. 1974; Quadrangle Press/The New York Times Book Company, New York.

New Edition of the Self-Help Sourcebook, Finding & Forming Mutual Aid Self-Help Groups. Edited by Ed Madara and Barbara White, the Fifth Edition of this spectacular book is the best ever. Every Medical Facility, Library and Faith Community should have their own copy. Up to date information of over 700 different support organizations. Give a copy to your favorite social worker, nurse, doctor or spiritual leader. $10 each, 25% discount to public libraries and book dealers: prepayment required. Make check payable to St. Charles-Riverside Medical Center and send it to American Self-Help Clearinghouse, Attn. Directory, St. Charles-Riverside Medical Center, 25 Pocono Road, Denville, New Jersey 07834-2995; 201/625-9565; Internet: http://www.cmhc.com/self-help/.

Resources for Young Adults

Medical Miracle—A 60 Minutes Production. A moving report on the life of David Jackson, son of Marjorie and Ian Jackson, which aired on "60 Minutes" on February 14, 1993. David and his parents give us an in-depth report of what life is like for a person who undergoes repeated facial reconstruction. David and his parents are role models for many of us. For your copy to use for educational purposes, send a contribution to Providence Hospital Foundation. Contact Eva Forman, Providence Hospital Foundation 800/423-5801.

Films/Videos and Audio Tapes

Cleft Lip and Palate—Feeding the Newborn. This dynamic 18-minute video developed in 1992 by the Hospital for Sick Children in Toronto, Canada, presents the appropriate methods to feed an infant with a cleft lip and/or palate. $95; preview fee of $10 applied toward purchase. (Lisa Sarsfield, Coordinator, Cleft Lip and Palate Program, The Hospital for Sick Children, 555 University Avenue, Toronto, Ontario M5G 1X8, make check payable to the Cleft Lip and Palate Fund; 416/813-7490).

They Don't Come with Manuals. By Paul Uzee with the National Council on Family Relations. This 29-minute documentary of parents of children with physical and mental disabilities tells it as it is. Parents share their deepest feelings and thoughts about life with their disabled children. One parent says "I love the child but hate the disability." The producers remind us that no two disabled children are alike and urge us to grow with these children. This film can empower parents, grandparents and professional caregivers to face the rigors of life with children who require extra care. $145.00, catalog number CB-038.

Face Facts Video Tapes. These outstanding videos are designed for parents and families to use after the birth of a child with Cleft Lip and Palate, Craniosynostosis, Hemifacial Microsomia, Orbital Hypertelorism or Treacher Collins syndrome. Narrated by Cliff Robertson, the tapes sensitively explore these five disorders. Each tape includes an overview of these disorders and features interviews with medical professionals, educators, family members and patients. $10.00 each for members, $15.00 each for nonmembers. All profits are used to develop future educational materials concerning craniofacial disorders and their treatment. (Toni Bao, Forward Face, 317 East 34th Street, 9th Floor, New York, NY 10016; 212/684-5860, 800/393-FACE; FAX 212/684-5864).

If Your Baby Has a Cleft. Nancy Smythe of the American Cleft Palate; Craniofacial Association introduced us to this wonderful resource produced in 1990 by the St. John's Hospital Cleft Palate Center in Santa Monica, California. It is an excellent tape for parents who have a baby with a cleft lip or palate and for use by genetic counselors. It provides information in a caring, professional style, 30 minutes in length. $25 to rent, $58 to buy (includes tax). (Contact Barbara Wasilewski, St. John's Hospital, Child Study Center, attention Cleft Palate Center, 1339 20th Street, Santa Monica, CA 90404; 310/829-8150).

"Rare" Should Not Mean Alone. An educational 35 minute video about Treacher Collins Syndrome. Parents, scientists, doctors and children tell the story that "Rare should not mean alone." Helpful to educate about all facial anomalies. A model film for other organizations to learn from. (Write the Treacher Collins Foundation, Box 683, Norwich, VT 05055).

Resources for People with Facial Differences

So Brightly Within. This 22-minute video has a mission close to all our hearts. We are urged to "look beyond the face to see the beauty that shines within." Four children with facial difference are filmed with their families doing the "normal" things children do. The children's and parents' honest feelings about life with a different face can spark thoughtful discussion. FACES is an organization that helps families with the nonmedical financial burdens of surgeries for children and some adults with facial disfigurement. Their commitment to raising funds for this noble work is part of this important film. Appropriate for Junior High to adult. For your copy send $20.00 to FACES, Box 11082, Chattanooga, TN 37403; 800/418/3223).

Understanding Craniofacial Syndromes. A 21-minute video by Dr. Ian Jackson. With before and after photos, Dr. Jackson describes and demonstrates treatment for major Craniofacial anomalies. With a $5.00 donation to the Providence Hospital Foundation you can use this excellent educational film. (Eva Forman, Providence Hospital Foundation, 16001 W. 9 Mile Rd, Fisher Center, 3rd Floor, Southfield, MI 48075; 800/423-5801).

What is Going to Happen to my Baby? This outstanding video has been produced for parents and professionals dealing with a cleft lip and plate to answer questions in the first months of a child's life. It builds confidence and competence into the parents' life. Write or call for a list of their award winning video tapes and booklets. Produced by the Center for Craniofacial Anomalies, University of Illinois Chicago Films. $95; $30 to preview. (University of Illinois Chicago Craniofacial Center M(C588), Box 6998, Chicago IL 60680; 312/996-7546, ask for Mark Steiner).

Chapter 53

Resources for Other Congenital Disorders

Organizations

American Academy for Cerebral Palsy and Developmental Medicine
P.O. Box 11086
Richmond, Va 23230-1086
(804) 282-0036

American Chronic Pain Association, Inc.
P.O. Box 850
Rocklin, CA 95677
(916) 632-0922

American Diabetes Association
National Center
1660 Duke Street
Alexandria, VA 22314
(703) 549-1500

American Foundation for Urologic Disease, Inc. (AFUD)
300 West Pratt Street
Baltimore, MD 21201
(800) 242-2382; (410) 727-2408

Information in this chapter was compiled from many different sources believed to be accurate as of January 1997. This list is intended to serve as a starting point on the search for further information; it is not comprehensive. Inclusion does not imply endorsement.

American Heart Association
7272 Greenville Avenue
Dallas, TX 75231-4596
(800) 242-1793
(214) 373-6300

American Pseudo-Obstruction and
Hirschsprung's Disease Society, Inc. (APHS)
P.O. Box 772
Medford, MA 02155
(617) 395-4255

Association for Retarded Citizens
500 East Border Street
Arlington, TX 76010
(817) 261-6003

Association of Birth Defect Children
827 Irma Avenue
Orlando, FL 32803
(407) 245-7035
(800) 313-2232

AVM (Arteriovenous Malformation) Support Group
P.O. Box 1261
Fernley, NV 89408
(702) 575-5421

CDC National AIDS Clearinghouse
P.O. Box 6003
Rockville, MD 20849-6003
(800) 458-5231

Center for Digestive Diseases
Central DuPage Hospital
25 North Winfield Road
Winfield, IL 60190
(708) 682-1600 ext. 6493

Resources for Other Congenital Disorders

Center for Substance Abuse Prevention (CSAP)
National Resource Center for the Prevention of
Perinatal Abuse of Alcohol and Other Drugs
9300 Lee Highway
Fairfax, VA 22031
(703) 218-5600
(800) 345-8824

Children with Special Health Care Needs Program
Division of Maternal and Child Health
Health Resources and Services Administration
U.S. Department of Health and Human Services
Parklawn Building, Room 6-05
5600 Fishers Lane
Rockville, MD 20857
(301) 433-2350

Children's Heart Link
5075 Arcadia Avenue
Minneapolis, MN 55436-2306
(612) 928-4860

Clearinghouse for Drug-Exposed Children
Division of Behavioral and Developmental Pediatrics
University of California, San Francisco
400 Parnassus, Room A203
San Francisco, CA 94143-0314
(415) 476-9691

Digestive Disease National Coalition
711 2nd Street, NE, Suite 200
Washington, DC 20002
(202) 544-7497

Division of Birth Defects and Developmental Disabilities
Mailstop F45
National Center for Environmental Health
Centers for Disease Control and Prevention
4770 Buford Highway, NE
Atlanta, GA 30341-3724
(404) 488-7150

Epilepsy Foundation of America
4351 Garden City Drive
Landover, MD 20785
(301) 459-3700
(800) EFA-1000

Fetal Alcohol Network
158 Rosemont Avenue
Coatesville, PA 19320-3727
(215) 384-1133

The Greater New York Pull-thru Network
62 Edgewood Avenue
Wyckoff, NJ 07481
(201) 891-5977

IVH (Intraventricular Hemorrhage) Parents
P.O. Box 56-111
Miami, FL 33256-1111
(305) 232-0381

Juvenile Diabetes Foundation
423 Park Avenue South
New York, NY 10016
(212) 889-7575

Klippel-Trenaunay Support Group
4610 Wooddale Avenue
Minneapolis, MN 55424
(612) 925-2596

La Leche League International (Breastfeeding)
9616 Minneapolis Avenue
P.O. Box 1209
Franklin Park, IL 60131-8209
(708) 455-7730

March of Dimes Birth Defects Foundation
1275 Mamaroneck Avenue
White Plains, NY 10605
(914) 428-7100

Resources for Other Congenital Disorders

National Black Child Development Institute
1023 15th Street, NW, Suite 600
Washington, DC 20005
(202) 387-1281

National Chronic Pain Outreach Association
7979 Old Georgetown Rd.
Suite 100
Bethesda, MD 20814-2429
(301) 652-4948

National Clearinghouse for Alcohol and Drug Information (NCADI)
P.O. Box 2345
Rockville, MD 20852
(301) 468-2600
(800)SAY-NO-TO (DRUGS)

National Coalition of Hispanic Health and
Human Services Organizations (COSSMHO)
1501 16th Street, NW
Washington, DC 20036
(202) 387-5000

National Coalition on Alcohol and Drug
Dependent Women and Their Children
1511 K Street, NW, Suite 926
Washington, DC 20005
(202) 737-9112

National Commission to Prevent Infant Mortality
Switzer Building, Room 2014
330 C Street, SW
Washington, DC 20201
(202) 472-1364

National Congenital Port Wine Stain Foundation
125 E. 63rd Street
New York, NY 10021
(516) 867-5137

National Diabetes Information Clearinghouse
1 Information Way
Bethesda, MD 20892-3560
(301) 654-3327

National Easter Seal Society
230 W. Monroe, 18th Floor
Chicago, IL 60606
(312) 726-6200
(312) 726-4258 (TDD)

National Eye Institute
Building 31, Room 6A32
Bethesda, MD 20892-2510
(301) 496-5248

National Institute of Child Health and Human Development
Building 31, Room 2A32
Bethesda, MD 20892-2425
(301) 496-5133

National Kidney and Urologic Diseases Information Clearinghouse
9000 Rockille Pike
Bethesda, MD 20892
(301) 654-4415

National Kidney Foundation (NKF)
30 East 33rd Street
New York, NY 10016
(800) 622-9010
(212) 889-2210

National Maternal and Child Health Clearinghouse (NMCHC)
8201 Greensboro Drive, Suite 600
McLean, VA 22102
(703) 821-8955 ext. 254

National Organization for Rare Disorders (NORD)
P.O. Box 8923
New Fairfield, CT 06812-8923
(203) 746-6518
(800) 999-6673

Resources for Other Congenital Disorders

Nevus Network
P.O. Box 1981
Woodbridge, Va 22193

NIH Neurological Institute
P.O. Box 5801
Bethesda, MD 20824
(301) 496-5751
(800) 352-9424

Pediatric AIDS Foundation
1311 Colorado Avenue
Santa Monica, CA 90404
(310) 395-9051

Spina Bifida Association of America
4590 MacArthur Blvd., NW
Suite 250
Washington, DC 20007
(202) 944-3285
(800) 621-3141

Sturge-Weber Foundation
P.O. Box 418
Mt. Freedom, NJ 07970
(201) 895-4445
(800) 627-5482

United Cerebral Palsy Associations and
The United Cerebral Palsy Research and Educational Foundation
1522 K Street, NW Suite 1112
Washington, DC 20005
(202) 842-1266
(800) USA-5UCP (outside Washington, DC)

Selected Sources of Information on the Internet

Administration for Children and Families
http://www.acf.dhhs.gov

Apgar Scoring for Newborns
http://www.childbirth.org/articles/apgar.html

British Columbia's Children's Hospital
http://www.childhosp/bc.ca/childrens/Ortho

Centers for Disease Control and Prevention
http://www.cdc.gov

Chiari Malformation Page
http://cpmcnet.columbia.edu/dept/nsg/PNS/ChiariMalformation.html

Food and Drug Administration
http://www.fda.org

National Center for Environmental Health (and Division of Birth Defects and Developmental Disabilities)
http://www.cdc.gov/nceh/i:/cehweb/nceb/Oncehhom.htm

The National Health Information Center
http://nhic-nt.health.org

National Institutes of Health
http://www.nih.gov/home.html

National Library of Medicine
http://www.nlm.nih.gov

The National Organization for Rare Disorders, Inc.
http://www.stepstn.com/nord/rdb_sum

Pediatric Database
http://www.icondata.com/health/pedbase/files

U.S. Department of Health and Human Services
http://www.os.dhhs.gov

Wide Smiles: Cleft-Links
http://www.widesmiles.org

Index

Index

Page numbers in *italics* refer to tables and illustrations; the letter "n" following a page number refers to a note.

A

Aase, J. M., MD *184,* 186, 187, 190, 192, 193, 194, 226, 240, 245, 246, 252, 256, 260, 269
ABDC *see* Association of Birth Defect Children (ABDC)
Abel, E. L. 186, 190, 193, 213, 215, 216, 219, 225, 235, 259, 268
Aboagye, K. 227, 229, 230, 231, 240
abortion, spontaneous 198
AboutFace 344, 541, 542, 553
AboutFace Newsletter 344
ABR *see* Auditory Brainstem Responses (ABR)
ACCH *see* Association for the Care of Children's Health (ACCH)
Accutane (isotretinoin) 7, 399–404
Achenbach Child Behavior Checklist 249
Achieving Zero Dioxin 390
acidemia 466
acidosis 291, 490

acne treatment 7, 400, 403
acquired heart disease, defined 291
Acta Obstetrica et Gynecologica Scandinavia 239
Acta Paediatrica Scandinavica Supplement 255
Acta Paediatr JPN 478
Adams, J. 417
Adams, M. L. 213, 217, 219, 220
Adamson, S. J. 494
ADHD *see* attention deficit hyperactivity disorder (ADHD)
adolescents, fetal alcohol syndrome 241, 243–45
adrenal function 517
Adsett, D. B. 472, 477
Aduss, Marcia 344
Advances in Alcohol and Substance Abuse 220
Advances in Substance Abuse 221
Advice to Parents of a Cleft Palate Child 345
AFO *see* ankle-foot orthosis (AFO)
AFP *see* alpha-feto-protein (AFP)
AFP-Plus test 21
African Americans
  alcohol consumption 227
  fetal alcohol syndrome 188
  sickle cell anemia 9

569

After Plastic Surgery: Adaptations and Adjustment 554
Agency for Children, Youth, and Families 507
Agency for Toxic Substances and Disease Registry (ATSDR) 364, 366
Ager, J. W. 198, 207
aggression *versus* assertiveness
  communication 27
  health care professionals 30
Agustsson, P. 479
A Handbook for Oral Fixation 553
AHEAD *see* Association of Hydrocephalus Education, Advocacy and Discussion (AHEAD)
AIDS (Acquired Immune Deficiency Syndrome) 463–64
  spina bifida 58
  toxoplasmosis 426
AJDC 478
AJNR 478
Alan R. Liss, Inc. 379
Albanese, Richard A. 389
Alcohol 255
alcohol, pregnancy 5–6, 8, 195–98, 223–26
Alcohol and Brain Development 257
Alcohol Health and Research World 254
Alcoholic Beverage Labeling Act (1988) 255
Alcoholism: Clinical and Experimental Research 194, 206, 207, 219, 220, 221, 222, 235, 237, 240, 253, 255, 256, 257, 268, 269
alcoholism, heredity 209–12
Alessandri, L. M. 494
Alexander, G. 455
allergies, spina bifida 54
The Alliance of Genetic Support Groups 64, 554
A los Padres de los Bebes Recien Nacidos con Labio Leporino / Paladar Hendido 343
alpha-feto-protein (AFP) 21, 60
  spina bifida test 36
Alterman, A. I. 210, 220
alveolar ridge 325–26, 327, 346
Amaro, H. 227, 229, 230, 231, 240

amblyopia 69, 353
ambulatory electrocardiography, defined 299
American Academy of Cerebral Palsy and Developmental Medicine 157, 559
American Academy of Dermatology 400, 403
American Academy of Pediatrics 135, 312, 392, 400
American Association of Neurological Surgeons 98, 100, 101
American Chronic Pain Association 559
American Cleft Palate-Craniofacial Association (ACPA) 340, 342, 542, 556
American College of Obstetricians and Gynecologists (ACOG) 19n, 479
  publications 24, 466
  ultrasound screening 23–24
American College of Physicians 304
American Cyanamid Company 373
American Diabetes Association 559
American Epilepsy Society 416
American Family Physician 315n
American Foundation for Urologic Diseases, Inc. 559
American Heart Association 290, 560
American Hirschsprung's Disease Association 313
American Journal of Anatomy 208
American Journal of Clinical Nutrition 237
American Journal of Diseases of Children 238, 478, 493, 494
American Journal of Epidemiology 371, 379, 387, 389, 457, 493
American Journal of Industrial Medicine 387, 388
American Journal of Medical Genetics 256, 456, 457, 458
American Journal of Medicine 406, 458
American Journal of Obstetrics and Gynecology 110, 207, 239, 478, 479, 493, 494, 495, 509, 510, 511
American Journal of Psychiatry 222
American Journal of Public Health 239, 379, 387, 389

Index

American Medical Association 407n
American Naturalist 222
American Neurological Association 416
American Pediatric Society 416
American Pseudo-Obstruction and Hirschsprung's Disease Society, Inc. 560
American Self-Help Clearinghouse 555
American Society of Pediatric Neurosurgeons 100, 101
Americans with Disabilities Act 56
America Online 533
Amiel-Tison, C. 480
amniocentesis 448, 451
  defined 60–61
  prenatal testing 20
  spina bifida 38
  twins 306
amniotic fluid 22, 38, 518
Anda, R. F. 224, 239, 266, 269
Andermann, E. 417
Andermann, F. 417
Anderson, H. 234, 237
Anderson, J. P. 481
Andrews, E. 509
Andrews, W. 511
anemia, fetal 22
anencephaly 11, 13, 34
  defined 61
  tests 21
aneurysm, defined 291
angenesis, lung *381*
angina pectoris, defined 291
angiocardiograms 291
angiocardiography, defined 291
angiogram, defined 353
angioid streaks, defined 353
angioplasy, defined 291
angiotensin-converting enzyme (ACE) inhibitors 405–6
angiotensin II 405
animal studies
  alcoholism 212–13
  chemicals and birth defects 363
  hypoxia 517
  insulin 514
  malnutrition 460
  premature birth 498
  see also studies

aniridia *381*, 382
ankle-foot orthosis (AFO), defined 60
Annales de Pediatrie 254
Annals of Medicine 208
Annals of the New York Academy of Sciences 194
Annegers, J. F. 417
anophtalmos *381*
anoxic brain damage 462–63
Answering Your Questions about Spina Bifida 33n
antibiotics 6, 442, 503–4
Anticonvulsant Drugs, Behavior, and Cognitive Abilities 95
anticonvulsant medications 352, 353
  hydrocephalus 87–88, *89, 91,* 92–93
  spina bifida 36
antiepileptic drugs 407–16
antiseizure medications 13, 144
aorta 275–76, 291
aortic valve, defined 291
aortopulmonary window 282
Apert Support and Information Network 546
Apgar, Virginia 127
Apgar scores 127, 144, 474, 487–89
aphasia, defined 291
Archives of Disease in Childhood 93, 94, 254, 479, 481, 492
Archives of Environmental Health 366, 371, 388, 389, 390
Archives of General Psychiatry 221, 222
Archives of Neurology 407n, 417
Archives of the Diseases of Children 207
Arnold Chiari Family Network 64
Arnold Chiari II malformation 41, 63
Aronsson, M. 242, 255
Arora, K. L. 457
arrhythmia 291, 298
arteriogram *see* angiogram
arteriography, defined 291–92
arterioles, defined 292
arteriosclerosis, defined 292
artery, defined 292
arthrogryposis *318,* 320, *381*
articulation, defined 346
articulation test, defined 346

571

asphyxia 126, 144, 465–77
   see also birth asphyxia
assistive devices 316
   braces, spina bifida 49
   cerebral palsy 139, 166
   standing frames 62
Association for Retarded Citizens 560
Association for the Care of Children's Health (ACCH) 64, 547, 549
Association of Birth Defect Children (ABDC) 546–47, 560
Association of Hydrocephalus Education, Advocacy and Discussion (AHEAD) 530
astigmatism 69, 353
Astley, S. J. 206, 228, 235
ataxia 71
ataxic cerebral palsy 122–23
atherosclerosis, defined 292
athetoid cerebral palsy 122–23
atresia 292, *381*
atria, defined 292
atrial fibrillation, defined 297
atrial septal defect (ASD) 277, 292, *381*
atrial septum (foramen ovale) 277, 292
atrioventricular (AV) node, defined 292–93
atrioventricular canal defect, defined 293
atrioventricular septal defect, defined 293
ATSDR *see* Agency for Toxic Substances and Disease Registry (ATSDR)
attention deficit hyperactivity disorder (ADHD) 186, 191
audiogram, defined 346
audiologists 334, 346
Auditory Brainstem Responses (ABR) 334
Avitable, N. 227, 240
AVM (Arteriovenous Malformation) Support Group 560
Azen, Stanley, PhD 416

B

Babinski's reflex, defined 353
Bachicha, J. 230, 238
Bachman, J. G. 212, 214, 221
Baclofen pump 157–58
bacterial endocartitis, defined 293
bacterial meningitis 125
bacterial vaginosis 504
Badawi, N. 494
Bain, R. 509
Baker, Dean B. 371
Baker, E. L. 268
Ball, Karen 546
balloon catheter 293, 303
   see also catheterization
Bannister, C. M. 92, 94, 107, 108, 109
Bao, Toni 556
Bard, A. 417
barium enema 311
Barkovich, A. J. 478
Barr, H. M. 198, 202, 207, 208, 226, 240, 250, 252, 257
Barrett, M. 227, 236
Barry, R. J. 323
Bartfai, T. 493
Bartholomew, M. 478
Bartlett, R. H. 480
Bartoshesky, L. E. 213, 221
Batchelor, Lori L. 313
Bauchner, H. 227, 229, 230, 231, 239, 240
Bauer, C. R. 477, 508, 509
Bayley Scales of Infant Development 231, 469, 473, 474, 475
BDMC *see* Birth Defects Monitoring Program (BDMP)
BDMP *see* Centers for Disease Control and Prevention (CDC), Birth Defects Monitoring Program (BDMP)
Beaudoin, A. R. 457
Beaumanoir, A. 92, 94
Becerra, J. E. *189*, 190, 193, 264, 268
Becker, J. R. 322
Becker, Leslie, Dr. 559
bed sores *see* pressure sores
Beginnings of Life 22

Index

Begleiter, H. 210, 219
behavioral audiometry 334
behavioral tests, fetal alcohol syndrome 186, 192, 202–4, 246
behavioral therapy, cerebral palsy 136, 163
Belai, I. 479, 495
Belai, Yitzak, MD 417, 418
Benedetti, P. 95
Bennett, F. C. 480
Berger, K. S. 208
Berger, M. S. 109
Berk, R. S. 213, 219
Berkelman, R. L. 260, 269
Berkowitz, Samuel, DDS, MS, FCID 334, 551, 552
Berney, J. 92, 94
Bertin, Joan E. 375
Bertollini, R. 417
Bettecken, F. 242, 255
B.F. Goodrich 374
Bien, E. 493
Bierich, G. R. 242, 255
Big Hearts for Little Hearts 290
bilateral, defined 354
bile pigments 126, 144
Bingol, N. 243, 253
Biochemistry and Pharmacology of Ethanol 221
Biostatics Coordinating Center (BCC) 502
birth asphyxia 483–92
  see also asphyxia
birth defects
  causes 6–7
  chemicals 7–8, 363–66
  hazardous waste sites 367–71
  increase 383–86
  prevention, folic acid 12–14
  spina bifida 3
  surveillance 260–61
  surveillance programs 11
  see also *individual diseases*
Birth Defects Monitoring Program (BDMP) 259
birthmarks 351, 356
birth weight
  brain damage 171–72
  cerebral palsy 151

birth weight, continued
  fetal alcohol syndrome *201*
  see also low birth weight
Blaauw, G. 90, 92, 94
Black, Timothy, MD 313
Blackard, C. 227, 240
bladder malfunction 44–47
  see also incontinence; urologic system
bladder tests 63
Blair, E. 477
Blake, Jeffrey N., BA 83n, 93, 94
Blakeslee, Sandra 375, 378
Blakey, D. H. 215, 216, 221
Blanc-Garin, A. P. 242, 253
Bland, J. 234, 237
blepharospasm 156
Blomqvist, Urban 388
blood clot, defined 294
blood flow regulation 466
blood pressure, AFP levels 21
blood pressure, defined 293
  see also hypertension
blood sugar levels 6
  see also diabetes
blood tests
  fetal 22, 505
  syphilis 441–42
blue babies, defined 293
BNBAS *see* Brazelton Neonatal Behavioral Assessment Scale (BNBAS)
Boden, Leslie I. 390
Bohlin, A. B. 196, 203, 204, 207, 243, 254
Bohman, M. 211, 212, 220
Bookstein, F. L. 202, 208, 250, 252, 257
Bordetella pertussis 71
Borland International 409
Borteyru, J. P. 181, 193, 207, 242, 254
Boss, L. 417
Boston City Hospital 229
Boston University School of Medicine 455
Bottoms, S. 511
Bourgeois, B. F. 95
Bowden, D. M. 206
bowel control 47–49
  see also incontinence

573

bowel obstructions 310
The Boy David 551
Boyle, C. A. 187, 193
Boyles, C. 227, 240
Bradley, Nancy 111, 111n, 112–15
bradycardia, defined 293
brain
　cerebrospinal fluid (CSF) 67
　ventricular system *42, 43*
　see also shunts
brain cell damage, jaundice 126
brain cysts
　cerebral palsy diagnosis 131
brain damage 462–63
　cerebral palsy 125, 142
Brain Development 110, 482
brain dysfunction
　fetal alcohol syndrome 191–92
brain formation
　spina bifida 41–44
brain injury
　aphasia 291
　asphyxia *484,* 485
　cerebral palsy 165
Brainstem Evoked Response (BSER) 334
brain tumor *318*
Branson, R. 232, 237
Brazelton Neonatal Behavioral Assessment Scale (BNBAS) 231
breast cancer 7
breast feeding, clefts 329–30
breech birth 487
Bremer, D. L. 210, 222
Brenneman, D. E. 493, 494
Brigham and Women's Hospital 455
Bright Promise 345
Brinciotti, M. 95
Brinsmade, A. B. 457
British Medical Journal 379, 417, 447, 457, 494
The Broken Cord 193
Broman, S. 493
Brooke, O. 234, 237
Brookline Books 551
Brooks-Gunn, J. 481
Brown, R. T. *200, 201, 203,* 204, 206, 226, 231, 235, 236
Bruell, Carol, MS 454

Bryce, R. L. 468, 477
BSER *see* Brainstem Evoked Response (BSER)
Bucher, H. U. 480
Budnick, Lawrence 390
Buffa, Debby 528
Building the Healing Partnership, Parents, Professionals and Children with Chronic Illness and Disabilities 551
buphthalmos 352, 354
Burack, J. A. 251, 253
Burman, A. 225, 238
Burns, K. 231, 235
Burns, W. 231, 235
Burris, Mary 545
Busch, S. G. 95
Butler, Jayne 534, 535
Butters, N. 210, 222
Byers, T. 224, 239, 266, 269

C

Cabili, S. 457
Cabral, H. 227, 229, 230, 231, 239, 240
caffeinated drinks 5
calcaneovalgus foot 317, 318
California: Birth Defects Study 389
California Birth Defects Monitoring Program (CBDMP) 171, 175, 176, 177
Cameron, H. 479
Campbell, D. 231, 239
Campbell, W. A. 479
Canadian Medical Association Journal 254, 255, 457
Canady, A. I. 94
capillries, defined 293
captopril 405
carbamazepine 407–16
cardiac, defined 293
cardiac arrest, defined 293
cardiac jelly 274, 275, 294
cardiology, defined 294
cardiomyopathy, defined 294
cardiopulmonary resuscitation (CPR) 294, 312
cardiovascular, defined 294

Index

cardiovascular function 517
Caring for Your Newborn 344
Caritis, S. N. 510, 511
Carlsson, C. 242, 255
Carmines, E. G. 480
Carpenter Syndrome Network 547
Carson, Benjamin S., Dr. 553
Carter, B. S. 490, 494
Cary, N. C. 94
Casarett and Doull's Toxicology 378
cataracts 354, *381*, 382
cat feces, toxoplasmosis 6, 425, 429
catheterization *46*
  cardiac 284, 289, 291, 299–300
  cardiac, defined 293
  defined 61
catheters, described 47
CAT scan *see* computerized axial tomography (CAT) scan
Catz, C. S. 508
CCA *see* Children's Craniofacial Association (CCA)
Cefalo, R. 510
Center for Craniofacial Anomalies 557
Center for Developmental Disabilities 549
Center for Digestive Dieases 560
Center for Substance Abuse Prevention (CSAP) 561
Center for Substance Abuse Treatment 507
Centers for Disease Control and Prevention (CDC) 190, 191, 260, 380, 421
  birth defects 13, 266, 376
  Birth Defects Monitoring Program (BDMP) 259, 260, 261, 264, *265*, 266, 267, 380
  grants 252
  guidelines 423
  Morbidity and Mortality Weekly Report 268, 366, 379, *381*, 383
  National AIDS Clearinghouse 560
  National Center for Environmental Health
    Division of Birth Defects and Developmental Disabilities 267, 561
    Fetal Alcohol Prevention Section 267
  publications 11n, 193

central nervous system (CNS)
  early puberty 53–54
  fetal alcohol syndrome 243, 244
  hydrocephalus *87*, 92
  infections 53
  spina bifida 34, 39
cerebellum, defined 205
cerebral, defined 120, 144
cerebral arteries 498
cerebral embolism, defined 294
cerebral palsy *318*, 468, 487, 488–89, 498
  acquired 125
  causes 125–26
  congenital 125
  described 120–21
  diagnosis 119–20, 130–32
  forms 121–23
  management 132–34
  prevention 128–29
  research 140–44, 165–73
  risk factors 127–28
  symptoms 129–30
  treatment 134–39
  twins 305
cerebral thrombosis, defined 294
cerebrospinal fluid (CSF) 103
  excessive accumulation 67, 68
  third vetriculostomy 97, 99–100
cerebrovascular regulatory mechanisms 498
Champus 341
Chance, P. F. 456
chancres 440
Charcot-Marie-Tooth disease *318*
Charkins-Drazin, Hope 550
Chasnoff, I. 227, 230, 231, 235, 236, 238
Chávez, G. F. *189*, 190, 193, 264, 268
chemicals, birth defects 7–8, 363–78, 380–86
Chen, Jianjua 379
Chiari II malformation 41, 42, 56, 63
Chicago Osteopathic Medical Center 229
Childbirth Graphics, Ltd. 344
Childhood Hydrocephalus 67n
Children's Craniofacial Association (CCA) 547

575

Children's Heart Link 561
Children's Hospital Medical Center, Boston 548
Children's Hospital of Michigan 527
Children's Hospital of Wisconsin 345
Children's Hydrocephalus Connection 524
Children's Medical Service 59
Children's National Medical Center 33n
Children with Facial Differences - A Parents Guide 550
Children with Special Care Needs Program 561
Childs Brain 94
Childs Nervous System 94, 109
The Child with Cleft Lip or Palate 344
Chinn, D. H. 109
Chisum, G. 231, 236
cholesterol, defined 294
chorionic villus sampling (CVS) 20–21, 518
Chrisman, Cindy 549
chromosome analysis 20, 22
chronic cerebellar stimulation 139
Churgay, Catherine A., MD 322
Ciba Foundation Symposium 254
Ciba-Geigy, grants 416
Cicero, T. J. 213, 217, 218, 219, 220, 222
cineangiography 291, 294
cineradiography 346
circulatory system, defined 294
circumcision, catheterization 47
Civil Rights Act (1964) 374
Clark, Carleen, RN 273n
Clark, Christine 546
Clark, Edward B., MD 273n
Clarkson, Thomas W. 387
Clarren, S. K. 186, 187, 190, 193, 194, 206, 225, 226, 228, 235, 240, 243, 244, 245, 253, 254, 256, 260, 262, 269, 317, 322, 452, 456
Clarren, Sterling K., Dr. 252
Clayton, P. J. 209, 211, 221
Clearinghouse for Drug-Exposed Children 561
cleft lip 325, *327, 381*
Cleft Lip and Cleft Palate: The First Four Years 325n, 343

Cleft Lip and Cleft Palate: The School-Aged Child 343
Cleft Lip and/or Palate: Will It Affect My Child? 345
Cleft Lip and Palate: Feeding the Newborn 555
Cleft Lip and Palate Fund 555
Cleft Lip and Palate Team 331
cleft palate 9, 326, *327, 381*
Cleft Palate-Craniofacial Journal 542
Cleft Palate Foundation (CPF) 325n, 326, 330, 331, 341, 548
 free information 343–44
 Parent-Patient Liaison Committee 340, 342–43
Cleft Palate Reflections 345, 551
The Cleft Palate Story 344, 551
Cleveland Clinic Children's Hospital 103n
Cleveland Clinic Foundation 107n
Clifford, E. 344
Clinical Obstetrics and Gynecology 236
Clinic in Developmental Medicine 109
Clinics in Plastic Surgery 546
Cloherty, J. P. 465, 478
Cloninger, C. R. 211, 212, 220
closed heart surgery, defined 294
Clostridium botulinum 155
clot, defined 294
clubfoot 9, 61, 315, 320
CMG/EMG tests, defined 63
CMV *see* cytomegalovirus
CNS *see* central nervous system
coarctation, defined 295
coarctation of aorta *381*
Coble, P. 228, 239
cocaine use during pregnancy 223, 228–32
Cockcroft, D. L. 455
cognitive delay 407, 468–69
Cohen, B. J. 457
Cohen, D. J. 251, 256
Cohen, F. L. 215, 220
Coles, C. D. 196, 198, 199, *200, 201, 203,* 204, 206, 208, 226, 230, 231, 235, 236, 262, 268
Collaborative Perinatal Project 465
collateral circulation, defined 295

Index

coloboma of eye *381*, 382
columella, defined 346
coma 475
communication disorder
  aggression *versus* assertion 27
  defined 346
Community Health Studies 386
Como Alimentar a un Bebe con Palendar Hendido 343
Complex Craniofacial Problems: A Guide to Analysis and Treatment 553
complex heart defects, defined 295
comprehension, defined 346
Compuserve 533
computerized axial tomography (CAT) scan
  cerebral palsy diagnosis 130–31
  defined 62–63, 144, 295, 354
computerized chromosome sorters 20
computers
  cerebral palsy 139
  pregnancy 8
  see also Internet addresses
Conceptualization and Measurement of Health of Children in the Health Insurance Study 481
congenital, defined 144, 295, 346, 354
congenital anomalies *413*
congenital convex pes valgus 318
congenital heart defect 273–90, 295
congenital malformations 8, 468
congenital megacolon 309
congenital rubella syndrome (CRS) 419–20
congestive heart failure *see* heart failure
conotruncal area, defined 295
conotruncal defects 275–76, 279–82
  tetralogy of Fallot 279–80, *280,* 290
  transposition 280–81
Consensus Development Conference on Antenatal Steroids 499
constipation 47
contracture, defined 144
contralateral, defined 354
convulsions 85
  see also seizures
Convulsions in Children with Hydrocephalus 94

Cook-Fort Worth Children's Medical Center 313
Cope, M. 480
Copper, R. 511
Cordero, José F., MD *189,* 190, 193, 261, 262, 264, 267, 268
Cordier, Sylvaine 388
Cornelia de Lange syndrome 188
Cornelius, M. 196, 198, 199, 207, 227, 228, 232, 234, 236, 237
Cornish, J. D. 480
coronary arteries 286–88
coronary arteries, defined 295
coronary artery disease, defined 295
coronary bypass surgery, defined 295
coronary thrombosis, defined 296
corpus callosum, defined 354
corrective shoes 320, 321–22
correlational studies, described 205
costs, spina bifida 11
Cottreau, C. 224, 227, 229, 232, 236
Council of Cardiovascular Disease in the Young *see* American Heart Association
cover tests 72
CPF *see* Cleft Palate Foundation (CPF)
CPR *see* cardiopulmonary resuscitation (CPR)
crack baby 235
cranial sutures 70
Craniofacial Anomalies Team 331
The Craniofacial Center 344
Craniofacial Foundation of America 542
Craparo, Frank, MD 22
Creighton University School of Medicine 21
Crépin, G. 242, 253
Crippled Children's Special Health Services 341
crossbite, defined 346
CRS *see* congenital rubella syndrome (CRS); rubella
CSF *see* cerebrospinal fluid (CSF)
CT scan *see* computerized axial tomography (CAT) scan
Cummins, S. 494
Cupid's bow 184, *328*

Current Developments in Psychopharmacology 95
Cusimano, M. D. 111, 115
cutaneous lesions, defined 354
CVS *see* chorionic villus sampling (CVS)
cyanosis 279–80, 296
cytomegalovirus (CMV) 6–7, 125, 435–37

D

Dahl, R. 228, 236
Daily Values
  folic acid 14, 15, 16
  see also minimum daily requirements
Daling, J. 235
Dam, M. 417
Dames, N. M. 207
Dandy-Walker malformation 70
Dandy-Walker syndrome 70, 86, 109, 112
Dansky, L. 417
Darby, B. L. 198, 207
Das, A. 511
Dasan Productions 345
databases
  antiepileptic drugs 409
  birth defects 380–83
Data Safety Monitoring Board 502
Davidson, Kathleen M. 527
Davis, Devra Lee, Dr. 377
Davis, J. A. 207
Davis, Margarett, MD, MPH 267
Dawson, Brenda V. 366
Day, Nancy L., PhD 196, 198, 199, 207, 224, 226, 227, 228, 229, 230, 231, 232, 234, 235, 236, 237, 239, 250, 252, 253
Decade of the Brain 177
decubitus, defined 61
  see also pressure sores
Deddish, R. 479, 494
defibrillator, defined 296
deformities, described 316
De Giorgio, Christopher M., MD 417, 418

Dehaene, P. 242, 244, 250, 251, 253, 256
De La Cruz, Patricia 416
Delia, Julian, MD 307
denasality, defined 346, 347
Denis Browne splint 320
Dennis, J. 494
dental arch, defined 346
dental care
  clefts 336–37
  hydrocephalus 72
Denver Developmental Screening Tool 71
Department of Agriculture 14
Department of Health, Education, and Welfare (DHEW) 232, 240
Department of Health and Human Services (DHHS) 425n, 561
  Healthy People 2000 259, 260, 264, 269
  publications 221, 238, 240, 255, 389
Depp, R. 510
Dermatalogic Drugs Advisory Committee 400
dermatologists 354, 400
Deroubaix, P. 242, 253
DeSanto, S. 107, 109
Dethero, Becky 559
Dethero Enterprises 559
The Developing Human 208
The Developing Person 208
Developmental Brain Dysfunction 254
developmental disabilities 129, 468–69
  cerebral palsy 152
  prenatal causes 459–64
Developmental Medicine and Child Neurology 94, 95, 151, 162, 163, 477, 478, 480, 493, 494
DHEW *see* Department of Health, Education, and Welfare (DHEW)
DHHS *see* Department of Health and Human Services (DHHS)
diabetes 514–15
  defined 296
  neural tube defects 13
  pregnancy 6

Index

diagnosis
  cerebral palsy 119–20, 130–32
  cytomegalovirus 436–37
  fetal alcohol syndrome 181–92, 251
  hemangiomas 357–58
  Hirschsprung's disease 311
  neonatal foot deformities 317–18
  neurologic system 62–64
  orthopedic decisions 315–16
  syphilis 441–42
  toxoplasmosis 427–28
Diagnosis and Treatment of Pediatric Foot Deformities 315n
diarrhea 47
  see also incontinence
diastole, defined 296
diastolic blood pressure, defined 296
diet and nutrition
  cerebral palsy 140
  folic acid 13–14
  folic acid and pregnancy 17
  pregnancy 4–6, 8
  see also foods
dietary supplements 5, 15
Di George syndrome 282
Digestive Disease National Coalition 561
digestive tract *48*
digitalis, defined 296
Dilantin 113
Dinner Through a Straw 553, 554
diplegia *122*
Disability in America 481
Discontinuing Antiepileptic Medication in Children with Epilepsy After Two Years Without Seizures 95
Diseases of Occupations 373
Disorders of the Placenta, Fetus and Neonate: Diagnosis and Clinical Significance 493
Distaval *see* thalidomide
Distinguished Federal Civilian Service Award 372, 395
diuretic, defined 296
Dobbing, J. 207
documentation, childhood behaviors 26–27
Dodge, Philip R., MD 93
Dolcourt, Joyce 549

Donald, C. A. 481
Donovan, C. M. 213, 221
Donovan, E. F. 509
Doppler-echocardiography *see* echocardiography
Doppler shift, defined 296
Dorris, M. 186, 193
double outlet right ventricle 281
Douglas, G. E. 215, 216, 221
Doull, John 378
Dow Chemical 364
Down syndrome 243
  chromosome cause 20
  described 9
  heart defects 275, 284
  tests 21
Dransfield, Jana 530
Drazin, David 550
drooling
  cerebral palsy 140
  surgery 163–64
Drug and Alcohol Dependence 235, 237, 238, 268
Drugs, Alcohol, Pregnancy and Parenting 235
drugs, birth defects 3–4, 7, 199, 210, 399
drug therapy, cerebral palsy 136–37, 143–44, 163
drug use during pregnancy 223–35
D'Souza, B. J. 95
d-transposition 280–81
Duc, G. 480
Duchenne's muscular dystrophy *318*
ductus arteriosus 277, 296
Dudell, G. 480
Dufresne, Craig R., Dr. 553
Dukelow, W. R. 455
Dunne, K. B. 317, 322
Dunne, P. M. 317, 322
Duration of Treatment for Childhood Epilepsy 95
Durham, F. M. 213, 220
Dykens, E. M. 251, 253
dysarthria 123, 144
dyskinetic cerebral palsy 122–23
dysmorphia 195, 262
dysmorphology, defined 326
dysrhythmia, defined 291

E

Ear Anomalies Reconstructed (EAR) 548
eardrum, defined 347
ear infections, clefts 333
Early Human Development 477
Easter Seal Society *see* National Easter Seal Society
Eaves, L. J. 212
echocardiography 300
　defined 297
　fetal 283
echo-Doppler *see* echocardiography
ectopia cordis 289–90
Edelin, K. C. 199, 208, 243, 255
edema, defined 297
EDF *see* Environmental Defense Fund (EDF)
Edmonds, Larry D. 266, 268, 366, 378, *381,* 383, 453, 456
education
　cerebral palsy 133, 168–69
　clefts 339–40
educational development, spina bifida 56–57
Edwards, A. D. 480
Edwards, M. J. 453, 455, 456, 457, 458
Edwards, M. S. B. 109
Edwards, W. 508
EEG *see* electroencephalogram (EEG)
Ehlers, C. L. 210, 220
Ehrenkranz, R. A. 509
Ehrlich, S. 231, 239
Einarson, T. 231, 238
Eisen, M. 481
Eisenhower, Dwight D. 395
elective referral, defined 297
electrical stimulation, spastic muscles 161–62, 168
electric blankets 447–55
electrocardiogram (EKG), defined 297
electrocardiography 299
Electroclinical Follow-up of Shunted Hydrocephalic Children 94
Electroencephalic and Clinicopathological Observations in Hydrocephalic Chldren 93

electroencephalogram (EEG)
　cerebral palsy diagnosis 131–32, *132*
　defined 144, 297, 354
　hydrocephalus 88, 92
　test, defined 63
Electroencephalography and Clinical Neurophysiology 220
electromanometry 311
electromyography, defined 145
electrophysiologic study (EPS), defined 297
Ellenberg, J. H. 478, 492, 493, 494
Elms, L. 344
Elvebeck, J. R. 417
embolus, defined 297
Emerson, R. 95
EMG test, defined 63
Emory University School of Medicine 206
enalapril 405
encephalitis, cerebral palsy 125, 151
encephalocele *381*
encephalopathy 466, 475, 483–92
encephalotrigeminal angiomatosis *see* Sturge-Weber syndrome
endocardial cushion defect 282–85, 293, *381*
　atrioventricular canal defect with hypoplastic ventricle 284–85
　complete atrioventricular canal defect 283–84
　ostium primum atrial septal defect 283
endocardial cushions, defined 297
endocardium *274,* 297
Endocrine Toxicology 379
endocrinologists 54
endogenous glutamate 462
endogenous opoids 217
endoscopy 97
endothelium 297, 500, 520
The Enduring Effects of Prenatal Alcohol Exposure on Child Development 257
Ens-Dokkum, M. H. 481
enterocolitis 310, 312
ENT specialists 333, 347
Environmental and Molecular Mutagenesis 221

Index

Environmental Defense Fund (EDF) 386
environmental factors
  birth defects 382
  clefts 326
Environmental Health Perspectives 208, 375, 379
Environmental Protection Agency (EPA) 364, 368, 386
Environmental Research 386
Environmental Research Foundation 363n
environmental toxins 375–76
  pregnancy 8, 150
Environment and Health Weekly 363n
enzyme, defined 297
EPA *see* Environmental Protection Agency (EPA)
Epidemiologic Reviews 389
Epilepsia 95, 417, 480
epilepsy 407
  cerebral palsy 123–24
  hydrocephalus 86, 108
  pregnancy 6
  spina bifida 53
Epilepsy, Pregnancy and the Child 417
Epilepsy Foundation of America 562
Erickson, J. David 261, 264, 267, 268, 453, 456
Erickson, S. *200, 201, 203,* 204, 206, 226, 231, 235, 236
Ericson, Anders 388
Erlanger Medical Center, Thompson Children's Hospital 542
Erlbaum Associates 493
Ernhart, C. B. 198, 207
Ernst, Cara C. 252
Escobar, G. J. 481
Essman, W. B. 95
Etches, P. C. 509
etretinate 403
European Journal Epidemiology 417
European Journal Obstetrics Gynecologic Reproductive Biology 479
eustachian tubes 333
Evans, J. 510
Everything You Want To Know About Your Child's Birth Defect 547
Exceptional Parent 64, 552
The Exceptional Parent Annual Directory of National Organizations 552
exercise testing, defined 297
expressive language, defined 347
extracorporeal membrane oxygenation (EDMO) 141
extrasystole, defined 297
eye problems 382
  cerebral palsy 124–25
  drooping eyelids *184*
  hydrocephalus 69, 79–81
  spina bifida 53
  Sturge-Weber syndrome 352
  see also vision impairment

F

Fabro, S. 207
Face Facts Video Tapes 556
FACES 543, 557
Faces 357n
facial clefts *381*
  see also cleft palate
Facial Deformities and Plastic Surgery 555
facial expressions, hydrocephalus 76–77
Faillace, W. J. 94
failure to thrive 124, 140
  defined 145
Falek, A. 196, 198, 199, *200, 201, 203,* 204, 206, 208, 226, 230, 231, 235, 236, 262, 268
Falk, M. 345
Fallot, Arthur 279
families
  cerebral palsy 133–34
  clefts 330–31
  reading list 551–55
Fanaroff, A. A. 508, 509
Farmer, Terri 542
Farrelly, Doris 529
FAS *see* fetal alcohol syndrome (FAS)
FDA Consumer 3n, 19n, 391n, 399n
FDA Drug Bulletin 400, 404
federal programs
  cerebral palsy information 146–47
  spina bifida resources 59

581

Fee, S. C. 479, 494
Feeding an Infant with a Cleft 330, 343
feeding issues, clefts 329–30
Feeding Your Special Baby 344
Feinstein, A. R. 480
Feldman, J. 250, 257
Feldman, Robert G. 366
Ferm, V. H. 455
Fernhoff, P. M. 196, 198, 199, 206, 262, 268
Fetal Alcohol Network 562
fetal alcohol syndrome (FAS) 5–6, 225–26
   consequences 245–49
   diagnosis 181–92
   parental alcohol consumption 195–205, 209–18
   prevention 259
   research 242–43, 249–52
fetal distress 465
fetal Doppler-echocardiography, defined 297
fetoscope 307
fetus
   hypotonia *317*
   prenatal hydrocephalus 107–9
   treatments 22
   see also pregnancy
fever 447–55
   neural tube defects 13
fibrillation, defined 297
fibrin, defined 297
Fields, Debbie 524, 525
Finer, N. N. 470, 478, 481, 482
Finkbine, Sherri 395
Finnegan, L. 231, 239
Fischetti, Michael 529
Fishbaugh, Michael 553
Fisher, N. L. 453, 456
Fisher's exact and chi square tests 85
Fishman, M. A. 94
fistulas
   defined 347
   heart defects 288–89
fits *see* epilepsy; seizures
Fits in Hydrocephalic Children 94
flatfoot, flexible 320–21
Fleming, Arthur W. 395
Flomenhaft, Brenda, MS 454

flourescent treponemal antibody absorption (FTA-ABS) test 442
Floyd, R. Louise, DSN, RN 267
flu shots *see* immunizations; vaccines
focal seizure, defined 354
folate *see* folic acid; vitamin B
Foley, J. 478
folic acid 3, 4–5, 11, 448
   defined 61
   sources 14–17
   spina bifida 38
   see also vitamin B
Food and Drug Administration (FDA)
   Accutane 399, 401, 402, 403, 404
   BOTOX for limb spasticity 156–57
   Drug Bulletin 255
   folic acid requirements 5, 15, 20, 38
   hydrocephalus shunt valves 105
   medication labeling 7
   Office of Food Labeling 17
   Office of Special Nutritionals 12, 15, 17
   Office of Women's Health 4
   thalidomide 392–96
   thalidomide application 371, 372
foods
   breakfast cereals 12
   caffeinated drinks 5
   citrus fruits 4
   continence 49
   folic acid 14–17, *16*
   fruits and vegetables
      folic acid 14
   grain products 5, 13, 38
   leafy green vegetables 4, 12, 38
   legumes 4, 12, 38
   magnesium 177
   toxoplasmosis 428–29
   see also diet and nutrition
Food Values of Portions Commonly Used 16
foot deformities 315–22
foramen ovale 277, 297
Forman, Eva 551, 555, 557
forme fruste, defined 354
For Parents of Newborn Babies wit Cleft Lip/Palate 343
Forsyth, J. S. 479
Forward Face 548, 556

Index

foscarnet 437
Foundation for Blood Research 21
Foundation for Nager and Miller Syndromes 543
Foundation for the Faces of Children 548–49
Fox, A. Mervyn, MD 25n
fractures, spina bifida 53
Frank, D. 227, 229, 230, 231, 239, 240
Fraser, F. C. 458
Freeman, J. M. 95
Freeman-Sheldon Syndrome Parent Support Group 549
Freier, C. 230, 231, 236
Freud, Sigmund 119, 120, 377
Fried, L. 227, 229, 230, 231, 240
Fried, P. 227, 228, 233, 234, 237
Friedler, G. 217, 220
Friedman, J. M. 107, 108, 110
Friedreich's ataxia *318*
frontal lobe, defined 354
Fuchs, M. 243, 253
Fudge, Emily 25n, 75n, 79n, 525
Fudge, Rachel 101
funduscopic examinations 72

G

Gado, M. 94
Gaily, E. 417
gait analysis, defined 145
Galbraith, R. S. 474, 478
ganciclovir 437
Gant, N. 225, 238
Garvin, Peg 543
gastrointestinal defects *381*
gastrostomy 140
  defined 145
Gay, G. 228, 237
gender factor, Hirschsprung's disease 310
General Motors 374
Genetic Counseling 552
genetic counselors, neural tube defects 36
genetic factors
  birth defects 8, 9–10, 17, 312, 382
  cerebral palsy 150, 154

genetic factors, continued
  clefts 326
  fetal alcohol syndrome 187, 188
  foot deformities 316
  neural tube defects 13
  spina bifida 36, 37
Genetic Information Via the Internet: Risks and Benefits 559
The Genetic Resource 552
genetics, defined 347
The Genetics of Cleft Lip and Palate 326, 343
genetic testing, pregnancy 9
Gennser, G. 232, 239
George Washington University, Rockville 511
Georgiade, N. 344
German, J. 458
German measles *see* rubella
Geschwind, Sandra A. 371
Geva, D. 199, 207, 226, 228, 237
gibbus, defined 61
Giffin, L. 321, 322, 323
Gilfallan, S. C. 378
Gill, A. B. 479
Gilligan, S. B. 211, 212, 220
Gilstrap, L. 3rd 225, 238, 479, 495
Giordano, A. 217, 219
glaucoma 352, 354, 356
  see also eye problems
Glick, P. L. 109
glucose intolerance 514
glutamate 142, 462
glycolipids 462–63
Gofman, John W. 386
Gold, E. O. 210, 222
Gold, M. S. 230, 238
Goldaber, K. G. 479, 495
Goldberg, M. 389
Goldberg, R. N. 477
Goldberg, Stanley J. 366, 388
Goldenberg, R. 511
Golden Har Parent Support Network 549
Goldman, Lynn R. 389
Goldschmidt, L. 199, 207, 228, 231, 232, 234, 236, 237, 239
Goodlet, C. R. 199, 204, 205, 208, 244, 251, 253

583

Goodwin, T. M. 479, 495
Gordon, N. 95
Gordon, T. 510
Gortmaker, S. 233, 240
Gott, Peggy S., PhD 417, 418
Goulet, L. 389
Gozes, I. 493
Grace, M. G. A. 482
gradient, defined 297
Graham, J. M. 198, 207, 454, 456, 458
Graham, K. 231, 238
Grannstrom, M. L. 417
Grant, A. 227, 237, 485, 492
Grathwohl, H. L. 254
Gray, R. A. 228, 233, 237
Gray, R. H. 387
The Greater New York Pull-thru Network 562
Greene, J. 231, 239
Greenhouse, Linda 375
Greenpeace 386, 390
Greenwood, N. 92, 94
Proceedings of Greenwood Genetics Center 268
Grenier, A. 480
Grennert, L. 232, 239
Grether, Judith K., PhD 171, 175, 176
Griffith, D. 230, 231, 236
Grigg, William 396
Grindulis, H. 473, 482
Grindulis, M. 488, 494
Gromisch, D. S. 243, 253
Gross, Jack 548
Grottos of America 341
growth rates 515
  cerebral palsy 124
  fetal alcohol syndrome 182–83, 187–88, 195, 199–202, 204, 242
  premature birth 499
  see also failure to thrive
Gruethner, Dawn 543
Guardians of Hydrocephalus Research Foundation 64, 529
Guiffre, R. 107, 109
Guinn, D. 511
Gunkel, H. 509
Guzinski, G. M. 254

H

Hack, M. 508, 509
Hadders-Algra, M. 488, 494
Hadeed, A. 231, 237
Halks-Miller, M. 109
Hall, Zach W., PhD 176
Halperin, M. E. 468, 477
Halperin, W. 268
Hamel, S. 231, 239
Handbook for the Care of Infants and Toddlers with Disabilities and Chronic Conditions 552
Handbook of Behavioral Teratology 221
handicapped children 339
handicaps 469–76
hand preferences, cerebral palsy diagnosis 130
Hanson, J. W. 198, 207, 252
Hansson, Evert 388
HANT *see* Hydrocephalus Association of North Texas (HANT)
Harada, Masazumi 387
Harbison, Raymond D. 378
hare lip, defined 347
Harousseau, H. 181, 193, 207, 242, 254
Harris, J. C. 246, 253
Harrison, G. 232, 237
Harrison, M. R. 22, 109, 110
Harrod, M. J. 107, 108, 110
Hartley, W. J. 455
Harvard Medical School 455
Harvard School of Public Health 455
Harvey, M. A. S. 452, 453, 456, 457
Hassoun, B. 227, 240
Haste, F. 234, 237
Hauser, W. A. 417
Hauth, J. 511
Hauth, J. C. 479, 495
Hazardous Waste and Hazardous Materials 389
hazardous waste sites 367–71
Hazelwood, M. E. 162
Hazlett, L. D. 213, 219
head injury, cerebral palsy 125, 128
health care providers
  cerebral palsy 133–34
  consultations 12

Index

health care providers, continued
  dietary supplements 5
  drug consumption 7
  hydrocephalus 68–69
  treatment of children 25
The Health Resource 547
health team, defined 297
Healthy People 2000 see under Department of Health and Human Services (DHHS)
Hearing and Behavior in Children with Cleft Lip and Palate 344
hearing impairment
  cerebral palsy 124–25
  clefts 333–34
  defined 347
hearing tests 72
heart, described 273, *274*
heart anomalies *381*
heart attack, defined 297
heart block, defined 297
heart development 273–90
heart failure, defined 299
heart flow defects 276–77
heart-lung machine, defined 299
heart malformations 9
heart murmurs 283–84, 286, 289
  defined 301
The Heart of A Child 273n
heart tumors 289
heart valves 278
  aortic *274*
  mitral *274*, 282, 283, 300
  pulmonary *274*
  tricuspid *274*, 282, 283
Heath, A. C. 212
Hegedus, A. M. 210, 220
Heinonen, Olli P. 387
Helge, H. 417
Helping Hearts 290
Helzer, J. 225, 238
hemangiomas 357–59
  defined 355
hemianopia 125, 145
hemiparesis 352
  defined 146, 355
hemiparetic tremors
  defined 145
hemiparetic tumors 122, 139

hemiplegia *122,* 355
hemispherectomy, defined 355
Henderson, G. I. 213, 220
Hendrickson, R. V. 455
Hendrickx, A. G. 455
Henerlau, Jennifer 525
herald spot 358
heredity
  alcoholism 209–12
  defined 299, 347
  see also genetic factors
Herha, J. 216, 221
Herman, C. S. 243, 256
Hernandez, P. 479, 495
herpes virus, cytomegalovirus 7
Herridge, P. 231, 238
Hessol, Nancy A. 379
Heston, L. L. 209, 211, 221
heterotaxy, defined 299
high blood pressure, defined 299
high-density lipoprotein (HDL), defined 299
High Risk: Children Without a Conscience 193
Hiilesmaa, V. 417
Hill, A. 472, 477
Hill, Washington, MD 21
Hillier, V. 92, 94
Hilton, M. 223, 224, 238
Hingson, R. 227, 229, 230, 231, 240
hip dislocations 319, 320
hippocampus 205–6, 459–60
Hirschberg examinations 72
Hirschsprung, Harold, Dr. 309
Hirschsprung's disease 309–13
Hirtz, D. J. 480
Hiscock, M. 251, 255
HIV (human immunodeficiency virus) 439, 463
Hixon, B. B. 95
Hochberg, E. 231, 239
Hodapp, R. M. 251, 253
Hoffmann-LaRoche 400, 401–2
Holden, K. R. 95
Hollander, D. I. 478
Hollowell, Joseph 267
Holmberg, P. C. 456
Holmes, L. 227, 240
Holmes, Sandra J. MD 93

holoprosencephaly 108
Holowach, J., MD 94
Holowach, Thurston J., MD 95
Holter monitoring, defined 299
homonymous hemianopsia, defined 355
Horbar, J. D. 508, 509
Hosking, G. P. 90, 92, 94
Hospital for Sick Children, Toronto 555
hotlines, Cleft Palate Foundation 342, 548
hot tubs 13, 447–55
Houchin, Pat 545
Hrbek, A. 242, 255
Huisjes, H. J. 488, 494
Hunter, A. G. W. 452, 457
Hunter, Donald 373
Hutzler, M. 232, 238
hydranencephaly 108
hydrocephalus 41, *42, 43, 381*
  children 67–73
  defined 61
  spina bifida 53, 56
  treatment 22, 98
  see also shunts
Hydrocephalus and Epilepsy 94
Hydrocephalus and Mental Retardation in Craniosynostosis 94
Hydrocephalus Association 25n, 30, 67n, 73, 78, 79n, 81, 101, 523n, 525–26
  Medical Advisory Board 75n
  National Directory 523–31
  publications 67n, 97n, 101, 533n
Hydrocephalus Association of North Texas (HANT) 530–31
National Hydrocephalus Foundation 525, 526–27
Hydrocephalus Network of Greater New York (HYDRONET) 529–30
Hydrocephalus News and Notes 103n, 105, 107n, 111n, 115
The Hydrocephalus Research Foundation 103n, 105, 110, 115
Hydrocephalus Support Group 523–31, 527–28, 528
hydronephrosis 114
HYDRONET *see* Hydrocephalus Network of Greater New York (HYDRONET)

Hymbaugh, K. J. 187, 190, 193, 267
hyperactivity, fetal alcohol syndrome 186, 190, 249
hypercarbia 466
hypernasality, defined 347
hypertension, defined 299
hyperthermia 447–55
hypertonia 129, 145
hypoglycemia 516
hypoplasia *381*
hypoplastic, defined 299
hypoplastic left heart syndrome *381*
hypoplastic ventricle 284, 303
hypotension 405, 485
hypotonia 129, 145
hypoxemia 485, 487, 498
hypoxia 281, 299, 463, 465, 466, 500, 517
  cerebral palsy 150, 151
hypoxic-ischemic encephalopathy 126, 142, 145

I

Iams, J. 511
Idelson, R. K. 187, 194, 262, 269
identical twins 306
Ieronimo, Margaret 543
Iffy, L. 493
IFSP *see* Individualized Family Service Plan (IFSP)
If Your Baby Has a Cleft 556
immune deficiency 432–33, 436
  see also AIDS (Acquired Immune Deficiency Syndrome)
immunizations
  Diphtheria, Tetanus, Pertussis (DPT) 71
  Haelmophilus influenzae type B 72
  measles 71–72
  mumps 72
  polio 72
  rubella 72, 420–22
  see also vaccines
incidence, defined 299
The Incidence of Seizure Disorder in Children with Acquired and Congenital Hydrocephalus 94

Index

incontinence 71
  cerebral palsy 139–40
  spina bifida 13, 44–49
Indian Health Service 191, 252
Individualized Family Service Plan (IFSP) 339
indomethacin 306
Infante, Peter F. 375
infants, first stool 309–10
infants, seizures 128
Information for the Teenager Born with a Cleft Lip and/or Palate 343
Institute of Medicine 470, 481
insulin 514–17
  pregnancy 6
  see also diabetes
insurance coverage, spina bifida 59
intellectual abnormalities, fetal alcohol syndrome 186
intellectual function, hydrocephalus 69
Intelligence in Epilepsy 95
International Fetal Medicine and Surgical Society 110
International Journal of Epidemiology 238
International Society of Exposure Analysis Newsletter 390
International Society of Plastic Surgery Journal 559
Internet addresses
  Administration for Children and Families 565
  American Self-Help Clearinghouse 555
  Apgar Scoring for Newborns 565
  British Columbia's Children's Hospital 566
  Carpenter Syndrome Network 547
  Centers for Disease Control and Prevention 566
  Chiari Malformation Page 566
  Department of Health and Human Services 566
  Food and Drug Administration 566
  HYCEPH-L 533, 534, 535
  Hydrocephalus Association 533, 534
  Let's Face It 541
  March of Dimes Birth Defects Foundation 18

Internet addresses, continued
  National Center for Environmental Health 566
  The National Health Information Center 566
  National Institutes of Health 566
  National Library of Medicine 566
  National Organization for Rare Disorders (NORD) 544, 566
  Olson, Gretchen (United Cerebral Palsy Association) 540
  Onyx, Pam (AboutFace) 542
  Pediatric Database 566
  United Cerebral Palsy Associations 537–40
  Wide Smiles: Cleft-Links 566
interrupted aortic arch, defined 299
Interventional Radiology 545
intestinal blockage 47
intimidation, health care providers 28–29
intracranial calcification, defined 355
intracranial CSF diversion 97
intracranial hemorrhage, cerebral palsy 126
intracranial pressure
  eye problems 79
  hydrocephalus 70, 90, 98
intractable seizure, defined 355
intrauterine growth retardation (IUGR) 498
invasive, defined 299–300
Iosub, S. 243, 253
ipsilateral, defined 355
IQ tests 202–3, 243–45, 461, 471, 474
Irwin, M. 210, 222
ischemia 300, 465
ischemic brain damage 462–63, 486
ischemic heart disease, defined 300
Ishikawa, T. 473, 482
Iversen, K. 242, 255
IVH (Intraventricular Hemmorhage) Parents 562
IVP test, defined 63
Iyasu, S. 493

J

Jackson, David 551, 555
Jackson, Ian, MD 551, 555, 557
Jackson, Marjorie 551, 555
Jackson, Patricia Ludder, RN 73
Jacob, T. 210, 222
Jacobson, Joseph L. 388, 389
James, Levy M. 366, 378
James, M. 230, 236
Jan, J. E. 477
Janz, D. 417
Jaskowiak, Melani 524
Jasperse, D. 196, 198, 207, 227, 228, 236
Jastek Wide Range Achievement Test 85
jaundice 145, 506
  cerebral palsy 120, 126, 128
Jessop, D. J. 481
Jick, Hershel, MD 455, 456
Jick, Susan S., MPH 455, 456
Joffe, J. M. 215, 220
Johansson, P. R. 242, 255
Johns Hopkins Hospital 290
Johns Hopkins University 394
Johnson, F. 511
Johnson, K. A. 417
Johnson, M. A. 494
Johnson, S. 345
Johnson Controls 374
Johnston, L. P. 212, 214, 221
Johnston, M. C. 208
Jones, K. L. 181, 182, 193, 207, 242, 244, 254, 256, 262, 269, 417
Jones, Kenneth Lyons, Dr. 252
Jones, Robert F. C., MD 98, 101
Journal of Child Psychology and Psychiatry 253
Journal of Developmental and Behavioral Pediatrics 236
Journal of Epidemiology and Community Health 379
Journal of Experimental Zoology 222
Journal of Neurosurgery 109
Journal of Occupational Medicine 378
Journal of Occupational Medicine and Toxicology 388
Journal of Pediatric Health Care 73
Journal of Pediatrics 49, 256, 389, 417, 456, 477, 482, 493, 494, 508
Journal of Perinatal Medicine 479
Journal of Pharmacology and Experimental Therapeutics 219, 220
Journal of Psychoactive Drugs 237, 238
Journal of Public Health Policy 269
Journal of Studies on Alcohol 208, 257
Journal of Substance Abuse 194, 269
Journal of the American Academy of Child and Adolescent Psychiatry 256, 257
Journal of the American College of Cardiology 366, 388
Journal of the American Medical Association 194, 212, 222, 239, 240, 256, 269, 395, 447n, 456, 478, 481, 493
Joyumpa, A. M. 213, 220
Juvenile Diabetes Foundation 562

K

KAFO *see* knee-ankle-foot orthosis (KAFO)
Kallen, B. 417
Kaminetzky, H. A. 493
Kanayama, M. 473, 482
Kantor, Arlene K. 379
Kapine, Amy 550
Kaplan, L. C. 187, 194, 262, 269
Kaplan, R. M. 481
Kaplan, W. 231, 236
Karchmar, E. J. 479
Kasten, Shirley 454
Kaufman Assessment Battery for Children (K-ABC) *203*
Kawasaki syndrome, defined 300
Kayne, H. 227, 229, 230, 231, 240
Kefauver, Estes 395
Kefauver-Harris drug law 372
Keith, L. 230, 238
Keller, A. J. 95
Kelly, J. F. 493
Kelsey, F. Ellis 393

Index

Kelsey, Frances O., MD 371, 372, 392–93, 395, 396–97
Kendler, K. S. 212
Kendrick, J. S. 224, 239, 266, 269
Kennedy, John F. 372, 395
Kenyon, Larry 535
Kero, P. O. 478
Kessler, R. C. 212
Kettinger, L. 213, 222
Khoury, Muin J. 261, 264, 268, 389
kidney malfunction, spina bifida 44–47
see also urologic system
kidney tests 63
Kilham, L. 455
King's College, London 307
Kitchen, W. H. 481
Klaucke, D. N. 261, 268
Klebanoff, M. 510
Kleinebrecht, J. 453, 457
Klepper, T. 228, 236
Kline, J. 232, 238
Klippel-Trenaunay Support Group 562
Klipstein, C. A. 488, 494
knee-ankle-foot orthosis (KAFO), defined 61
Knight, George J., PhD 21
Knights, R. 227, 237
Koepke, T. 475, 477
Kohler's disease 321
Kok, J. H. 172
Koller, S. 453, 457
Kopra-Frye, Karen, Dr. 252
Koren, G. 231, 238
Korones, S. B. 508, 509
Kouvailanen, K. 457
Kreye, M. 227, 240
Kricker, Anne 386
Kristensen, Petter 387
Kullander, S. 232, 239
Kuosma, E. 456
Kurisaka, M. 107, 108.110
Kurland, L. T. 417
Kurtzweil, Paula 18
Kwok, Bernard C. T., MD 101
Kyllerman, M. 242, 255

L

labeling
 dietary supplements 15
 drugs 400
Labio Hendido y Paladar Hendido: Los Cuatro Primeros Anos 343
labor unions 374
Lacro, R. V. 417
lactic acidemia 466
LaDue, Robin A., Dr. 186, 187, 194, 226, 240 ,245, 246, 252, 254, 256, 260, 269
La Leche League 329, 562
Lam, B. C. C. 474, 478
Lammer, E. J. 261, 264, 268
Lancaster, J. S. 198, 208
Lancaster Cleft Palate Clinic 344, 345
The Lancet 15, 193, 207, 221, 254, 256, 269, 375, 447, 456, 457, 458, 482, 494, 509
Landesman-Dwyer, S. 186, 193
Landis, J. R. 478
Landon, M. 510
Landress, H. 227, 236
Landwehr, J. B., Jr. 111, 115
Lanes, Marsha Thomas, MS 454
language disorder, defined 347
language therapy
 cerebral palsy 133
 clefts 332
 studies 195
Laor, A. 492
Larrick, George P. 395
Larsson, G. 196, 203, 204, 207, 243, 254
laryngoscopy, defined 63
latex allergy, spina bifida 54
Latham, Jeanne 17
Lawless, Edward W. 375
Lawrence, K. M. 93
Layde, P. M. 453, 456
The Layman's Guide to Sturge-Weber Medical Terminology 351n, 353–56
Leach, J. 318, 322
lead poisoning 8, 375, 461
Learner Managed Designs, Inc. 552

learning disabilities
  hydrocephalus 76
  spina bifida 13
Leavitt, Richard 8
LeBaron, Pam 543
Lee, J. A. 213219
Leff, Patricia Tanner 551
left-heart flow defect, defined 300
Leiber, B. 242, 255
Lemoine, P. H. 181, 193, 207, 242, 244, 247, 248, 251, 254
Lemons, J. A. 509
Lenz, Widuking, Dr. 372, 393, 394
leprosy 396
Let's Do Lunch (and Other Meals) 559
Let's Face It 541n, 552, 559
Let's Face The Music, A Story of Our Lives 548
leukemia 363
Levene, M. I. 473, 474, 482, 488, 494
Leveno, K. J. 479, 495
Levenson, S. 227, 229, 230, 231, 240
Leviton, A. 478, 485, 493, 494
Lewis, Christine, PhD 15
Lewis, Ricki, PhD 22
Liakos, Ann Marie 103n, 105, 110, 526
Lie, Rolv Terje 152, 383
Lieber, R. L. 323
Lieberman, E. 493
life expectancy, spina bifida 54–56
lifestyles, pregnancy 10, 223–35
Ligelis, Calliope 544
Lindbohm, Marja-Lusa 379
lipids 300, 500
lipoproteins 299, 300
Lipp, A. E. 480
Lippek, Sue 252
Lipson, A. H. 458
lissencephaly 108
Littenberg, B. 481
Little, B. 225, 230, 238
Little, Ruth E., Dr. 119, 121
lobectomy, defined 355
Loeb, Alan 390
Loffredo, C. 388
Long, W. 509
Looking Forward, Guide for Parents of the Child with Cleft Lip and Palate 345

looping, defined 300
looping defects of heart 275, 285
Lorber, J. 92, 94
Lord, E. M. 213, 221
Los Angeles County/University of Southern California (LAC/USC) Medical Center 408, 409, 416, 418
Los Angeles Times 384
Löser, H. 242, 255
Low, J. A. 474, 478, 479
Low Achieving Children: The First Seven Years 493
low birth weight 142, 497–507
  AFP levels 21
  see also birth weight
low density lipoprotein (LDL), defined 300
l-transposition 281
Lucey, J. F. 508
Luciano, Mark, MD, PhD 103, 103n, 104
lumen, defined 300
Lupton, B. A. 477
Lutiger, B. 232, 238
Lykken, D. T. 209, 211, 221
Lyn, L. 210, 222
Lynberg, M. C. 261, 264, 266, 268

M

MacBride, M. C. 488, 494
MacDowell, C. G. 213, 221
MacDowell, E. C. 213, 221
MacGregor, S. 229, 230, 238, 239
MacPhail, S. 479
Madara, Ed 555
Magid, K. 189, 193
magnesium, cerebral palsy 175–77
magnetic resonance imaging (MRI) 300, 466
  cerebral palsy diagnosis 130
  defined 63, 145, 300, 355
  fetal alcohol syndrome 191–92
  hydrocephalus 98
  spina bifida 52
Majchrowicz, E. 221
Majewski, F. 242, 244, 248, 254, 255
Major Research Programs (MRP) 513

Index

Making the Difference: An Orientation Package for Health Care Providers 552
Malee, K. 479, 494
Mallory, Lou 416
Malloy, M. H. 508
malnutrition 140, 150, 459–61
malocclusion, defined 347
mandible, defined 348
Mann, S. L. 254
Manning, F. A. 109, 110
manometry 311
Manual of Neonatal Care 478
March of Dimes
　alcohol 5
　Birth Defects Foundation 18, 64, 341, 344, 562
　publications 552
　Tay-Sachs disease 9
Marfo, K. 253
marijuana use during pregnancy 223, 226–28, 487
Marsh, J. L. 94
Martier, S. 198, 207
Martin, M. Louise, DVM, MS 267
Massengill, R. 344
Mast, T. J. 387
Mastrioacovo, P. 417
Matayoshi, K. 455
maternal alcohol use 181–82, 210
　see also fetal alcohol syndrome
Maternal and Child Health Clearinghouse 17
Maternal Fetal Medicine Units Network Publications 510–11
Maternal Health Practices and Child Development Project (MHPCD) 225, 227, 228, 230, 232, 233, 234, *234*
Maternal Lifestyle Study (MLS) 507
The Maternal Shunt Dependency Database 111n
Matricardi, M. 95
Mauldin, D. 323
maxilla, defined 348
May, P. A. 193
May, Rita M. 545
Mayfield, Lynn 543
McAllister, J. Pat, II, PhD 107n
McBride, W. G., Dr. 372

McCarrell, Vicki 543
McCarthy's Scale of Children's Abilities 228, 475
McCormick, M. C. 481
McDaniel, K. 251, 255
McDonald, E. 345
McDonald, S. 344, 345
McEvoy, L. 225, 238
McGill Journal of Education 253
McGue, M. 209, 211, 221
McKelvey, C. A. 189, 193
McKinlay, S. 199, 208, 243, 255
McKinstry, Robert E., Dr. 551
McLachlan, J. A. 207
McNellis, D. 510, 511
McRorie, M. M. 453, 457
Means, L. W. 251, 255
measles *see* rubella
mechanical aids *see* assistive devices
Mechanisms of Alcohol Damage in Utero 254
meconium 309–10, 465
Medicaid 341
Medical Birth Registry (Norway) 382
Medical Care 481
Medical College of Wisconsin 307
Medical Economics Company, Inc. 193, 268
Medical Genetics 387
Medical Miracle: A 60 Minutes Production 551, 555
Medical Research Council 220
Medical Sciences Bulletin 405n
Medtronic Neurological 159
Megliola, Maryanne, RN 454
Meis, P. 511
Mekdeci, Betty 546
Mellits, E. D. 95
Mello, N. K. 221
memingomyelocele 70
meningitis, cerebral palsy 151
Ment, Laura, Dr. *131*
mental health care, clefts 341–42
mental impairment, cerebral palsy 121, 123
mental retardation 468–69
　fetal alcohol syndrome 188, 202, 243–45
　hydrocephalus 86

mental retardation, congenital
  prenatal causes 459–64
  spina bifida 13
Menuet, J. C. 181, 193, 207, 242, 254
Mercer, B. 511
Merikangas, K. R. 209, 211, 221
metabolic acidemia 466
metabolic disorders, cerebral palsy 150
metatarsus adductus 315, 316, 317, 319–20
metatarsus varus 317, 319–20
Metropolitan Atlanta Congenital Defects Program (MACDP) 261, 262, 263, 266
Meyer, E. R. 209, 213, 220, 222
Meyer, L. S. 209, 221
MHPCD *see* Maternal Health Practices and Child Development Project (MHPCD)
Michaelis, H. 453, 457
Michaelis, J. 453, 457
Michaelis, R. 242, 255
microcephalus *381*
microcephaly 127, 202
middle ear, defined 348
Miettinen, O. S. 457
Miller, Anthony B. 366, 371
Miller, B. T. 217, 219
Miller, M. W. 208
Miller, P. 456
Milunsky, Aubrey 455, 456
mineral supplements 12
  folic acid and pregnancy 14
  see also vitamin supplements
Minerva, A. 344
minimum daily requirements
  folic acid 13, 14, 38
  see also Daily Values
Mintz, Morton 372, 394, 397
Miodovnik, M. 511
Mires, G. J. 479
Mirsky, A. F. 204, 208, 250, 257
miscarriages
  amniocentesis 21
  computers 8
  smoking 9
mitral valve *274,* 282, 283, 300
Mittendorf, R. 493
Mizrahi, E. M. 480

Moawad, A. 511
Mobius Syndrome Foundation 543
Moller, K. 345
monozygotic twins 306
Monson, R.R. 268
Montgomery, I. N. 213, 219
Moore, C. 213, 219
Moore, J. R. 473, 482, 488, 494
Moore, Julia 390
Moore, K. L. 208
Morgan, D. 323
Morgan, K. Z. 386
Mori, Koreaki 107, 108, 110
Moron, P. 198, 207
Moro reflex 130, 474
morphine studies 217
Morse, B. A. 187, 194, 262, 269
Moscoso, P. 477
Moss-Wells, S. 198, 208
motor control
  cerebral palsy 165
  cerebral palsy diagnosis 130
  fetal alcohol syndrome 202
  hydrocephalus 69–70
Moya-Moya Foundation 543
MRI *see* magnetic resonance imaging
mucocutaneous lymph node syndrome *see* Kawasaki syndrome
Muir, D. W. 474, 478, 479
Mulley, R. 457
multiple births, cerebral palsy 127, 151
multivitamins 3, 38
  see also vitamin supplements
Münchener Medizinische Wochenschrift 255
murmur *see* heart murmur
Murphy, M. G. 490, 494
Murray, J. 230, 231, 236
muscle relaxants 157
muscle spasms 155
  see also spasticity
muscle tone, cerebral palsy 129
muscular dystrophy, Duchenne's *318*
musculoskeletal defects *381*
musculoskeletal examinations 315
musculoskeletal system, spina bifida 39, 49–52
Mustonen, A. 457

Index

mutagens 373
Mutch, L. M. 494
myelomeningocele 35–36, *51, 317*
 brain formation 41
 see also spina bifida
myelomeningocele, defined 61
myocardial infarction 298, 301
myocarditis 291
myocardium *274,* 303
myometrium 518, 520
myotonic dystrophy 320
myringotomy, defined 348

N

Nadler, D. 198, 207
Naeye, R. L. 233, 238, 478, 493
Nagey, D. A. 478
Najem, G. Reza 389
Nakane, Y. 417
Nakayama, D. K. 109
Nanson, J. L. 251255
Narod, S. A. 215, 216, 221
nasal alae 325, *327, 328*
nasal emission, defined 348
nasopharyngoscope, defined 348
National Advisory Child Health and Human Development (NACHHD) 497n, 513n
National AIDS Clearinghouse 560
The National Association for the Craniofacially Handicapped 341, 357n, 543
National Black Child Development Institute 563
National Center for Education and Maternal and Child Health 65
National Chronic Pain Outreach Association 563
National Clearinghouse for Alcohol and Drug Information 563
National Cleft Palate Association 340
National Coalition of Hispanic Health and Human Services Organizations 563
National Coalition on Alcohol and Drug Dependent Women and Their Children 563

National Collaborative Perinatal Project 489
National Commission to Prevent Infant Mortality 563
National Congenital Port Wine Foundation 563
National Council on Family Relations 556
National Diabetes Information Clearinghouse 564
National Easter Seal Society 341, 344, 345, 564
National Eye Institute 505, 564
National Foundation for Facial Reconstruction (NFFR) 544
National Household Survey on Drug Abuse (1990) *224, 232*
The National Hydrocephalus Foundation 103n
National Information Clearinghouse (NIC) 549
National Institute of Allergy and Infectious Diseases (NIAID) 421, 425n, 431, 432, 435n, 443
 publications 419n, 439n
National Institute of Child Health and Human Development (NICHHD) 20, 140, 507, 513, 564
 clinical trials 501, 502
 Mental Retardation and Developmental Disabilities (MRDD) Branch 430, 459, 459n, 461, 462, 463
 Neonatal Research Network 499, 508, 509
 Pregnancy and Perinatology Branch 497n, 513n
 publications 508–11
 reports 465n, 483n
National Institute of Neurological Disorders and Stroke (NINDS) 119n, 120, 126, *132,* 140, 143, 146, 171, 175, 175n, 176, 177, 454
 Antiepileptic Drug Development Program 143–44
 Neuroepidemiology Branch (NEB) 175, 175n, 492
 Office of Scientific and Health Reports 147
 publications 67n, 119n, 147

National Institute on Alcohol Abuse and Alcoholism (NIAAA) 181n, 219, 223, 242
   grants 252
   publications 181n, 195n, 209n, 223n, 241n, 259n
   Research Scientist Award 219
   special reports 255
National Institute on Drug Abuse (NIDA) 219, 221, 238, 240, 507
   surveys 223, 226, 228, 229
National Institutes of Health (NIH) 75, 120, 146, 172, 173, 177, 425n
   Consensus Development Conference 508
National Kidney and Urologic Diseases Information Clearinghouse 564
National Kidney Foundation 564
National Maternal and Child Health Clearinghouse 564
National Oral Health Information Clearinghouse (NOHIC) 544
National Organization for Rare Disorders (NORD) 544, 553, 564
National Research Council (NRC) 377
National Resource Center for the Prevention of Perinatal Abuse of Alcohol and Other Drugs 561
National Society of Genetic Counselors 65
National Vascular Malformation Foundation 544–45
Native Americans, fetal alcohol syndrome 188, 189, 191, 266
Neale, M. C. 212
Neerhof, M. 229, 239
Neill, Catherine, A., MD 273n
Nelson, Karin B., MD 171, 175, 176, 478, 492, 493, 494
neocortex, defined 206
neonatal encephalopathy *see* encephalopathy
neonatal foot deformities 317
neonatal intensive care 504–7
Neonatal Research Network Publications 508–9
nerve development
   spina bifida 49
   thalidomide 372

nervous system
   cerebral palsy 125, 127–28
   regeneration 167
   spacticity 158
   spina bifida 51–52
   sprouting 166–67
Nesmann, E. R. 215, 216, 221
neural crest cells 276
neural tube defects (NTD) 4–5, 407, 415–16
   defined 61
   folic acid 11–17
   heat exposure 447–55
   spina bifida 34
   see also *individual defects*
Neurobehavioral Toxicology and Teratology 193, 220
Neuroendoscopic Third Ventriculostomy 101
neuroendoscopy 97
Neuroepidemiol 477
neurofibromatosis 114
Neurological Assessment During the First Year of Life 480
Neurological Institute 147, 565
neurologic development 486
   cerebral palsy 127
neurologic disorders
   hydrocephalus 67
   immunizations 71–72
   research 120
   Sturge-Weber syndrome 351, 352
neurologic examination 468, 474
neurologist, defined 355
Neurology 83n, 417
neuropsychology
   hydrocephalus 77
   tests 203
Neuropsychopharmacology 222
neurosurgeons
   brain shunts 42
   defined 61, 355
   immunizations 71
   spina bifida 41
neurosyphilis 441
Neurotoxicology and Teratology 206, 208, 219, 235, 236, 237, 239, 388, 389
Neuspiel, D. 231, 239

Index

Nevus Network 565
New England Journal of Medicine 20, 94, 95, 110, 152, 153, 172, 193, 236, 240, 253, 382, 383, 417, 509, 510, 511
New Solutions 375
New Technologies in the Treatment of Hydrocephalus 101
New York State Congenital Malformation Registry 368
New York State Department of Health (NYDOH) 367
New York Times 372, 375, 379, 384, 394
New York University Medical Center 529–30, 544
NFFR *see* National Foundation for Facial Reconstruction (NFFR)
NIAAA *see* National Institute on Alcohol Abuse and Alcoholism (NIAAA)
NIAID *see* National Institute of Allergy and Infectious Diseases (NIAID)
NIC *see* National Information Clearinghouse (NIC)
NICHHD *see* National Institute of Child Health and Human Development (NICHHD)
Nilsen, N. O. 457
NINDS *see* National Institute of Neurological Disorders and Stroke (NINDS)
nitric oxide 462, 500, 520
Noble, E. P. 213, 221
Nock, B. 213, 217, 219, 220
Noel, Pat 529
Noetzel, Michael J., MD 83n, 93, 94
NOHIC *see* National Oral Health Information Clearinghouse (NOHIC)
NORD *see* National Organization for Rare Disorders (NORD)
nosocomial infection 505
nuclear magnetic resonance *see* magnetic resonance imaging (MRI)
Nurminen, M. 456
Nursing Clinics of North America 220
Nursing Your Baby with Cleft Palate or Cleft Lip 344

nutrition information
  folic acid 13
  see also diet and nutrition
nystagmus 69

O

Obe, G. 216, 221
obesity, defined 301
O'Brien, Maggie 530
Obstetrics and Gynecology 115, 238, 479, 492, 495, 508, 510
occipital lobe, defined 355
occlusion, defined 348
occupational health 373
Occupational Safety and Health Act (OSHA) 372
occupational therapist, defined 355
O'Connell, M. A. 234, 237
O'Connor, L. 213, 217, 219, 220
Odem, R. R. 217, 222
Oeschsli, F. W. 494
Ogawa, Y. 473, 482
Oh, W. A. 508, 509
O'Hara, Barbara 252
Ohry, A. 457
Okah, F. 509
Okuma, T. 417
Olds, Betsy 548
O'Leary, Debby 93
O'Leary, J. 94
Olegård, R. 242, 255
oligodendrocytes 462–63
oligohydramnios 405
Olin Corporation 374
Olivas-Ho, Regina, RN 416
Olshan, Andrew F. 379, 388
Olson, Heather Carmichael, Dr. 250, 252, 257
Olson, J. 234, 239
Olson, S. 234, 239
O'Mally, P. M. 212, 214, 221
oncocytic cardiomyopathy 289
Onstad, L. 508
open heart surgery, defined 301
ophthalmologist 355
  hydrocephalus 72, 79
  strabismus 53

oral cavity, defined 348
orofacial, defined 348
oromotor training 163
orthodondists 337
orthodontics, defined 348
orthopaedic issues, spina bifida 49–52
orthopaedic surgeon
   defined 61
   spina bifida 50, 52
orthopedics, pediatric 315
orthopedic surgeon 315–16
orthopedist, cerebral palsy 133
orthotic devices, defined 145
OSHA *see* Occupational Safety and Health Act (OSHA)
osteochondrosis 321
ostium primum defect *see* atrial septal defect
otitis media, defined 348
otolaryngologists 333, 348
Ottawa Prenatal Prospective Study 228, 233
Ouest Medical 193, 207, 254
Our Child with a Cleft Lip and Palate 344
Outcome After Discontinuation of Antiepileptic Drug Therapy in Children with Epilepsy 95
ovarian cancer 7
oximetry, defined 301
Ozonoff, David 390

P

pacemaker node, defined 301
Paediatric and Perinatal Epidemiology 237, 481
palatal insufficiency, defined 348
palate, defined 349
Palkes, H. S. 94, 95
palsy 120, 145
   see also cerebral palsy
Pamlanye, Jackie 530
Pampiglione, G. 93
Paneth, N. 486, 493
Papanicolaou, G. 212, 222
Papile, L. A. 509

papilledema 69
paralysis, spina bifida 11, 13, 49
paraparesis, defined 146
paraplegia 69, *122*
parapodium, defined 62
parents
   alcohol consumption 195–205, 209–18
   clefts 330–31, 335–36, 340–41
   hydrocephalus 73
   involvement in treatment 25–30
   reading list 551–55
   spina bifida 56–60
   teaching social skills 77
A Parent's Guide to Cleft Lip and Palate 345, 553
paresis, defined 122, 145
parietal lobe, defined 356
Parker, S. 227, 229, 230, 231, 239, 240
Partners in Intensive Care 550
Pastores, F. S. 107, 109
Patel, N. B. 479
patent ductus arteriosus 278, *381*, 406
Pater, E. A. 479
paternal alcohol consumption 209–18
pathologic fetal acidemia 466
Patwardhan, R. V. 213, 220
Paul, R. H. 510
Paulozzi, L. 254
Paz, I. 492
PC SAS 85
Peabody Picture Vocabulary Test 85
Peacock, J. 234, 237
Peckinpah, Sandra Lee 345
Pediatric AIDS Foundation 565
Pediatric Clinic North America 322
pediatric dentistry 349
pediatrician, defined 349
Pediatric Neurology 477, 478
Pediatric Neurosurgery 115
Pediatric Research 239, 480
Pediatrics 171, 172, 175, 206, 235, 236, 237, 239, 240, 323, 456, 477, 480, 481, 492, 508
penicillin 442
Pennington, S. N. 251, 255
Pennsylvania Hospital 22
perceptual problems, hydrocephalus 80

Index

percutaneous umbilical blood sampling (PUBS) 22
Pereira, A. 234, 239
pericarditis, defined 301
pericardium *274,* 301
perinatal asphyxia 463–64, *472*
  cerebral palsy 126
  see also asphyxia
Perinatal Emphases Research Centers (PERC) 513
Perinatal Research Program (PRP) 513
peristalsis 310
Perlman, J. M. 474, 477
Persson, P. 232, 239
Peters, E. C. 233, 238, 478
Peters, John M. 367
Petitti, D. B. 481
PET scan *see* positron emmission tomography (PET) scan
Pharmaceutical Information Associates, Ltd. 405n
pharyngeal flap, defined 349
phenobarbital 113–14, 407–16
phenytoin 72
phenytoin sodium 407–16
Phillips, E. A. 508
Phillips, J. B. 508
phocomelia 372, 391, 393–94
Phoenix Chlidren's Hospital 524
physical examinations, pregnancy 3–4
physical therapist, defined 356
physical therapy
  cerebral palsy 133, 134–36, 166
  children 71
  spina bifida 52
Physicians for Social Responsibility (PSR) 386, 390
Physicians' Guide to Rare Disorders 553
Pickens, R. W. 209, 211, 221
Pileggi, Anna 542
Pinkert, T. M. 240
pituitary function 517
placenta
  abnormalities 21
  cerebral palsy 169–70
  twins 306–7
placenta previa 487
plastic surgery 349

platelets, defined 301
Platzman, K. A. *200, 201, 203,* 204, 206, 226, 230, 231, 235, 236
Pleet, H. 454, 456
plegia, defined 122, 145
plural septa, defined 302
Polakoski, K. L. 217, 222
Polan Adele 389
Poland, R. L. 508
polyhydramnios 305–6
Ponseti, I. V. 322
porencephaly 70
Portman, R. J. 490, 494
port wine stain 351, 356
  see also birthmarks
positron emmission tomography (PET) scan 356
Powell, Nancy, BSN 454
PPG Industries 364
precocious puberty
  hydrocephalus 70
  spina bifida 53–54
preeclampsia 498, 503
pregesterone insufficiency 150
pregnancy
  alcohol use 195–98, 223–26
  anencephaly 34
  antiepileptic drugs 407–16
  asphyxia 486–87
  cerebral palsy 127–28, 141, 149–51
  cocaine use 223, 228–32
  drug use 400–402
  folic acid 12–14
  hydrocephalus 111–14
  marijuana use 223, 226–28
  spina bifida 34, 36, 39–41
  streptococcal infections 423–24
  syphilis 442–43
  thalidomide 371–74
  tobacco use 8, 9, 223, 232–33
  twins 211, 305–7
  unplanned 4
Pregnancy and Maternal Hydrocephalus Survey 115
Premarket Approval pathway 105
premature delivery 497–501
  AFP levels 21
  cerebral palsy 127, 172–73
  twins 306

597

premaxilla, defined 349
prenatal alcohol exposure 195–205, 223
  see also fetal alcohol syndrome
prenatal testing 9
  hydrocephalus 107–9
  methods 19–23
Prensky, A. L. 95
Prescription Parents, Inc. 344, 345, 550
pressure sores
  spina bifida 55
  see also decubitus
prevention
  cerebral palsy 120–21
  cytomegalovirus 437
  fetal alcohol syndrome 259
  neural tube defects 11–14
  spina bifida 38–39
  syphilis 443
primary care management,
  hydrocephalus 70–72
Primary Care Needs of Children with Hydrocephalus 67n
Principles and Practice of Obstetrics and Perinatology 493
Proceedings of the Society for Experimental Biology and Medicine 221
prognosis, defined 356
Prognosis for Seizure Control and Remission in Children with Myelomeningocele 94
Prognosis of Childhood Epilepsy 94, 95
Projesz, B. 210, 219
prolabium *328*
prolapse, cord 487
prolapse, rectum 47
prosthesis, defined 349
  see also assistive devices
prosthetic speech aid, defined 349
prosthodontists, defined 349
Providence Hospital Foundation 551, 555, 557
Pryds, O. 480
PSR see Physicians for Social Responsibility (PSR)
psychological issues
  cerebral palsy 133
  clefts 337–38
  fetal alcohol syndrome 192
  spina bifida 57–58

Psychological Medicine 221
psychologist 349
psychometric evaluations,
  hydrocephalus 85
Psychopharmacology 222
psychosocial issues, birth defects 315, 497
puberty, early onset see precocious puberty
Public Health Service (PHS) 5, 243, 423, 425n, 432, 439
  Agency for Toxic Substances and Disease Registry 389
  Centers for Disease Control and Prevention (CDC) 400
  folic acid recommendations 12, 14
  grants 454
  Surgeon General's advisory 255
Public Health Surveillance 268
PUBS see percutaneous umbilical blood sampling (PUBS)
Pueschel, S. M. 253
pulmonary, defined 301
pulmonary artery 275–76, 286, 302
pulmonary artery anomaly *381*
pulmonary atresia, defined 302
pulmonary blood flow, defined 302
pulmonary function 500
  see also respiratory distress syndrome
pulmonary hypoplasia 406
pulmonary stenosis *280*
pulmonary valve, defined 302
pulse oximetry, defined 301
Putting the Lid on Dioxins 390
pyrimethamine 428

Q

quadriparesis, defined 146
quadriplegia *122*
Quantitative Applications in the Social Sciences Series 480

R

Rabinowic, I. M., MA, RRCS, DO 79n

Index

RACHEL *see* Remote Access Chemical Hazards Electronic Library (RACHEL)
RACHEL's Hazardous Waste News *see Environment and Health Weekly*
racial factor, drug use 188, 227
Rader, Jeanne, PhD 17
radiation, pregnancy 8
Radiation and Human Health 386
radiography, defined 349
Ragan, H. A. 387
Ragozin, A. S. 186, 193
Randall, C. L. 213221
The Rand Corporation 481
Randels, Sandra P. 186, 187, 194, 226, 240, 245, 246, 254, 252, 256, 257, 260, 269
Rann, Patti 553, 554
rapid plasma reagin (RPR) test 441
"Rare" Should Not Mean Alone 556
reflexes
 cerebral palsy diagnosis 130
 defined 146
Regier, D. 225, 238
Reich, T. 211, 212, 220
Rekate, Harold, MD 98, 101
Remote Access Chemical Hazards Electronic Library (RACHEL) 363n
renal failure 405, 474–75
renal function 517
renal scan, described 63
renal sonogram, described 63
Reproduction: The New Frontier in Occupational and Environmental Health Research 379
reproductive system, male 375–78
Research Society on Alcoholism 193
resonance, defined 349
Resources for People with Facial Differences 541
respiratory acidemia 466
respiratory distress syndrome 405, 499, 504
respiratory syncytial virus 284
Restrepo, M. 386
Retin-A (tretinoin) 403
Retzky, S. 229, 239
Reuss, M. L. 172

Reviews of Environmental Contamination and Toxicology 387
Revue l'Alcoölisme 253
rhabdomyomas 289
rheumatic heart disease 291, 302
Rh incompatibility 126
 cerebral palsy 128–29, 151
 defined 146
rhizotomy 143, 157, 159–61
Rhoads, George G., MD 20–21
Richardson, G. 196, 198, 199, 207, 224, 226, 227, 228, 229, 230, 231, 232, 234, 236, 237, 239
Richardson, Gale A., PhD 235
Richens, A. 417
Rickards, A. 481
right-heart flow defect, defined 302
Rikonen, R. S. 478
Riley, E. P. 209, 221, 251, 255
Riley Hospital 553
Ring, S. 457
Risch, C. 210, 222
risk factors
 cerebral palsy 127–28, 149–54
 chemical exposure 368
 foot deformation *317*
 heat during pregnancy 449–50
Ristow, H. 216, 221
Rita, P. 386
Ritz, C. R. 472, 477
Robert, E. 417
Roberts, J. 511
Robertson, C. M. T. 470, 473, 474, 478, 481, 482, 556
Robins, L. 225, 238
Robles, N. 196, 198, 199, 207, 226, 227, 228, 232, 234, 236, 237
Robson, S. 479
Rocco, L. 510
Rodeck, C. 109, 110
Rodis, J. F. 479
Roland, E. H. 477
Romero, R. 510, 511
Rosa, F. W. 3–4, 417
Rosen, M. 510
Rosenfeld, C. 225, 238
Rosett, H. L. 199, 208, 243, 255
Rosey...the Imperfect Angel 345
Ross, Martha, Scheele 33n

Rothman, Kenneth J., DrPH 455
Routine Antenatal Diagnostic Imaging with Ultrasound (RADIUS) 23
Rowley, D. L. 493
rubella 150
  birth defects 6
  cerebral palsy 120, 129
  defined 146, 302
  pregnancy 125
  prevention 420–21
  research 421–22
  symptoms 419–20
Rübsaamen, H. 457
Rush, Cathy 549
Rutledge, J. 107, 108, 110
Ryan, L. 231, 239
Ryan, M. M. 481

S

Saaftlas, A. K. 493
Sabel, K. G. 242, 255
Sabo, V. 510
Sachs, W. H. 187, 194, 262, 269
sacral agenesis *318*
sacral lipoma *318*
sacral nerves, spina bifida 47
Sainte-Rose, Christian, MD 98, 101
St. Charles-Riverside Medical Center 555
St. John's Hospital Cleft Palate Center, Santa Monica 556
St. Louis Children's Hospital 84, 85
Salter, R. B. 322
Samaille, P. P. 242, 253
Samaille-Villette, C. 242, 253
Sambamoorthi, U. 196, 198, 207, 227, 228, 236
Sameroff, A. 486, 493
Samet, J. M. 190, 193
Sampson, P. D. 202, 208, 226, 235, 240, 250, 252, 257
Sandin, B. 242, 255
Sands, C. 473, 482, 488, 494
Sanotskii, I. V. 375
Santos-Ramos, R. 107, 108, 110
Sargent, Larry A., MD 359

Sarsfield, Lisa 555
SAS Institute Inc. 94
SAS/STAT Guide for Personal Computers 94
Sato, K. 107, 108, 110
Sato, Susumo, Dr. 132
saunas 447–55
Saunders, M. 417
Savitz, David A. 379
Saxen, L. 456
Scandinavian Journal of Work Environment and Health 367, 379, 386, 387, 388
Scheiner, A. P. 213, 221
Schenker, S. 213, 220
Scher, M. 196, 198, 199, 207, 227, 228, 236, 239
Schleifer, Maxwell 552
Schmidt, D. 417
Schmidt, William E. 375
school settings, hydrocephalus 78
Schreuder, A. M. 481
Schuckit, M. A. 210, 220, 221, 222
Schultzberg, M. 493
Schwartz, David A. 387
Scialli, A. R. A. 208
Science 367, 372, 389
Science, Technology & Human Values 390
Scientific American 395
scoliosis 13, 58
  defined 62
Scott, H. 492
Scott, M. 250, 257
Scranton, P. E., Jr. 323
Seattle Foundation 252
second opinions 29
Seidman, D. 492
seizures 468, 473
  cerebral palsy 121, 123–24, *132*
  defined 356
  hydrocephalus 70, 83–93
  medications 72
  spina bifida 53
  Sturge-Weber syndrome 352, 354
Seizures in Children with Congenital Hydrocephalus 83n
selective dorsal root rhizotomy, defined 146

Index

Self-Help Sourcebook, Finding & Forming Mutual Aid Self-Help Groups 555
Seminars in Perinatology 220, 480, 481
sensory deficits, fetal alcohol syndrome 202
sensory nucleus, defined 206
septal defects of heart 276–77
septation 276–77
  defined 302
septum, defined 302
Serdula, M. 224, 239, 266, 269
Sever, Lowell 379
sexual function, spina bifida 58–59
sexually transmitted diseases (STD) 440
Shadyside Maxillofacial and Cleft Palate Prosthetics Center 345, 551
Shaer, Catherine, MD 33n
Shankaran, S. 475, 477, 508, 509
Shannon, Linda 545
Shapiro, Y. 457
Shaw, Gary M. 388, 389
Shaywitz, B. A. 251, 256, 468, 480
Shaywitz, S. E. 251, 256
Shen, Perry, MD 417, 418
Shepard, T. H. 456
Shimada, J. 107, 108, 110
Shinnar, A. 95
Shiota, K. 456
Shoenfeld, Y. 457
short stature, hydrocephalus 70
Shotan, A. 406
shunts 53
  defined 62
  eye problems 79
  failure 42, 44, 112
  hydrocephalus 41–44, 68, 69, 70–71, 83, *87,* 98, 100
  variable pressure valves 103–5
  venticuloatrial (VA) 111
  ventriculoperitoneal (VP) 111
Shy, K. K. 480
Siamese twins 306
Sibai, B. M. 510, 511
Sibling Information Network 65
sickle cell anemia 9
Siegel, S. 231, 237

Sierra Club 386
signature mark 35
Sigvardsson, S. 211, 212, 220
Sillanpaa, M. 92, 94
Silverstein, J. 226, 235
Simell, O. G. 478
Sims, M. 231, 240
Sinclair, J. E. 468, 477
sinus node, defined 301
Sixty (60) Minutes (TV) 551, 555
Sjogren's Syndrome Foundation 545
Skelton, J. 458
skin problems 354
  spina bifida 54
  see also birthmarks
sleep study, defined 64
Slotkin, T. A. 236, 253
slurred speech 71
Smellie-Decker, Mary, RN 527
Smith, Charlene 547
Smith, David F., Dr. 186, 187, 194, 245, 246, 252, 256, 257, 260, 269
Smith, David W., Dr. 181, 182, 190, 193, 207, 242, 243, 252, 253, 254, 256, 452, 453, 454, 456, 457
Smith, Deborah, MD 4
Smith, I. E. 196, 198, 199, *200, 201, 203,* 204, 206, 208, 226, 230, 231, 235, 236, 262, 268
Smith, M. K. 366
smoking, pregnancy 8, 9, 223, 233–35
Smythe, Nancy 542, 548, 556
Snell, L. 225, 230, 238
Snyder, E. Y. 465, 478
Sobol, A. 233, 240
So Brightly Within 557
Social Biology 193
social development
  hydrocephalus 75–78
  spina bifida 57
Social Security Supplemental Income (SSI) 59
socioeconomic factors
  alcoholism 210
  fetal alcohol syndrome 189–90
  neural tube defects 14
soft palate *see* velum
Sohar, E. 457
Sokol, R. A. 225, 235, 240

Sokol, R. J. 190, 194, 198, 207, 260, 262, 266, 268, 269
Someone Like Me: A Booklet for Children Born with Cleft Lip and Palate 553
Sonderegger, T. B. 254
sonogram *see* ultrasound
Soriano, Katherine 529
Soyka, L. F. 215, 220
spastic cerebral palsy 122
spastic diplegia 119, 121, *122*
  defined 146
spastic hemiplegia *122*
  defined 146
spasticity, cerebral palsy 152, 155–62
spastic paraplegia *122*
  defined 146
spastic quadriplegia *122*
  defined 146
spatial relationships, hydrocephalus 76
Specialized Training of Military Parents (STOMP) 550
special needs children, hydrocephalus 76
Special Olympics 52
Speck, G. 323
Spectrum (1981) 95
speech defect, defined 350
speech development, clefts 333, 334–36
speech-language pathologist, defined 349
speech therapy, cerebral palsy 133
sphincter, defined 62
sphincter muscle 48
spina bifida *318*
  antiepileptic drugs 415
  defined 62
  described 4–5, 34–36
  level 39
  medical issues 34–56
  non-medical issues 56–59
  prevention 3–6
  spared function 41
  tests 21
Spina Bifida Association of America 52, 59, 60, 65, 79n, 565
spina bifida occulta, defined 35
spinal column, development 34–35
spinal cord
  open 56
  spina bifida *34–35*, *37,* 39–41, *40,* 49
spinal cord tumor *318*
spine bending 13
spiramycin 432
Spirits of Survival (S.O.S) 524–25
Spohr, H. L. 244, 248, 249, 251, 256
Sponsler, Cathy 547
sports activities, spina bifida 52
Spragget, K. 458
squinting 79, 81
Staffer, D. 196, 198, 199, 207
Staheli, L. T. 315, 321, 322, 323
standing frame, defined 62
Stanford-Binet Intelligence Test 228, 471
Stanley, F. J. 477
Stark, A. R. 478
Starr, C. 345
Starr, P. 344, 345
state programs
  fetal alcohol syndrome surveillance 260–61
  spina bifida resources 59
State University of New York (SUNY), Albany 22
statistics
  alcohol use during pregnancy 223–25
  antiepileptic drugs 409–10
  birth defects 376, *381*
  cerebral palsy 121, 151–54
  chemicals and birth defects 363–64
  fetal alcohol syndrome *189, 265*
  pregnancy and folic acid 14
  spina bifida 3, 33, 36
Stedman's Medical Dictionary 465, 478
Stein, R. E. K. 481
Stein, Z. 232, 238
Steiner, Mark 557
Steinhausen, H. C. 244, 248, 249, 251, 256
Stellman, G. R. 92, 94
Stening, Warwick A., MD 101
stenosis 302, *381*
stereognosia 125, 146
stereotaxic thalamotomy 139

Index

sterilization 374
steroids 499
Stevenson, D. K. 509
Stickler Involved People 545
Stockard, C. R. 212, 222
Stoffer, D. 227, 228, 236, 237, 239
Stoll, B. J. 509
STOMP *see* Specialized Training of Military Parents (STOMP)
Stone, G. W. 455
Stone, R. K. 243, 253
Stopping Medication in Children with Epilepsy 95
strabismus 69, 124, 146, 156
   spina bifida 53
Streissguth, Ann P., PhD 182, 186, 187, 193, 194, 198, 202, 207, 226, 240, 242, 243, 244, 245, 246, 250, 252, 254, 256, 257, 260, 262, 269, 208
streptococcal infections 302, 423–24
strokes, cerebral palsy 126, 151
Stroup, D. F. 260, 269
studies
   adoptees 211
   alcoholism 211, 212–18
   amniocentesis 20–21
   antiepileptic drugs 407–16
   birth defects 152–53, 377–78, 389
   cerebral palsy 120, 175–77
   drug use during pregnancy 223–35
   epilepsy 85
   fetal alcohol syndrome 190–91
   folic acid and pregnancy 14
   hazardous waste sites 367–71
   health insurance 481
   heat exposure during pregnancy 447–55
   hydrocephalus 111–14
   hydrocephalus and seizures 84–85
   maternal lifestyles 507
   prenatal issues 228, 233
   twins 211
   ultrasound 23
   ultrasound screening 23
   Yale Universtity 368–71
Sturge-Weber Foundation 351n, 352–53, 545–46, 565
Sturge-Weber syndrome 351–53

Sturge-Weber Syndrome 351n
Substance Abuse 220
sudden infant death syndrome (SIDS) 519
sulfa drugs 392, 428
Sulik, K. K. 208
Sullivan, T. 229, 239
sunsetting 79, 81
Superneau, D. W. 458
support groups
   cerebral palsy 537–40
   clefts 340–41, 541–57
   hydrocephalus 523–31, 533–35
surgery
   cerebral palsy 137–39, 159–61
   clefts 331–33
   endocardial cushion defects 282
   endoscopy 97
   foot problems 320
   Norwood procedure 285
   spina bifida 41
Svikis, D. S. 209, 211, 221
Swanson, M. W. 480
Sweeney, Melanie Morrison 550
symptoms
   brain shunt failure 44
   cerebral palsy 121
   Chiari II malformation 42
   hydrocephalus 67, 68
   rubella 419–20
   syphilis 440–41
   toxoplasmosis 426–27
syndrome, defined 303
syphilis 439–43
   birth defects 6
syrinxes 52, 62
systemic blood flow, defined 303
systole, defined 303
systolic blood pressure, defined 303

T

tachycardia 289, 303
Tack, E. D. 474, 477
Taha, T. E. 387
Takashashi, R. 417
Talent, B. K. 95
talipes equinovarus *see* clubfoot

Tan, S. E. 213, 219
Tartar, R. E. 210, 220, 222
Taskinen, Helena 367, 379
Taussig, Helen, B., MD 394
Taxol (pacitaxel) 7
Taylor, Frances 147
Taylor, N. B. 478
Taylor, P. 199, 207, 227, 228, 232, 234, 236, 237
Tay-Sachs disease 9
TCE *see* trichoroethylene (TCE)
Team Approach to the Cleft Lip and Palate Child 345
Tegison (etretinate) 403–4
Tegretol 113
telangiectasia 358
temperature factors, pregnancy 8, 447–55
temporal lobe, defined 356
tendon contracture 161
Tennes, K. 227, 240
Tennessee Craniofacial Center 359, 542
Teo, Charles, MD 101
Teratogenesis Carcinog Mutagen 456
teratogens 4, 223–35, 371–74, 406, 453
Teratology 206, 236, 238, 269, 366, 387, 388, 455, 456, 457, 458
tethered cord 51–52
see also spinal cord
tethered cord, defined 62
tetralogy of Fallot 279–80, *280,* 290, 303, *381*
Tew, B. 107, 108, 109
Thacker, S. B. 260, 269
thalidomide 371–74, 391–96
They Don't Come with Manuals 556
The Young Person with Down Syndrome 253
Third Ventriculostomy 101
Thom, E. 510, 511
Thomas, J. A. 379
Thornton, Joe 390
thrombosis, defined 303, 356
Thurnau, G. 511
Thurston, D. L. 94, 95
Thurston, Jean Holowach, MD 93
thyrotoxicosis 150
thyrotropin 499

Tikkanen, Jorma 387
Tilson, Hugh A. 388
Timperi, R. 227, 229, 230, 231, 240
tobacco use during pregnancy 223, 232–33, 487
Tomlin, P. J. 379
tomography *see* computerized axial tomography; positron emmission tomography
Torfs, C. P. 494
Tosca, M. 262, 268
touch impairment 125
see also stereognosia
Touwen, B. C. L. 488, 494
toxemia, AFP levels 21
toxins
  alcohol 212
  birth defects 8
  see also chemicals
Toxoplasma gondii 426
toxoplasmosis 6, 125, 425–33
trabeculectomy, defined 356
Transformation and Identity: The Face of Plastic Surgery 555
Treacher Collins Foundation 550, 556
treatment
  cerebral palsy 132–39
  clefts 329–31, 341
  cytomegalovirus 437
  hemangiomas 358–59
  Hirschsprung's disease 311–12
  hydrocephalus 103–5
  Sturge-Weber syndrome 352
  syphilis 442–43
  toxoplasmosis 428–29
tremors 122–23
Treponema pallidum 439
Treponema pallidum hemagglutination assay (TPHA) 442
tretinoin 403
trichoroethylene (TCE) 363–65
tricuspid atresia, defined 303
Trimble, M. 95
Trisomy-13 114
truncus arteriosus 281–82, 303
trust, health care professionals 30
Truwit, C. L. 478
TTTS *see* twin-twin transfusion syndrome (TTTS)

Index

Tucker, J. M. 479
Tucker, M. 495
tumors
  brain *318*
  heart 289
  hemiparetic 122, 139
  spinal cord *318*
Tunell, R. 196, 203, 204, 207, 243, 254
Turner, J. E. 386
Twenty/twenty (20/20) (ABC-TV) 384
twins, alcoholism 211
Twins Magazine 305n
twin-twin transfusion syndrome (TTTS) 305–7
Tyson, J. E. 508, 509

U

Uauy, R. D. 508
Uhari, M. 457
Uhl, C. N. 243, 254
Ulcickas, Marianne, MPH 455
Ulleland, C. N. 181, 182, 193, 194, 242, 254
ultrasonography
  cerebral palsy diagnosis 131
  defined 146
ultrasound 428
  hydrocephalus 107, 108
  prenatal testing 19
  recommendations 23
  spina bifida 38
  twins 306
Umpierre, C. C. 455
unbalanced atrioventricular canal 284
Understanding Craniofacial Syndrome 557
unilateral, defined 356
United Cerebral Palsy Associations 121, 565
  Program Services Department 537
  publications 537n
  Technology Projects Group 537
United Cerebral Palsy Research and Educational Foundation 140, 152, 154, 161, 162, 164, 169, 170, 171, 172, 173, 565
  fact sheets 538

United Cerebral Palsy Research and Educational Foundation, continued
  Research Fact Sheets 149n, 155n, 156, 158, 163n, 165n, 170, 423n, 424
United Ostomy Association 309n, 313
University of Alabama, Birmingham 511
University of California, San Francisco 22, 73, 561
University of Illinois, Chicago 344, 557
University of Michigan Medical School 322
University of New Mexico, Albuquerque 192
University of Rochester Medical Center 290
University of South Carolina School of Medicine 549
University of Southern California (USC) 416, 418
University of Tennessee College of Medicine 359
University of Toronto 533, 534
University of Utah School of Medicine 307
University of Washington, Seattle 252
University of Western Ontario 25n
urinary tract infections, infants 45
urine backflow 45
  fetal genitourinary system 22
urine flow 45–47
urodynamic testing, defined 63
urologic system, spina bifida 39, 44–47
urologists 45, 62
uvula 326, *327,* 350
Uzee, Paul 556

V

VABS *see* Vineland Adaptive Behavior Scales (VABS)
vaccines
  pregnancy 6
  rubella 420–21
  see also immunizations

605

The Validity of Psychometric Testing in Children with Congenital Malformations of the Central Nervous System 94
valvuloplasty, defined 303
Valzelli, L. 95
Van de Bor, M. 231, 240
Van der Berg, B. J. 494
Van Dorsten, J. 511
Varfis, G. 92, 94
vascular, defined 303
vascular lesions 357
   see also birthmarks; hemangiomas
Vaters syndrome 114
Vaucher, Y. 232, 237
VCUG test 63
Veen, S. 481
vein, defined 303
vein of Galen 288–89
velopharyngeal closure, defined 350
velopharyngeal incompetence 350
velopharyngeal insufficiency 350
velum (soft palate) 326, *327,* 349, 350
Venereal Disease Research Laboratory (VCRL) test 441
ventrical septal defects (VSD) 277
ventricles, defined 62, 303
ventricular fibrillation, defined 297
ventricular hypertrophy 280, *280,* 303
ventricular septal defect 303, *381*
ventricular septum, defined 303
ventriculostomy, third 97–100
verbal and non-verbal clues, hydrocephalus 76–77
vermilion *327, 328*
vertebrae *37*
   see also spinal cord
Verter, J. 509
vesicoureteral reflux *45*
Vianna, Nicholas 389
video display terminals, pregnancy 8
villi cells 20
   see also chorionic villus sampling (CVS)
Vinci, R. 227, 229, 230, 231, 239, 240
Vineland Adaptive Behavior Scales (VABS) 246
Vineland Social Maturity Scale 85
Vining, E. P. 95
Vintzileos, A. M. 479
viral myocarditis, defined 303
vision impairment
   cerebral palsy 124–25, 168
   hydrocephalus 69
   see also eye problems
vitamin A 5, 399, 403–4
vitamin B 11, 61
   safe quantities 15–16
   spina bifida 38
vitamin D 5
vitamin supplements 3
   folic acid 12, 14
voice synthesizers 139
Von Hippel Lindau Family Alliance 546
Von Knorring, A. L. 211, 212, 220
Voyce, Lisa K. 389
Vreman, H. J. 509
Vulsma, T. 172

W

Wachendorf, Diane 553
Wada, Y. 473, 482
Walbaum, R. 242, 253
Wald, Niel 386
Walizer, Elaine 551
Walker, Marion L., MD 100, 101
Walker-Warburg syndrome 86
Walkinshaw, S. 479
Wall, T. L. 210, 220
Waller, K. O. 261, 264, 268
Walther, J. 231, 240
Wanner, R. A. 457
Ward, Kenneth, MD 307
Ware, J. E. 481
Warkany, J. 447, 455
Washington Post 372, 394, 397
Washington Star 396
Washington University School of Medicine 218
Wasilewski, Barbara 556
Watanabe, K. 107, 108, 110
water on the brain *see* hydrocephalus
water on the kidney *see* hydronephrosis
Waters, Cheryl H., MD 417, 418
Watkinson, B. 227, 228, 233, 237

Index

Webb, K. 163
Webster, W. S. 457, 458
weight factor, neural tube defects 13
Weinberg, A. 107, 108, 110
Weindling, A. M. 479
Weiner, L. 187, 194, 199, 208, 243, 255, 262, 269
Weitzman, M. 233, 240
Welker, Elizabeth 530
Wenger, D. R. 318, 322, 323
Werner, E. E. 250, 257
Wertelecki, W. 458
West, J. R. 194, 199, 204, 205, 208, 244, 251, 253, 257
Western Australia Research Unit for Child Health 490
Western Psychiatric Institute and Clinic 235
What is Going to Happen to My Baby? 557
What Is Hirschsprung's Disease? 309n
wheelchairs
　pressure sores 54
　spina bifida 49, 50
Whelan, Cathleen 530
White, Barbara 555
Whitfield, M. F. 480
Wibberley, D. J. 387
Wicka, D. 345
Wide Smiles Newsletter 345
Wiegmann, Paul *122, 138*
Willett, Walter, MD 455
Williams, M. A. 493
Williams, Rebecca 10
Williamson, D. F. 224, 239, 266, 269
Willis, Judith 404
Willms, J. 244, 248, 249, 251, 256
windblown feet 319
Winkler, C. L. 479, 495
Witter, F. 510
Woldt, E. 475, 477
Wolf, A. 198, 207
Wolk, Rochelle B., PhD 75n
women's rights movement 374
Wong, P. K. 477
Woods, H. M. 213, 220
Workman-Daniels, K. 481
World Health Organization (WHO) 261, 269, 387
World Wide Web pages *see* Internet addresses
Wozniak, D. F. 213, 220, 222
Wright, E. C. 508
Wright, L. L. 478, 508, 509
Wright, R. G. 457
Wu, Paul, MD 416
Wyatt, J. S. 480
Wynn, S. 345

X

X-rays
　angiocardiograms 291
　barium enema 311
　heart 286
　pregnancy 8
　shunts 104
　VCUG test 63
　see also computerized axial tomography

Y

Yakes, Wayne F. J., Dr. 545
Yale/NYDOH study 368–71
Yale University School of Medicine *131*, 367
Yazigi, R. A. 217, 222
Yetley, Elizabeth, PhD 12
Yeung, C. Y. 474, 478
Younes, N. 509
Young, A. 243, 254

Z

Zachary, J. 509
Zagon, I. S. 236, 253
Zeller, R. H. 480
Zenick, Harold 379
Zhang, Jun 387
Zigler, E. 251, 253
Zinreich, S. James, Dr. 553
Z Kinderchir 94
Zuckerman, B. 199, 208, 227, 229, 230, 231, 239, 240, 243, 255